Veterinary Toxicology

Veterinary Toxicology

Vijay Kumar Matham, M.V.Sc
(Pharmacology & Toxicology)
Assistant Professor
Department of Pharmacology & Toxicology
Veterinary College, KVAFSU
Bidar - 585 401, Karnataka

New India Publishing Agency
Pitam Pura, New Delhi- 110 034

Published by
Sumit Pal Jain *for*
New India Publishing Agency
101, Vikas Surya Plaza, CU Block, L.S.C. Mkt.,
Pitam Pura, New Delhi- 110 088, (India)
Phone: 011-27341717, Fax: 011-27341616
E-mail: newindiapublishingagency@gmail.com
Web: www.bookfactoryindia.com

ISBN : 978-81-90723-74-9

Composed and Designed by NIPA

NOTICE

Medicine is an ever-changing science. As new research and clinical experience broaden our knowledge, changes in treatment and drug therapy are required. The author and the publisher of this work have checked with sources believed to be reliable in their efforts to provide information that is complete and generally in accord with the standards accepted at the time of publication. However, in view of the possibility of human error or changes in medical sciences, neither the author nor the publisher nor any other party who has been involved in the preparation or publication of this work warrants that the information contained herein is in every respect accurate or complete, and they disclaim all responsibility for any errors or omissions or for the results obtained from use of the information contained in this work. Readers are encouraged to confirm the information contained herein with other sources. For example and in particular, readers are advised to check the product information sheet included in the package of each drug they plan to administer to be certain that the information contained in this work is accurate and that changes have not been made in the recommended dose or in the contraindications for administration. This recommendation is of particular importance in connection with new or infrequently used drugs.

ABBREVIATIONS

1. ADI : Acceptable daily intake
2. ALARA(P) : As low as reasonably achievable (practicable) In GBR regulations relating to worker exposure. In USA goal of risk management (USNRC regulations).
3. ATP : Adenosine triphosphate
4. BAL : British anti-Lewisite
5. BATNEEC : Best available technology not entailing excessive cost BCF Bioconcentration factor
6. BEM : Biological effect monitoring
7. BOD : Biochemical oxygen demand
8. BPEO : Best practicable environmental option (GBR)
9. b.w. : Body weight
10. CLn : *See* LC
11. COD : Chemical oxygen demand
12. DEn : *See* EDn
13. DNA : Deoxyribonucleic acid
14. DNn : *See* NDn
15. EC : Enzyme classification number *or* effective concentration
16. ECn : Median effective concentration to n % of a population
17. EDI : Estimated daily intake
18. EDn : Median effective dose to n % of a population
19. EEC : Estimated exposure concentration
20. EED : Estimated exposure dose
21. EEL : Environmental exposure level
22. EMDI : Estimated maximum daily intake

23. EQO : Environmental quality objective
24. EQS : Environmental quality standard
25. ERL : Extraneous Residue Limit
26. ETS : Environmental tobacco smoke
27. GAP : Good agricultural practice
28. GLP : Good laboratory practice
29. GMP : Good manufacturing practice
30. HSG : Health and Safety Guide (IPCS)
31. HQ : Hazard quotient
32. IC : Inhibitory concentration
33. IDLHC : Immediately dangerous to life or health concentration
34. i.m. : Intramuscular
35. inhl : By inhalation
36. i.p. : Intraperitoneal
37. IPD : Individual protective devices
38. I-TEF : International Toxicity Equivalency Factor
39. i.v. : Intravenous
40. KOC : Organic carbon partition coefficient
41. KOW : Octanol water partition coefficient
42. LCn : Median concentration lethal to n % of a test population
43. LDn : Median dose lethal to n % of a test population
44. LEL : Lowest effect level, same as LOEL
45. LOEL : Lowest observed effect level
46. LOAEL : Lowest observed adverse effect level
47. LTn : Median time for death of n % of a test population
48. LV : Limit value
49. MCL : Maximum contaminant level (Safe Drinking Water Act)
50. MCLG : Maximum contaminant level goal (Safe Drinking Water Act)
51. MAC : Maximum allowable concentration
52. MEL : Maximum exposure limit
53. MF : Modifying factor
54. MOE : Margin of exposure
55. MRL : Maximum residue limit

56.	mRNA	:	Messenger ribonucleic acid
57.	MSDS	:	Material safety data sheet
58.	MTC	:	Maximum tolerable concentration
59.	MTD	:	Maximum tolerable dose, Maximum tolerated dose
60.	MTEL	:	Maximum tolerable exposure level
61.	NADP(H)	:	Nicotinamide adenine dinucleotide phosphate (reduced)
62.	NDn	:	Median dose narcotic to n % of a population
63.	NEL	:	No effect level, same as NOEL
64.	NOAEL	:	No observed adverse effect level
65.	NOEL	:	No observed effect level
66.	OEL	:	Occupational exposure limit
67.	OES	:	Occupational exposure standard
68.	PEL	:	Permissible exposure limit
69.	PMR	:	Proportionate mortality rate, ratio
70.	p.c.	:	Per cutim (Latin) = Through the skin
71.	p.o.	:	Per os (Latin) = By mouth
72.	POW	:	Octanol water partition coefficient
73.	PPD	:	Personal protective device
74.	PPE	:	Personal protective equipment
75.	PTWI	:	Provisional tolerable weekly intake QSAR Quantitative structure activity relationship
76.	RD	:	Rate difference
77.	RfC	:	Reference concentration
78.	RfD	:	Reference dose
79.	RME	:	Reasonable maximum exposure (USEPA)
80.	RNA	:	Ribonucleic acid
81.	RR	:	Rate ratio
82.	SAR	:	Structure-activity relationship
83.	s.c.	:	Subcutaneous
84.	SCE	:	Sister chromatid exchange
85.	SMR	:	Standard mortality ratio
86.	SNARL	:	Suggested no adverse response level

87. STEL : Short term exposure limit

88. t1/2 : Half-life

89. TCDD : 2,3,7,8-tetrachlorodibenzo-p-dioxin

90. TDI : Tolerable daily intake

91. TEF : Toxicity equivalency factor

92. TEQ : Toxicity equivalent

93. TLn : *See* LTn

94. TLV : Threshold limit value

95. TMDI : Theoretical maximum daily intake

96. TSEL : Tentative safe exposure level

97. TWA : Time-weighted average

98. TWAC : Time-weighted average concentration

99. TWAE : Time-weighted average exposure UF Uncertainty factor.

❑❑❑

PREFACE

"All substances are poisons; there is none which is not a poison. The right dose differentiates a poison and a remedy" ***- Paracelsus (1493-1541)***

The Veterinary toxicology, in recent years, has acquired greater importance than ever before because of increasing and indiscriminate use of farm chemicals and drugs accompanied by rapid degrading impact of environmental pollution on health of animals. The indiscriminate feeding habits of domestic animals especially in developing countries make them more prone to the impact of natural toxicants especially Phytotoxins and Mycotoxins. Toxicology has been recognized as a separate discipline in veterinary sciences both at undergraduate and post graduate levels for the last four decades and a lot of emphasis has been given on its teaching, research and practical utility from clinical point of view.

This was written with two goals in mind i) to provide a textbook for veterinary students that would supplement their classroom instruction and ii) to supply a valuable aid to practicing Vet Clinicians. The book has been prepared in a most comprehensive manner with up to date reference which offers invaluable, clinically oriented guidance on numerous potentially toxic substances. In addition, to covering traditional and non-traditional areas of toxicology it provides a wealth of quick reference charts and tables that put vital information at your finger tips in seconds. It is needless to say that the intent of the author is to primarily provide a comprehensive information on the basic and applied principles of toxicology including clinical toxicology.

This volume has been designed primarily as a textbook for, or adjunct to, courses in toxicology. However, it should also be of interest to those not directly involved in toxicologic education. For example, the research scientist in toxicology will find sections containing current reports on the status of circumscribed areas of special interest. Those concerned with community health, agriculture, food technology, pharmacy,veterinary medicine, and related disciplines will discover the contents to be most useful as a source of concepts and modes of thought that are applicable to other types of investigative and applied sciences. For those further removed from the field of toxicology or for those who have not entered a specific field of endeavor, this book attempts to present a selectively representative view of the many facets of the subject. Toxicology: The Basic Science of Poisons has been organized to facilitate its use by these different types of users. The book describes the elements of method and approach that identify toxicology. It includes those principles most frequently invoked in a full understanding of toxicologic events, such as dose-response, and is primarily mechanistically oriented. Mechanisms are also stressed in the subsequent sections of the book, particularly when these are well identified and extend across classic forms of chemicals and systems. However, the major focus in the book is on the systemic site of action of toxins. The intent therein is to provide answers to two questions: What kinds of injury are produced in specific organs or systems by toxic agents? What are the agents that produce these effects? A more conventional approach to toxicology has been utilized in describing, the toxic agents by chemical or use characteristics. An attempt has been made to illustrate the ramifications of toxicology into all areas of the health sciences and even beyond. This is intended to provide perspective for the non toxicologist in the application of the results of toxicologic studies and a better understanding of the activities of those engaged in the various aspects of the discipline of toxicology. It will be obvious to the reader that the contents of this book represent a compromise between the basic, fundamental, mechanistic approach to toxicology and the desire to give a view of the broad horizons presented by the subject. While it is certain that the author's selectivity might have been more severe, it is equally certain that it could have been less so, and I hope that the balance struck will prove to be appropriate for both toxicologic training and the scientific interest of our colleagues.

Vijay Kumar Matham

CONTENTS

Chapter 1

INTRODUCTION

Toxicology is defined as the study of chemical or physical agents which interact with biologic systems to produce a response in the organisms. Toxicity is the relative ability of a substance to cause injury to biologic tissue. Given the broad range of toxicities any substance might eventually invoke in an organism, it is easy to understand the wisdom of Paracelsus (1493-1541) when he said, "*All substances are poisons; there is none which is not a poison. The right dose differentiates a poison and a remedy*".

Toxicology is the study of the harmful effects of chemical compounds on biologic systems, including their properties, actions, and effects. The toxic agent is referred to as a toxicant or poison. The term toxin refers to poisons produced by a biologic source (eg, venoms, plant toxins); the redundant term biotoxin is occasionally used. Toxicosis, poisoning, and intoxication are synonymous terms for the disease produced by a toxicant. Toxicity (sometimes incorrectly used instead of poisoning) refers to the amount of a toxicant necessary to produce a detrimental effect. Hazard describes the likelihood of poisoning under conditions of use.

If 2 poisons act via similar mechanisms on the same organs, their combined effects may be additive. Synergism is the amplification of the combined actions of 2 or more agents having the same biologic effects. Antagonism is the inhibition or elimination of the effect of one agent by another; it may be chemical or functional.

Toxicant accumulation and biomagnification occurs when absorption exceeds the capacity of the body to destroy or excrete a xenobiotic (foreign) compound. Likewise, the terms are applied to the environment, an ecosystem, species, etc, when a compound increases because of increased application or decreased destruction or disappearance. These elements are used with ecotoxicology, the study of the relation of potentially toxic chemicals in living organisms and their environment. When residual compounds are introduced into plant or animal species early in the ecosystem food chain, the levels tend to be successively higher in the next species that feeds on the contaminated plant or animal; eg, predatory birds, which are at the "end" of the food chain, often have the highest levels of certain residual chemicals.

The dose determines if the effects of any substance are toxic, non-toxic, or beneficial. Dose is the quantity of a substance to which an organism is exposed. In toxicological studies, the dose given to test animals is expressed in terms of quantity administered:

- Per unit weight, usually expressed as milligrams of substance per kilogram of body weight (mg/kg).
- Per area of skin surface, also expressed as mg/kg.
- Per unit volume of air inhaled, usually expressed as parts of vapor or gas per million parts (ppm) of air by volume. Solids would be expressed as milligrams of material per cubic meter of air (mg/m3). Inhaled doses can also be expressed by time.

Toxicity Tests

The design of any toxicity test incorporates selection of:

- A test organism, which can range from cellular material and selected strains of bacteria through higher order plants and animals.
- The response or biological endpoint, which can range from subtle changes in physiology and behavior to death.
- An exposure or test period.
- Dose or series of doses.

The objective is to select a test species that is a good model of humans, a response that is not subjective and can be consistently determined, and a test period that is relatively short. Often tests must be selected that yield indirect measurements or responses that supposedly correlate well with the response of interest — for example, determining carcinogenic potential by measuring mutagenic potential.

Dose-Response Relationship

A particular toxicity test exhibits a dose-response relationship when there is a consistent mathematical relationship between the proportion of individuals responding and a given dose for a given exposure period. For example, the number of mortalities increases as the dose of chemical given to a group of organisms increases.

Measurement of Response

Different species of test organisms differ in how they respond to a specific chemical. In addition, there are variations in response to a given dose within a group of test organisms of the same species. Typically, this intraspecies variation follows a normal (Gaussian) distribution when the number of organisms responding is plotted against the degree of response for a given dose.

Several basic relationships can be readily identified from the plots. A dose is often described as either a lethal dose (LD) in a test where the response is mortality, or effective dose (ED) in a test where the response is some other observable effect.

Constructing an ultimate dose-response curve enables the identification of doses which affect a given percent of the exposed population, e.g., the LD_{50} is that dose which is lethal to 50 percent of the test organisms.

Dose-Response Terms

The National Institute for Occupational Safety and Health (NIOSH) defines a number of dose-response terms:

- Lethal dose fifty (LD_{50}) calculated dose of a substance which is expected to cause the death of 50 percent of an entire defined experimental animal population.

- Lethal dose low (LDLo) The lowest dose of substance introduced by any route other than inhalation which has been reported to have caused death in humans or animals.
- Toxic dose low (TDLo): The lowest dose of a substance introduced by any route other than inhalation, over any given period of time, and reported to produce any toxic effect in humans or carcinogenic, neoplastigenic, or teratogenic effects in animals or humans.
- Toxic concentration low (TCLo) The lowest concentration of a substance in air to which humans or animals have been exposed for any given period of time that has produced any toxic effect in humans or carcinogenic, neoplastigenic, or teratogenic effects in animals or humans.
- Lethal concentration low (LCLo): The lowest concentration of a substance in air which has been reported to have caused death in humans or animals.

Use of Dose-Response Relationship

Comparing the LD_{50} of chemicals in animals gives a relative ranking of acute toxicity of each. For example, DDT (LD_{50} for rats = 113 mg/kg) would be considered more toxic than ethyl alcohol (LD_{50} for rats = 1400 mg/kg). Using this LD_{50} (mg/kg) and multiplying by 70 kg (average mass of human) gives a rough extrapolation to humans, assuming they are as sensitive as the species tested to the substance tested. However, LD_{50} serves only as a rough estimate of one aspect of the toxic potential of a substance.

Toxicity Rating Chart (Oral)

Toxicity Rating	Oral Acute LD_{50} for Rats
Extremely toxic	1 mg/kg or less (e.g., dioxin, butulin toxin)
Highly toxic	1 to 50 mg/kg (e.g., strychnine)
Moderately toxic	50 to 500 mg/kg (e.g., DDT)
Slightly toxic	0.5 to 5 gm/kg (e.g., morphine)
Practically nontoxic	5 to 15 gm/kg (e.g., ethyl alcohol)

Shortcomings of Dose-Response Data

Several shortcomings must be recognized in utilizing LD_{50} dose-response data for assessing the overall toxicity of a compound. One is that an LD_{50} is a single value and does not indicate the shape of the curve — that is, what the dose-response interval is, which is as important as how high or low the LD_{50} is. Thus, comparing these values can give the wrong impression.

Second, the LD_{50} measures only acute toxicity. The full range of toxicity testing includes subacute, chronic, carcinogenic and reproductive toxicity, amongst others. Therefore, while useful, the LD_{50} must be used with considerable discretion and caution.

Routes of Exposure

There are three main pathways for substances to enter the body:

- Absorption (through contact with skin, and eyes)
- Inhalation
- Ingestion

The primary function of the skin is to act as a barrier against entry of foreign materials into the body. If this protective barrier is overcome, toxic chemicals enter. The barrier is greatly diminished by lacerations and abrasions. Also, many organic solvents greatly increase the permeability of the skin to materials that would otherwise not pass through it. Another factor is that the skin provides a large surface area for contact with toxic agents.

Inhalation is the most rapid route, immediately introducing toxic chemicals to respiratory tissues and the bloodstream. Once admitted to the blood through the lungs, these chemicals are quickly transported throughout the body.

Health hazards to animals from *ingestion* of materials are a lesser concern than skin and respiratory hazards. The number of substances that can be ingested are limited – that is, it is difficult to swallow vapors and gases.

Types of Toxic Hazards

Systemic Poisons - chemical agents which act on specific target organs or organ systems.

Asphyxiants – agents which deprive the tissues of oxygen, a condition called anoxia. This group is divided into simple and chemical asphyxiants. The *simple* asphyxiants act by diluting or displacing atmospheric oxygen, which lowers the concentration of oxygen in air.

Chemical asphyxiants act in one of two ways. Some prevent the uptake of oxygen in the blood. Carbon monoxide, for example, interferes with the transport of oxygen to the tissues by strongly binding with hemoglobin to form carboxyhemoglobin, which leaves inadequate hemoglobin available for oxygen transport.

A second type of chemical asphyxiant does not permit the normal oxygen transfer either from the blood to the tissues or within the cell itself. Hydrogen cyanide is an example of this type.

Irritants – materials that cause inflammation of membranes. The mechanism of irritation is either by corrosive or drying action, and may affect the eyes, skin, respiratory membranes, or gastrointestinal tract. The irritant must come in direct contact with the tissue to cause an inflammation reaction.

Allergic Sensitizers – sensitization to a chemical involves immune mechanisms. When a foreign substance called an antigen enters body tissue, it triggers production of antibodies, which react with the antigen to make it innocuous. Upon first exposure to a specific chemical, there are no antibodies in the body. After subsequent exposures, the concentration of antibodies increases until a threshold is reached. At this point, the antibody level is high enough that upon exposure to the chemical the antigen- antibody reaction, also called an allergic reaction, is severe enough to manifest itself as one or more symptoms. The body has become "sensitized" to that chemical.

Carcinogens – a substance that is known or suspected to cause cancer in an organism. The following characteristics apply to carcinogens:

- Chemical carcinogens have distinct mechanisms compared to other toxic agents. The biologic effect is persistent, cumulative, and delayed, and repeated doses can be more effective than large doses.
- They are defined by their ability to induce neoplasms. An organism can respond to a carcinogen by:
  1) an increase in the incidence of one or more types of tumors compared to controls;
  2) development of tumors not seen in controls;
  3) the occurrence of tumors earlier than controls; and
  4) an increase in the number of tumors in individual animals compared to controls.
- Carcinogens are diverse chemical (and physical, e.g., ionizing radiation) agents such as organic (benzene) and inorganic (arsenic compounds) chemicals, solid-state materials, and hormones. The widely divergent properties of these chemicals appear to produce neoplasms by different mechanisms.

- Some react directly with DNA and as a result are mutagenic, others do not bind covalently to DNA, but produce neoplasms after the reaction with DNA.

Reproductive Toxins (Mutagens, Teratogens) – chemicals which affect reproductive capabilities, including chromosomal damage (mutations) and effects on fetuses teratogenesis). A mutagen changes a gene in a sperm or egg cell of the parent. The parent is not affected, but the offspring suffer the consequences. Teratogenesis is also manifested in offspring but differs from mutagenesis in that it results from exposure of the embryo or fetus to the agent itself.

Most of the information we have about reproductive hazards comes from testing animals. Most known reproductive toxins have similar effects in laboratory animals. Therefore, we usually assume that most agents which adversely affect reproduction in animals also have the potential to harm human reproduction.

Summary

The field of toxicology is evolving at a rapid rate. Considerable strides both in terms of elucidating the mechanism of toxicity, as well as the specific effects of individual chemicals are being made. However, the vast majority of chemicals have had little, incomplete or inadequate testing done on them. Newer tests are often of greater sensitivity, thereby indicating effects at levels previously thought safe.

The result of our increasing knowledge is increasing caution - we see that the more we know the more we realize how little we know. The message for us is this– minimize all exposure by reducing time, frequency and concentration of exposures, and substituting less toxic materials whenever possible.

Important Chronological Events

1. 4500 B.C. : Gula first god connected to poisons
2. 2000 B.C. : Shen nung treatise on herbal medical experiment poisons
3. 850 B.C. : Homer wrote of arrows poisoned with venom in the iliad and odyssey

4. 384-322 B.C. : Aristotle described preparation of poison arrows

5. 370-286 B.C. : Theophrastus wrote "de historia plantarum"

6. 470-399 B.C. : Socrates philosopher executed with poison hemlock for corrupting the youth of Athens

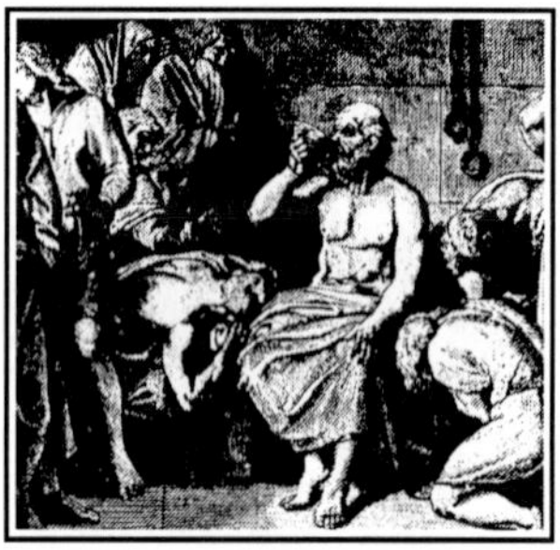

Socrates drinking hemlock, the American state poison

7. 204-135 B.C. : Nicander of Colophon wrote poetry about poisons and antidotes in two poems "Theriaca" and "Alexipharmaca" Theriaca concerns poisons and Alexipharmaca is about antidotes

8. 132-63 B.C. : Mithridates VI of Pontus developed the mithradatum, 1st universal antidote experimented with acute toxicity on criminals, allegedly ingested 36 ingredient mixtures to "innoculate" himself against all poisons

9. 81 B.C. : Sulla issued "Lex cornelia" 1st law against poison

10. 69-30 B.C. : Cleopatra experimented with poisons on prisoners and allegedly committed suicide with asp

11. 54-55 A.D. : Locusta infamous poisoner who used cyanide

12. 37-68 A.D. : Nero used prisoners as food tasters to distinguish poisonous from edible mushrooms 37-68 A.D. Andromachus refined mithradatum (theriac of andromachus)

13. 40-80 A.D. : Dioscorides wrote Materia Medica and classified poisons as vegetable, animal, or mineral types.

14. 129-200 A.D. : Galen prepared "Nut theriac" wrote "De antidotis I, II"

15. 801 A.D. : Ibn wahshiya arabic toxicologist wrote book on poisons

16.	1135-1204	:	Moses maimonides wrote "treatise on poisons and their antidotes" wrote of poisons from insects, snakes and mad dogs
17.	1250-1315	:	Petrus abbonus wrote "De Venenis" on poisons
18.	1300	:	Heironyma spara developed cosmetics that contained arsenic, which she dispensed for money
19.	1400	:	Cesare borgia poisoner used arsenic to kill for political gain
20.	1495-1555	:	Georgius agricola (georg bauer) agricola wrote "De re metallica" (of metal matters) documenting the health effects of mining book VI or the enormous volume described two kinds of arsenic poisoning; black foot disease & acute poisoning that causes swelling without pain
21.	1493-1541	:	Paracelsus developed theory of dose response and coined the phrase, "the dose makes the poison"
22.	1510-1590	:	Ambroise pare spoke out against the use unicorn horns and bezoars as therapy
23.	1519-1589	:	Catherine medici infamous poisoner who experimented on the poor
24.	1640	:	Hieronyma spara infamous poisoner used arsenic
25.	1650	:	Marchioness de brinvillier infamous poisoner experimented on the sick and poor documenting time to onset, symptoms and potency
26.	1611-1678	:	William Piso 1st to study ipecacuanha
27.	1633-1714	:	Bernardino ramazzini wrote "de morbis artificum diatriba"
28.	1673-1754	:	Richard mead wrote book of poisons
29.	1680	:	Catherine deshayes poisoner used aconite, arsenic
30.	1700	:	Guilia toffana poisoner used arsenic in preparation known as "aqua toffana"
31.	1714-1788	:	Percivall pott related disease to occupation with scrotal cancer in chimney sweeps

32.	1730-1805	:	Felice Fontana 1st scientific study of venomous snakes
33.	1752	:	Mary Blandy poisoned father with arsenic
34.	1767-1837	:	Philip physick early promoter of orogastric lavage
35.	1777-1835	:	Baron guillaume dupuytren studies on orogastric lavage to remove poisons
36.	1787-1853	:	Bonaventure orfila father modern toxicology wrote "traite de poisons"
37.	1797-1882	:	Robert christison wrote "treatise on poisons" and described acute renal failure from renal involvement in response to poisons
38.	1783-1855	:	Francois magendie discover emetine studied strychnine cyanide
39.	1794-1846	:	James marsh developed marsh arsenic test
40.	1813-1878	:	Claude bernard -mechanism of carbon monoxide and curare
41.	1807	:	Anna maria zwanizer poisoner used antimony and arsenic
42.	1820	:	Edward jukes self-experimented orogastric lavage
43.	1813	:	Bertrand confirmed charcoal use in arsenic poisoning
44.	1831	:	Touery confirmed charcoal use strychnine ingestion
45.	1839	:	Marie lefarge poisoner used arsenic (1st marsh test)
46.	1845	:	John tawell poisoner used cyanide
47.	1846	:	Garrod 1st study of charcoal in animal studies
48.	1848	:	Howard Rand 1 st study of charcoal in humans
49.	1855	:	William palmer, poisoner used strychnine
50.	1857	:	Madeline smith alleged poisoner used arsenic
51.	1848	:	O.H. Costill wrote 1st book- poison symptom treatment
52.	1826-1897	:	Theodore wormley wrote "microchemistry of poisons"
53.	1842	:	Hugo reinsch developed qualitative arsenic and Hg test
54.	1847-1915	:	Max gutzeit quantitative test for small qty arsenic

55. 1860 : Albert nieman isolated cocaine
56. 1854-1918 : Rudolf kobert studied digitalis and ergot alkaloids
57. 1850-1929 : Louis lewin studied numerous biological toxins
58. 1863 : Edmond de la pommarais, poisoner used digitalis
59. 1865 : Edward pritchard, poisoner used antimony
60. 1869-1970 : Alice hamilton worked to improve worker safety
61. 1881 : George henry lamson, poisoner used aconite
62. 1886 : Adelaide bartlett allegedly poisoned chloroform
63. 1889 : Florence maybrick poisoner used arsenic
64. 1891 : Thomas neville cream, poisoned prostitutes with strychnine
65. 1892-1905 : Johann hoch poisoner used arsenic
66. 1898 : Cordelia botkin put arsenic in chocolate
67. 1898 : Roland molineux poisoned using cyanide of Hg
68. 1910 : Hawley harvey crippen, poisoned using hyoscine
69. 1911 : Frederick henry seddon poisoned using arsenic in flypaper
70. 1912 : Henri girard poison mushroom amanita phalloides
71. 1914 : Harrison narcotics act 1st law criminalize non-med use xenobiotics
72. 1920 : Arsenic compounds developed for treating syphillis
73. 1921 : Robert armstrong poison arsenic in weed killer
74. 1922 : Landru poisoned with cyanide
75. 1927-1972 : Louis james casarett co-edited the first modern textbook of toxicology with john doull "toxicology; the basic science of poisons" in 1975
76. 1929 : Julias fazekas and susanna olah poisoned with arsenic obtained from boiling fly paper
77. 1948 : Sadamichi hirasawa poisoned bank employees with KCN

78.	1954	: Christa ambros lehmann poisoned with parathion laced chocolate truffles
79.	1954	: Nannie doss poisoned relatives with arsenic
80.	1960	: Sheldon murphy studied the toxicology and metabolism of organophosphorous compounds
81.	1962	: Founding of the society of toxicology & first formal meeting on april 15.
82.	1962	: The official journal "toxicology and applied pharmacology" in atlantic city; there were 9 founders and 183 charter members
83.	1965	: Carl coppolino, poisoned wife with succinylcholine
84.	1971	: Graham frederick young mother poisoned co workers with thallium
85.	1971	: Judias buenoano poison husband & son with arsenic
86.	1974	: Ronald clark o'bryan poisoned his son with cyanide laced candy "pixy stix" at halloween
87.	1978	: Georgi markov diplomat murdered with ricin delivered in a pellet gun disguised as an umbrella
88.	1978	: Jim Jones orchestrated mass suicide with cyanide in Guayana
89.	1974-1998	: Harold shipman, poisoned over 250 patients with heroin and morphine hanged himself in prison
90.	1980	: Founding of the american board of toxicology
91.	1983-1987	: Donald harvey poisoned patients with arsenic and cyanide
92.	1988	: George trepal poisoned his neighbours with thallium nitrate in coca cola
93.	1980-1990	: Michael swango, poisoned people with succinylcholine, kcl, arsenic

contd...

HISTORY OF TOXICOLOGY

Word Origins

- Toxin derived from
  - *Toxon* (Greek) for bow and arrow
  - *Toxikon* related to poison dipped arrows
- Poison derives from *poi*, to drink and becoming *potare* in Latin (potion)
  - Venomous nature derived from wen to win, and led to venus/venerate through "love potions" (called venin)

Antiquity : Prehistoric Man

- Knowledge of poisonous plants and animals
- Hunting, warfare, assassination

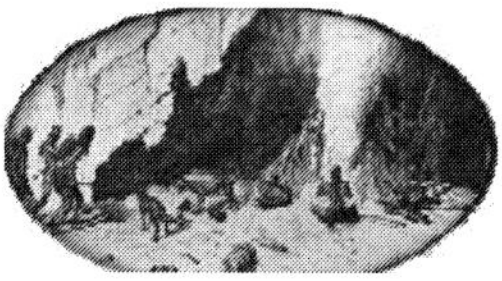

First "Mention"

- 3100-3000 BC : Menes
- Egyptian pharoah of the 1st dynasty
  - United upper and lower Egypt
  - Founded Memphis as capital
  - Building of dams
  - Founding of many new cults and temples
- Cultivated and studied effects of poisonous and medicinal plants

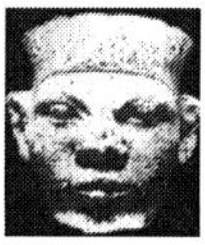

First Written Record

- 2700 BC (actually published in 1600 AD)
- Shen Nung, early emperor of China
- Shen-nung pen ts'ao ching (Divine Husbandman's Materia medica)
  - Contained lists of poisonous and medicinal plants and drugs
  - Included Effects and antidotes
  - E.g., iodine, opium, canabis, mercury

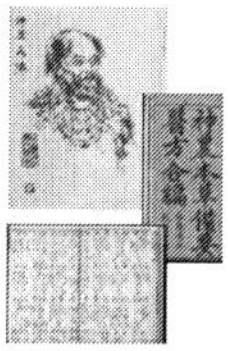

Antiquity : The Vedas

- 900 BC : Hindu Scriptures
- Atharva Veda
  - First indian text dealing with medicine
  - Mention of poisoning for use in warfare e.g., arrows with ducts, castor bean poison, poisoned nets and hook traps

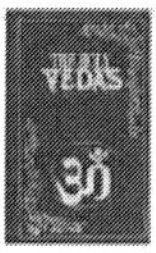

Antiquity : Bible

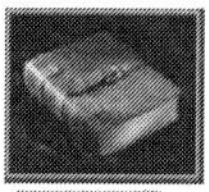

- 400 BC
- Deuteronomy
  - "with the venom of reptiles gliding in the dust
  - "poisonous are their grapes and bitter their clusters"
- Book of Job
  - "for the arrows of the Almighty pierce me, and my spirit drinks their poison"
  - The poison of asps he shall drink in; the viper's fangs shall slay him"

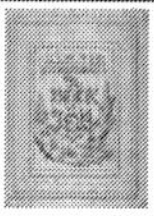

Antiquity

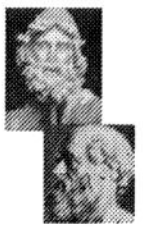

- 600 BC : Homer
- Odysseus obtains poison for his arrows
- 460-355 BC : Hippocrates
- Introduced principles of clinical toxicology related to bioavailability of toxicants
- Oath to 'not poison'
  - "to please no one will I prescribe a deadly drug nor give advice which may cause his death"

Antiquity : Theophrastus

- 370-286 BC
  - Born in Eresus, on the island of Lesbos
- Student of Aristotle
- Considered the father of Botany
  - Most relevant work is *De Historia Plantarum*
- Included numerous references to poisonous plants

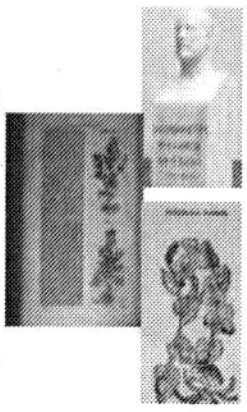

Antiquity

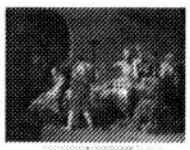

- 469-399 BC : Socrates
- Execution/suicide death of by hemlock
- 197-130 BC : Nicander
- Greek poet, physician to attalus, King of Bathynia
- *Alexipharmaca*
  - Discribes poisons in general, analyses of 19 specific persons and cures
- *Theriaca*
  - Describes poisonous animals, the effects of their poisons and proper remedies
  - First recorded reference to the use of letches
  - Term theriac come to mean antidose

Antiquity

- 385-322 BC : Demosthenes
  - Great Greek orator
  - "All speech is vain and empty unless it be accompanied by action"
  - Suicide by poisoned pen
- 69-30 BC : Cleopatra
  - Suicide by poisonous snake

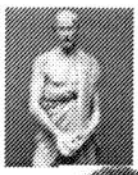

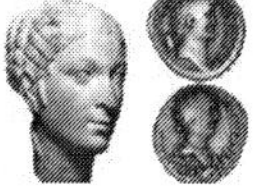

HISTORY OF TOXICOLOGY

Antiquity

- 132-83 BC : King Mithridates VI of Pontus
  - Poison paranola
  - Conducted poison experiments on criminals
  - Regularly ingested poisons to develop an "immunity"
  - Attempted suicide by poison but failed at attempt

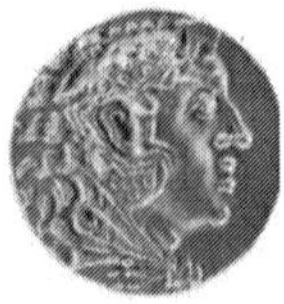

First Poison Law

- Circa 82 BC: Dictator Lucius Cornelius Sulla - *Lex Cornelia*
  - Growing conspiracy to kill men for profit
  - Provisions for both the poisoner and the provider of the poison

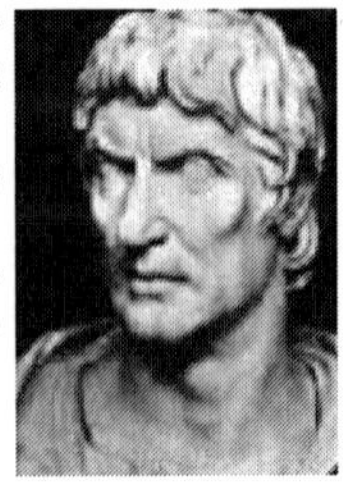

Dioscorides

- 40-90 AD
  - from Anazarbus (south-central Turkey)
- Greek surgeon with the Roman army of Emperor Nero
- Compiled medicinal herbs, later translated into Latin as *De Materia Medica*
- Classification standard of poisons into plant, animal, and minerals
- Remained the authority in medicinal plants for over 1500 years

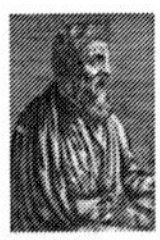

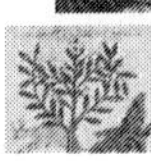

Dioscorides : Therapeutics

- *Arum maculatum*
  - Arum, or Cuckoo-Pint
- Ancient physicians called this plant the Drakontaia Mikre, or "small dragon", because central stalk resembles a serpent
- According to Dioscorides, its shape revealed its purpose as an antidote for snakebite
  - Rubbing one's hands with Arum root was supposed to make one unbiteable.

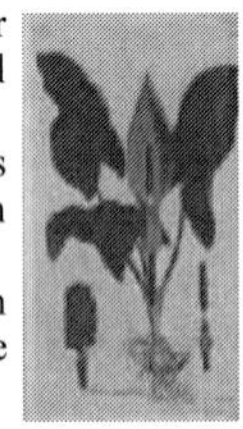

Nero

- 37-68 AD
  - Mother (Agrippina) consults with skilled poisoner (Locusta) to poison Emperor Claudius such that her son from a previous marriage (Nero), seize power
  - Cleverly poisoned step-brother Brittanicus
  - Used slaves as food tasters to differentiate poisonous mushrooms from edible ones

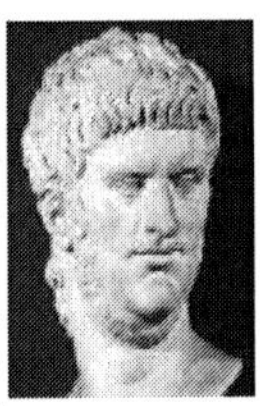

Galen

- 129-199 AD : Claudius Galen of Pergamum
- Greek physician, philosopher
- Believed therapeutics should be in the hands of physicians rather than herbalists
- *Galena:* a remedy or antidote for poison

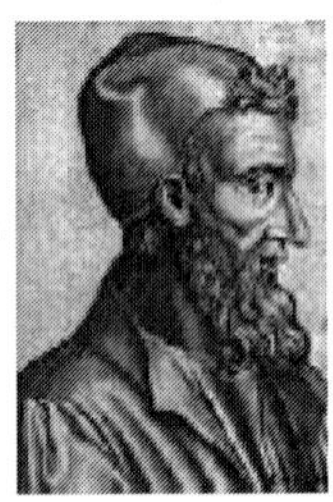

Middle Ages

- 980-1037: Avicenna (Ibn Sina)
  - Persian Physician, Philosopher, Scientist
  - Wrote 450 books
    - The Canons of Medicine
  - At an early age turned to medicine and then determined treatments for the sick

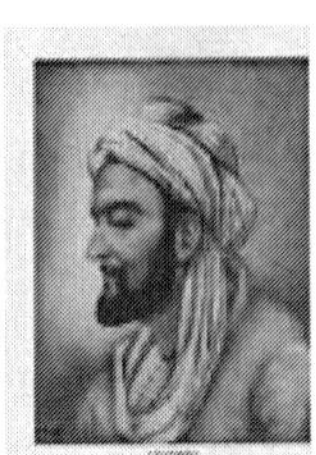

Middle Ages - Early Renaissance

- 1135-1204: Moses ben maimon Poisons and Their Antidotes (1198)
  - treatment of poisonings from insects, snakes, and mad dogs
- Wrote on the subject of bioavailability
  - noting milk, butter, cream could delay intestinal absorption of substances
- 1200s : Alchemists
  - Fermented product to yield 60% ethanol beverage

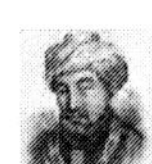

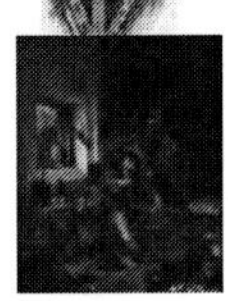

Chapter 2

GENERAL TOXICOLOGY

Definitions

- *Toxicology*: Knowledge (or science) of poisons, including their *chemical properties, identification, biological effects,* and the *treatment* of conditions they cause.
- *Poison*: Any solid, liquid, or gas that, when introduced into or applied to the body, can interfere with the life processes of cells of the organism - by its own inherent chemical properties - without acting mechanically and regardless of temperature.
- *Poison = Toxicant*: The term poison is now used less often. Reason: Historical application of the term (malicious) vs. a compound used as a feed additive, agricultural, or other chemical - manufactured to fulfill a perceived human need.
- *Xenobiotic*: Any substance, harmful or not, that is foreign to the body.

Toxicity: refers to the amount of poison that, under a specific set of conditions, will cause a detrimental effect. It indicates the relative potency of the toxic compound.

Example: The toxicity of aldicarb is > the toxicity of carbaryl. Usually agents are compared on a mg/kg basis; but toxicity can alternatively be compared on a molecule/kg basis.

Illustration

Toxicant	M.W.	LD_{50} in mg/mouse	LD_{50} in molecules/mouse
Botulinus toxin	9×10^6	0.01	6.75×10^{12}
Tetrodotoxin	319	0.0087	1.63×10^{16}
DDT	352	6	1.03×10^{19}

Note: Toxicity is not the condition produced by the toxicant.

Toxicosis is the condition (*disease state*) produced by the toxicant.

- Ecosystem Health: involves comprehensive evaluations of the environment, including the interactions among abiotic and biotic elements from a range of stressors, and considers strategies to protect its resources for the long term. Especially focused on the *long range* health and utility of both natural and human-altered ecosystems. Considers people a part of the ecosystem and integrates input from many stakeholders and various experts to endeavor to bring about ecological health. This term implies sustained provision of ecological services (clean air, clean water, climate control, food production); and it is achieved in significant part through maintenance of high levels of biodiversity.

Values for the terms listed below (i.e., mg of toxicant/kg of BW) pertain to the *species and strain of animal, as well as the route of administration tested.* They are often used for extrapolation in considering the potential hazard to other species such as man.

TD = toxic dose

TDL = toxic dose low: lowest dose that produces an adverse effect and, by definition, 2 x the TDL = a nonlethal dose.

HNTD = the highest nontoxic dose: the largest dose that does not exert a detrimental effect.

NOAEL = similar to HNTD. NOAEL: the "no-adverse-effect" (no detected adverse effect) level from a specific study, except that the NOAEL is more often used to refer to repeated, e.g., lifetime, exposures.

RfD = Reference dose: the highest dose expected to have no effect on the species of interest (often human beings) despite a lifetime of exposure. The RfD may be set at 1/10 of the HNTD or 1/10 of the NOAEL.

TDH = toxic dose high: a dose that will produce an effect and 2 x this dose is a lethal dose.

LD = lethal dose.

LD LO = lethal dose low: lowest dose that produced deaths in animals during the period of observation (sometimes expressed as LDmin). Often percentages are attached to the LD to indicate the fraction of the animals that would be expected to die from a given dose.

LD_{50} = median lethal dose. This is a calculated dose that is projected as being likely to cause death in half of the exposed animals of the species/strain/age/sex exposed. Thus often times, many animals would still be expected to die at doses less than the LD_{50}.

LC = lethal concentration. It pertains to lethal concentration of a toxicant in feed, water, soil or other "matrix" to which the animals are exposed. As in the case of LD, various percentages are attached to indicate the fraction of the animals expected to die.

TC = toxic concentration. Toxic concentrations relate to the first recognition of a toxic effect. The specific (threshold) toxic effect(s) should be identified when a toxic concentration is given.

MTD = maximum tolerated dose. It is sometimes used to indicate maximum tolerated dose (highest dose not causing death). Other times it is used to indicate minimum toxic dose (lowest dose causing any abnormality). Thus, it is best to ask what is meant by MTD.

ED or EC = imply effective dose or effective concentration. These terms are typically applied to xenobiotics or feed additives. Percentages are used to indicate the fraction of individuals of the test species/strain/age/sex expected to respond.

Chronicity factor = the ratio of the acute LD_{50} to the chronic or 90 day LD_{50}.

May be influenced by the tendency to accumulate vs. being rapidly eliminated or detoxified.

May be influenced by cumulative damage that occurs from repeated toxic insults to a target tissue e.g.: *Warfarin* - on a repeated basis is more toxic to dogs than on a single dose basis.

Chronicity Factor (Warfarin) = (Acute LD_{50}) / (90 day LD_{50}) = 1.5 mg/kg / 0.08 mg/kg = 18.75

Therefore, the C.F. for warfarin is approximately 19.

Many toxicants do not accumulate or have much of a cumulative effect.

e.g.: C.F. for *caffeine* = 1.3.

Toxicants with a C.F. > 2.0 are considered relatively cumulative

Some toxicants induce a degree of tolerance in the animal when it initially receives low doses e.g.: *Potassium cyanide*: The acute LD_{50} is 10 mg/kg, but pre-exposed animals tolerate 250 mg/kg. Therefore, the C.F. for KCN = 0.04.

Hazard : The *likelihood* of poisoning *under the conditions of usage* and the *probability of exposure.*

- Hazard and toxicity arenot the same; toxicity is the ability of a given dose to have a particular effect, but hazard also considers the likelihood of a person or animal ever being exposed to that dose.

  Hazard depends on:
  - Volume available,
  - Concentration,
  - Location,
  - Use restrictions,
  - Label warnings,
  - Users allowed access
  - Other factors.

Risk: An *estimate* of the likelihood of adverse effects assuming that a chemical exposure of a population has occurred.

- Risk is expressed in terms of the *estimated frequency* of a problem in the exposed population (*i.e., one in a million*)....
- ....*or in terms of relative risk*, that is, the probability of a disease in an exposed vs. an unexposed population (i.e., *twice the rate of the unexposed population*).

Risk Assessment is Comprised of Stages Including

- *Hazard identification* - which asks whether a particular chemical can cause an adverse health effect.
- *Dose-response evaluation* - which considers the relationships between dose and the incidence of the adverse health effected in the population. Considers thresholds, shape of dose-response curves, etc.
- *Exposure assessment* - involves estimation of level and uniformity of exposure of the population.
- *Risk characterization* - the last stage involves a prediction of the frequency and severity of effects in the exposed population.
  - When 95% confidence limits are given in the risk characterization, you have an idea of the reliability of the prediction.
- *Note: Risk assessment involves currently evolving methods. There are a large number of assumptions typically involved and there can be considerable differences in the calculated risk depending upon these assumptions and the risk model employed. An astute risk assessor states the assumptions used and attempts to indicate their level of confidence in the risk calculation.*

Risk Management

- Regulatory agencies often isolate risk assessment from risk management. The latter pertains to the measures taken to reduce risk. In toxicology, this is commonly focused on reducing exposure of the population of concern.
- Environmental cleanups at waste sites may rely upon bioremediation, vitrification, mechanical removal and incineration, capping, soil incineration, water pumping and activated carbon binding or "air stripping."
- In veterinary practice risk management may involve changing the feed and water or removing animals from the site until the source of exposure is known and eliminated.

Deposition - Implies removal of particles from inhaled air because of impact with and retention by an airway surface.

Clearance - Implies elimination of deposited particles from their initial deposition site

Retention - Pertains to quantity of particles that remain in the respiratory tract at a particular time after exposure.

Branches of Toxicology

1. *Forensic toxicology*: concerned with identification and analysis of suspected materials at the scene of crime to identify the actual cause of death
2. *Occupational toxicology*: concerned with study of poisons in working/ occupational environment
3. *Environmental toxicology*: deals with the study of environmental pollutants on different forms of life
4. *Laboratory toxicology*: study involved with invitro and invivo tests in laboratory animals
5. *Pharmacological toxicology*: study related with the toxicity of drugs
6. *Regulatory toxicology*: concerned with controlling the availability and use of chemicals either for industry or domestic use by mandatory testing before it enters in to market.
7. *Clinical toxicology*: deals with the cause, diagnosis, treatment and clinical management of conditions that are caused by or associated with toxic substances
8. *Formal toxicology*: deals with the formal toxicological studies which are pre requisite for release of new drug
9. *Genetic toxicology*: deals with the study of interaction of toxicants with the hereditary process
10. *Industrial toxicology*: deals with the clinical studies of workers of industries and environment around them
11. *Aquatic toxicology*: deals with assessing the toxicity on aquatic organisms/ marine life
12. *Geographical toxicology*: deals with the geographical distribution of toxicants/ toxicity
13. *Toxinology*: deals with assessing the toxicity of substances of plant and animal origin and those produced by bacteria.

Classification of Toxicants/Poisons

1. Based on target organs
2. Based on use
3. Based on source
4. Based on effect

5. Based on physical state
6. Based on chemistry
7. Based on analytical behaviour of toxicants.

I. Based on Target Organs

- on CNS: eg- anaesthetics, organomercurials, strychnine, Pb etc
- on CVS : eg- CO, digitalis, cyanide, radio active substances
- On GIT : eg- heavy metals, acids, alkalies
- Kidney : eg- Ochratoxin, Cd, Hg etc
- Liver : eg- CCl_4, Paracetamol, chlorpheniramine maleate etc.

II. Based on Use

Pesticides

- *Insecticides*: Organophosphates, organochlorines, pyrethroids etc.
- *Fungicides*: pentachlorophenol,captan,
- *Herbicides*: triazine, paraquat, 2,4 -D.

Rodenticides: Warfarin, Fluoroacetate

- Feed additives : antibiotics, coccidiostats, hormones
- Solvents: benzene, ether, methanol etc.
- Food additives: mono sodium glutamate
    1. *Preservatives*: ascorbic acid, sodium bisulphate
    2. *Antioxidants*: ascorbic acid
    3. *Emulsifying agents* : cholic acid, desoxycholic acid
    4. *Colouring agents*: amaranth, tartrazine
    5. *Anticaking agents*: aluminium calcium silicate.

III. Based on Source of Toxicants

- *zoo toxins*: snake venom
- *plant toxin*: HCN
- *Bacterial toxin*: *E.coli* endotoxin
- *Fungal toxin* : aflatoxin
- *Minerals* : Cu

- *Industrial poisons*: As, Pb, HCN, Radio active materials Man made industrial effluents: minimata disease, Bhopal tragedy
- *Environmental contaminants*: Methyl iso cyanate, chlorofluro carbons, dioxins, poly chlorinated biphenyls, polybrominated phenyls

IV. Based on Effects

- Poisons causing anoxia and respiratory insufficiency
  1. Poisons inhibiting oxygen uptake from pulmonary alveoli: Eg- paraquat, alpha naphthyl thiourea(ANTU)
  2. Poisons hindering oxygen transport to tissues: eg- nitrites, CO, Chlorate etc
  3. Poisons inhibiting oxygen utilization by tissues: eg- cyanide, H_2S, fluoroacaetate
  4. Poisons affecting haemopoeitic organs: eg- radio active materials
  5. Poisons inhibiting haeme synthesis : eg- Pb
- Poisons affecting nervous system
  1. Poisons directly damaging brain and spinal cord ;Eg- salt, organomercurials
  2. Poisons acting on specific receptors in nervous system: eg- organophasphates, carbamates, strychnine, snake venom
  3. Poisons altering neuronal conduction and ionic permeability: eg- pyrethroids, organochlorines
- Poisons causing abdominal distress and colic : eg- urea, arsenic, corrosives etc.
- Hepatotoxins: eg- aflatoxins, rubratoxins
- Nephrotoxins: eg- oxalates, ochratoxins, carbamates
- Poisons causing lameness: eg- Selenium, Flourine
- Poisons causing photosensitization: eg- lantadine A , Hypericine etc
- Poisons causing coagulatiuon defects: eg- bee venom
- Poisons inducing free radical generation : eg- Nitrogen dioxide, diquat
- Poisons irritant to mucous membrane: eg- sulphur dioxide, ozone, NO_2

V. Based on Physical State

- *Solids*: eg- metals
- *Liquids*: eg- benzene
- *Gases*: eg- CO, cyanide, SO_2, oxides of nitrogen
- *Dust toxicant* : eg asbestos, silicon dust.

VI. Based on Chemistry

Inorganic toxicants

- *Metals*: lead, copper, mercury
- *Non-metals*: phosphorous, sulphur, chlorine, nitrate etc.
- *Acids and alkalies*: hydrochloric acid, sulphuric acid etc.

Organic Toxicants

- *Alcohols and phenols*: eg- methyl alcohol, ethyl alcohol, phenol
- *Ethers*: eg- diethyl ether
- *Hydrocarbons*: eg- cyclopropane, benzene, paraffin, napthalene
- *Halogen derivatives of hydrocarbons*: eg-Chloroform DDT, BHC
- *Aldehydes and ketones*: eg- formaldehyde, acetaldehyde
- *Organic acids*: eg- formic acid, salicylic acid
- *Esters*: eg- organophosphates, succinyl choline
- *Amines*:eg- adrenaline, ephedrine, aphetamine
- *Amides*: eg- phenacetin
- *Glycosides*: eg- digitoxin
- *Alkaloids*: eg- nicotine, atropine
- *Proteins*: eg- ricin, crotin, abrin
- *Aromatic amines*: eg- organochloroines
- *Coumarin derivatives*: eg- warfarin.

VII. Based on Analytical Behaviour of Toxicants

Volatile toxicants : eg- HCN, alcohols, acetone, phenol

Extractive toxicants : eg- alkaloids, organic acids, nitro compounds

Metals and metalloids : eg- Cu, Hg, Zn, Ag

Factors Influencing Toxicity/Poisoning

Dose

The three types of doses commonly used are

1) Therapeutic dose: the dose meant for treating disease
2) Toxic dose: increased therapeutic dose producing toxic effect
3) Lethal dose: high toxic dose resulting in death of the animal,which is subcategorized into
   a) Minimal lethal dose: inducing any death in a population,
   b) Median lethal dose: based on LD_{50} values chemicals are classified into different classes by giving rating on 6 point scale,
   c) Maximal lethaldose: death of 100% population eg: morphine

Route of Exposure

There are primarily three routes of exposure i.e.,Skin, GIT and lungs .the amount of poison absorbed is inversely proportional to the number of layers (skin -3 layers,epidermis,stratified,germinal and dermis;GIT-2 layers-mucosa and submucosa;lungs 2 layers alveolar epithelium and capillary epithelium)

a. *Skin* : the absorption in the intact is less than skin which is having the abrasions or loss of continuity. Absorption is faster for oily solutions compared to the powder and aqueous forms

b. *GIT* : small intestines in the monogastric animals and rumen and reticulum in the ruminants are the major site of entry into the blood stream following the oral route. Unionised andlipophyllic substances are better absorbed through highly vascularised large surface area of intestines the absorption is faster on an empty stomach than full stomach which results in the dilution of poisons leading to delay in onset of poisons Eg: Zinc phosphide is absorbed faster in empty stomach whereas ANTU is absorbed faster in full stomach

c. *Lungs* : eg: CO,volatile aneasthetics etc.

Physical and Chemical Nature

1. Toxic substances may be in the form of gases,aerosols,liquids,fine particles and coarse solids eg: arsenic trioxide absorption is more in finely divided forms and oily forms
2. Particle size can influence toxicity. Compared to larger particles, small particles may more readily reach the lungs when inhaled or be absorbed

in the gut when ingested; large particles in suspension may cling to hair and accumulate on the skin.

3. Lipid soluble compounds that are non-polar and non-ionized are more readily absorbed and moved across biological membranes than are polar, water soluble and ionized particles.
4. Chemical nature: Eg: CO is more toxic than CO_2, nitrate is less toxic than nitrite, methanol more toxic than ethanol, arsenic trioxide is more toxic than arsenic pentoxide,barium chloride and carbonate is more toxic than barium sulphate.

Sources

Sources of Natural Toxicants and those Produced Outside of Living Organisms.

Naturally Occurring Toxicants

- Naturally occurring elements and compounds in the atmosphere, soil, and water. e.g., carbon dioxide, nitrate, fluoride, copper, lead, selenium.
- Toxins
  - *Toxin* and *biotoxin* are synonyms. The term implies only a toxic compound which has been manufactured by a living organism.
  - *Bacterial toxins* (endotoxins, exotoxins).
  - *Mycotoxins* (in veterinary medicine, usually implies toxins from mycelial fungi); but in human medicine, the term mycotoxin is more often taken to mean a toxin from a mushroom.
  - *Plant toxins* also known as *phytotoxins.*
  - *Algal toxins* such as from blue-green algae as well as marine organisms such as dinoflagellates are collectively called *phycotoxins.* Blue-green algae are also termed cyanobacteria which are photosynthetic bacteria. Some of the phycotoxins of the marine dinoflagellates are known to bioaccumulate in food chains.
  - *Animal toxins* also known as zootoxins.

    Note: Some poisonous gases are produced by bacteria (e.g., ammonia, hydrogen sulfide).

Produced Outside of Living Organisms

a. Produced through chemical manufacturing.

b. *Produced on purpose*: (e.g., synthetic xenobiotics such as acetaminophen, or pesticides such as the now banned herbicide 2,4,5-T).

c. *By-products not produced on purpose*: (e.g., contaminants of products or waste effluents released into air, water, soil, etc.). An example would be polychlorinated dibenzodioxins, which were never produced on purpose, but are nevertheless important pollutants (including being an inadvertent contaminant in 2,4,5-T).

d. *Produced as a result of minimally controlled reactions.* (e.g., carbon monoxide from incomplete combustion).

Hazardous Wastes

- Hazardous wastes often include both"used chemicals" (such as used solvents, metals, commercial products such as paints, and often polychlorinated biphenyls [PCBs]). They also often contain contaminant by-products (particularly troubling examples include chlorinated dibenzodioxins). *Complex mixtures* of a range of compounds are *often* encountered in hazardous wastes. Biodegradation, photodegradation, hydrolytic, fire-associated, and other products of chemical reactions among chemicals on site may also be included in the mix. *Across a hazardous waste site, multiple permutations may be encountered.* Chemical analyses are one way of assessing the presence of some of the compounds present. Such assays are best combined with bioassays to characterize the effects and to avoid grossly underestimating the hazards present.

Source

Plants : The Toxicity Resulting from Plants is Governed by Three Factors

1. *Stage of plant*: Immature jowar has increased cyanide content
2. *Part of plant :* Seeds and fruits have high amount of toxins eg:castor seeds and cotton seeds
3. *Storage conditions* : high humidity with optimal temperature favors the rapid fungal multiplication to produce toxin eg: aflatoxins.

Frequency of Exposure

1. Single lethal dose =LD_{50} may be sufficient to kill eg:cyanide, OP compounds, rodenticides, radiation
2. Sub-lethal dose resulting in

   a) Tolerance : eg: Phytotoxins

b) Immunosuppression
c) Mutagenecity
d) Carcinogenicity
e) Reproductive abnormality
f) Accumulation Eg; lead and fluoride.

Animal Factors

Species, Breed or Strain

a. Ivermectin more readily penetrates the blood brain barrier (BBB) of collies compared to the other breeds of dogs making them more prone for ivermectin toxicity
b. Rabbits are less susceptible to atropine toxicity due to the presence of atropinase enzyme
c. Norbomide is lethal to rats whereas harmless to others
d. Ruminants are least susceptible to HCN toxicity since acid hydrolysis place a major role in hydrolysis of cyanogenic glycoside
e. DDT is less toxic in mammals than insects due to increased metabolism in mammals.

Age

Very young and very old animals are more prone to toxic substances as detoxification and excretory mechanisms are not fully developed in young ones and decreased immune status and wasting conditions in aged /geriatric animals accompanied by low functional ability of liver and kidneys.

Eg: Carbon monoxide - neonates are especially sensitive due in part to increase CO binding by neonatal hemoglobin

Gender

Generally females are more prone to toxic effects of chemical than males due to the protective action of testosterone in males

a. Chlorpyrifos - bulls are especially sensitive due to testosterone influence on biotransformation to a toxic metabolite
b. Females are more sensitive to Redsquill rodenticide toxicity

Stage of Development

Eg: Teratogens, such as *Veratrum californicum* in lambs exposed *in utero*

Physiologic State

In pregnancy there is increased metabolism of poisons due to enzymatic degradation by placental enzymes thus reducing toxicity .some toxic agents which cross placentla barrier can cause abortions and other teratogenic effects.

a. Nitrate poisoning forming methheamoglobinemia
b. Lead lowering the cognitive abilities in the exposed neonates
c. Lead and DDT are excreted in milk in lactating animals
d. White snakeroot in lactating vs. non-lactating cows - excreted via milk protecting the lactating dam but putting the nursing animal at great risk.

Health at Time of Exposure

Presence of diseases and debilitating animals are more prone for toxicity.

a. Bufo toad poisoning is more hazardous to old animals with preexistent heart disease.

Individual Variation

Any population of the same species has a normally distributed variation in response to individual toxicants due to change in genetic component and individual idiosyncracies.

Environmental Factors

Air Circulation

Eg: silo gases accumulate in confined spaces and settle to low spots.

Season, Temperature

Eg: digitalis toxicity is increased when temperature is increased and soman toxicity is more when temperature is less.

Light Factors

Biological rhythms and circadian cycle influence susceptibility

a. CCL_4 and chloroform toxicity is less in evenings while cyclosporine and methotrexate toxicity is higher in morning
b. Photosensitization from poisonous plants or xenobiotics develops only after sufficient exposure to UV light. Some toxicants readily photodegrade following exposure to bright sunlight.

Water Factors

Quantity

a. Freezing

b. Overcrowding

c. System or human failures.

Quality

a. Palatability

b. Constituents including medications,

c. Salts

d. Bacteria,

e. Algae, etc.

Dietary factors

Nutrients

Malnourished animals are more susceptible for toxicity due to low level of synthesis of metabolising enzymes.

a. High protein diets reduces fluoride and lead toxicity

b. Too little carbohydrate increases susceptibility of ruminants to urea toxicosis.

Contaminants

Natural toxins such as aflatoxin, feed additives such as monensin, and manmade toxicants such as pesticides may contaminate feed or food products

Quantity

Too little feed increases tendency to ingest toxic amounts of poisonous plants, and also increases susceptibility to some mycotoxins. However, inadequate nutrition actually protects against toxic effects of some other toxicants that are bioactivated by enzymes in the liver, such as carbon tetrachloride.

Palatability

Toxicant may enhance or decrease palatability; or, alternatively, other foods present may mask toxicant.

Housing Factors

- Size (influences crowding, ability to get away from a toxicant, stress, etc.).
- Construction materials (e.g., lead, PCBs, formaldehyde, etc.).
- Heating and ventilation equipment (malfunctions may set the stage for toxicoses from poisonous gases such as carbon monoxide or natural gas which contains methane).
- Bedding materials (e.g., improper bedding materials sometimes with leaves of poisonous plants produces? laminitis in horses).

Miscellaneous

- People (Caretakers, children, visitors, other animals).
- Other factors.

Toxicokinetics

- It is a term derived from the Greek word 'kinesis' meaning a movement. It deals with the time course of xenobiotic absorption, distribution, metabolism and excretion. In other words, it means "What the body does to the xenobiotic".

Absorption

Movement of xenobiotics molecules from point of exposure site into circulation.

Movement of Xenobiotics Across Biological Membranes (Biotransport)

Biotransport is the translocation of a solute from one phase to another phase without a change in the form of the solute. The phases are separated by a biological barrier usually anatomic.

The barrier surrounding a cell as well as many cellular organelles are characterized by a lipoidal membrane. Likewise, the barrier surrounding the various tissues and organs is lipoidal and differs in that it may be from one to several cell layers in thickness. Whether the biologic membrane be a tissue or organ, the wall of the intestine, a capillary or a particular cell, the solute passes through by first penetrating the cell membrane. The characteristics of the cell membranes are basically the same for all barriers.

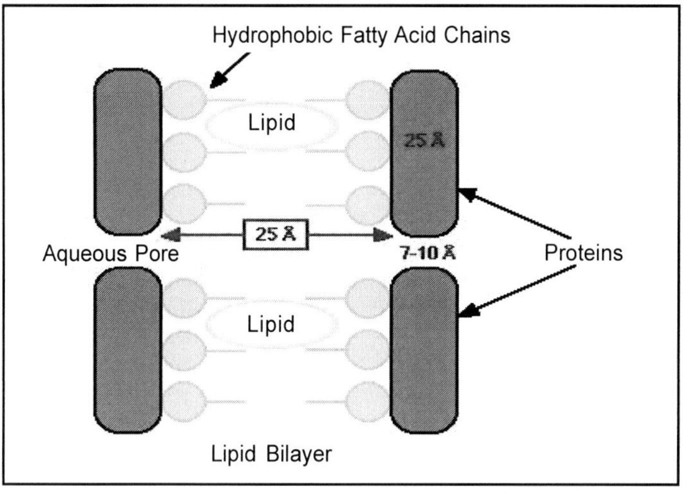

Schematic drawing of a section of cell membrane depicting the phospholipid bilayer, with the hydrophilic heads as circles and hydrophobic fatty acid chains as wavy lines. Globular proteins dispersed throughout the membrane penetrate the lipid phase, providing channels of communication between the external environment and the cell interior. The cell membrane showing a double layer of lipid molecules covered by a protein coat. The hydrophobic end of each molecule is directed inward, while its hydrophilic end faces outward toward the protein coat.

Mechanism of Biotransport

The various routes of xenobiotic absorption are

1. Passive diffusion
2. Carrier mediated active transport A) active transport B) active efflux
3. Filtration
4. Facilitated diffusion
5. Pinocytosis

Passive Diffusion

Passive diffusion is the direct movement of a solute through a biologic barrier from the phases of higher concentration to a phase of lower concentration. There is no requirement of energy. This is the most common mechanism of transport. The rate of diffusion is related to lipid solubility and polarity, pH, etc.. The concentration gradient is the most important factor in determining rate. The rate of diffusion can be expressed by the following equation.

(Ficks Law of Diffusion)

Rate of diffusion = KA (C1 - C2)/d

K	=	diffusion constant, (M.W., shape of molecule degree of ionization, lipid solubility).
A	=	surface area available
d	=	thickness of membrane
C1-C2	=	concentration gradient

Note : For a given membrane A will be constant

Factors effecting passive diffusion

Permeability Coefficient

a) *Lipid water partition coefficient* : greater the Lipid water partition coefficient greater is the solubility of the xenobiotics and greater will be the absorption of the xenobiotics

b) *Diffusion coefficient* : it is the movement of xenobiotic molecules within the cellular compartment and at any given point of time it is constant (hence it is not significant).

Concentration gradient

Greater the concentration of the xenobiotic greater will be the movement of the xenobiotic and greater will be the absorption.

Degree of ionization

It is indirectly proportional to the absorption process. It is based on pH of the media and pKa of the xenobiotic.

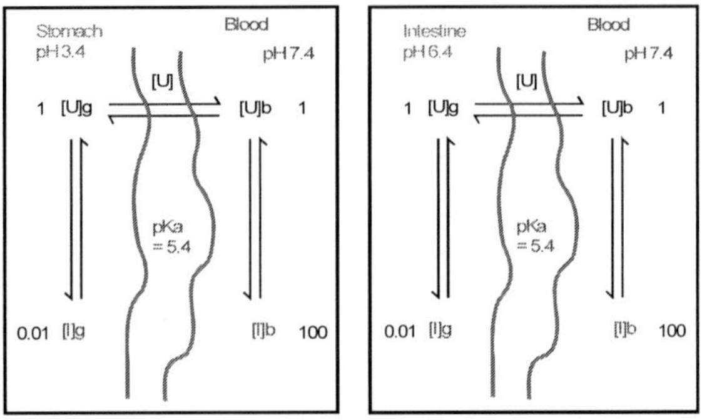

Each substance has a value called pKa which represents the pH at which the substance is 50% ionized. From the Henderson-Hasselback equation, one can derive the following formulae to determine the degree of ionization, remembering that the unionized particle is lipid soluble and the one that crosses the cell membrane.

For calculating the Total no. of ionized ions

For acids, pKa = pH + log (unionized/ionized)

For bases, pKa = pH + log (ionized/unionized)

Or

Weak acid (I) = (U) x $10^{(PH-pKa)}$

Weak base (I) = (U) x$10^{(pKa - PH)}$

S.No	Type of Xenobiotic	Type of PH	U/I	Rate of absorption
1	Acidic	Acidic	U	↑
2	Acidic	Basic	I	↓
3	Basic	Basic	U	↑
4	Basic	Acidic	I	↓

Ion trapping is used in the treatment of some poisoning conditions. The Henderson-Hasselbalch relationship is clinically important when it is necessary to accelerate the excretion of xenobiotics by the kidney, eg, in the case of an overdose. Most xenobiotics are freely filtered at the glomerulus, but sufficiently lipid soluble xenobiotics can be reabsorbed from the tubular urine. When a patient takes an overdose of a weak acid xenobiotic, its excretion may be accelerated by alkalinizing the urine, eg, by giving bicarbonate. This is because a weak acid dissociates to its charged, polar, form in alkaline solution and this form can not readily diffuse from the renal tubule back into the blood. Conversely, excretion of weak bases is accelerated by acidifying the urine, eg, by administering ammonium chloride,. For such compounds the pH will influence the % of ionized and unionized ions.

Filtration

Involves the bulk flow of water related to osmotic and hydrostatic pressures. Small water soluble, polar and non-polar, substances are transported by this process. It is most probable that these substances pass through spaces between cells rather than across the cell membrane. It is a purely physical process and the most important force is a pressure gradient. Examples include water and urea.

Specialized Transport Mechanisms

Specialized transport mechanisms give the membrane selectively so that it can control the transport of specific substances into and out of the cell or across the cell membrane.

Facilitated Diffusion or Transport

This is a carrier mediated transport system characterized by:

- Selectivity
- Competitiveness
- Saturability
- Concentration gradient

No energy is required for this transport. The rate of transport is at first related to the concentration gradient but as the gradient increased, the rate reaches a limiting or maximal rate.

Ex: Glomerular membranes, cerebrospinal fluid junction, hepatic sinusoids.

Carrier Mediated Transport

a) *Active transport*: This is a carrier mediated transport system, but energy is required and the transport is against a concentration gradient. However, it is characterized by saturability, selectivity, and competitiveness.

b) *Active efflux*: P glycoprotein is involved in this. p-glycoprotein is also called as Multi drug resistance factor.

Features

- Energy is utilized
- Transport maximum/ saturability is seen
- Non competitive inhibition is observed
- Competitive inhibition is also observed

Ex: nerve terminals, renal brush border membrane, BBB, placental barrier etc.

Pinocytosis

A transport mechanism which requires energy. The transport mechanism is by invagination of the cell membrane to form a vesicle and the engulfing of the invagination.

Stages of pinocytosis. Macromolecular solutes in contact with the membrane are trapped in microscopic cavities or cups - invaginations - formed on the surface of the membrane. The membrane fuses around and completely encloses the fluid to form a vesicle. The vesicle is pinched off, passing some fluid and solutes, across the membrane into the interior of the cell.

Factors Which Modify Absorption

The movement of the solute (xenobiotic) from the site of administration into the blood stream or the lymphatic system unchanged is defined as absorption. The rate of absorption is important since this determines the onset of xenobiotic action and course of xenobiotic effect. Absorption rate will also influence the toxicity.

Physicochemical Factors of Transport Mechanism

Xenobiotic Product

Form of xenobiotic, solubility, concentration exposed etc.

Site of Absorption

- Area of absorbing surface
- Blood supply to absorbing surface.

Route of Exposure

The route of exposure determines the absorbing surface. Xenobiotics exposed exerts a local effect or a systemic effect. When the local effect is observed,the xenobiotic is exposed appropriately in a local area and usually no systemic effect is observed.ex: local effect of a preparation of a xenobiotic exposed to the skin, or a mucous membrane. Some xenobiotics enters orally for a local effect on gastrointestinal tract (corrosive chemicals) or urinary tract (urinary poisons/toxins).

a. Molecular size and shape
b. Lipid solubility
   i. Partition coefficient - relation to lipid solubility
   ii. Weak acids - weak bases

For acids, pKa = pH + log (unionized/ionized)

For bases, pKa = pH + log (ionized/unionized)

Lipid diffusion: A large number of xenobiotics are weak bases or weak acids. The pH of the medium determines the fraction of molecules charged (ionized) if the molecule is a weak acid or base. If the pKa of the xenobiotic and the pH of the medium are know, the fraction of ionized molecules can be predicted by means of the Henderson-Hasselbalch equation:

"Protonated" means *associated with a proton* (a hydrogen ion); this form of the equation applies to both acids and bases. *Ionization of weak acids and bases:* Weak bases are ionized-and therefore more polar and more water soluble→when they are protonated; weak acids are not ionized→and so less water soluble→when they are protonated.

Plasma Protein Binding

Xenobiotics will be in the blood stream partly as free xenobiotic and partly as bound xenobiotic. Most xenobiotics are bound to some extent to plasma proteins. Many plasma proteins can bind xenobiotics, however, albumin is the most important. Both acidic and basic xenobiotics bind but acidic xenobiotics are bound more extensively. Since only free xenobiotic diffuses into extravascular space, xenobiotics tightly bound have limited distribution. There is a limited number of binding sites on proteins. These sites can become saturated and additional xenobiotic will exist as free xenobiotic and varying consequences result. Xenobiotics vary in their affinity for proteins. Those having a strong affinity will displace those of a lesser affinity (xenobiotic interaction). All acidic xenobiotics binds to albumin and all basic xenobiotics binds to α1-acid glycoprotein.

Plasma protein binding more → distribution is less → time taken for action is more → metabolism is less → elimination is slow → half life of the xenobiotic is more.

Factors effecting plasma protein binding

1. *Concentration of the plasma proteins* : greater the concentration greater is binding
2. Binding affinity of the xenobiotic
   - >80% high affinity
   - 50-80% moderate affinity
   - <50% low affinity
3. Disease conditions
   a) *Low plasma proteins*: renal failure.gastrointestinal disorders,hepatic cirrhosis etc.
   b) *High plasma proteins*: benign tumours, hypothryoidism

4. Age ; very young and very old have low protein concentration
5. *Xenobiotic interactions* : exposure of two or more xenobiotics at a time having varied plasma protein binding affinity will have significant impact on the overall response produced by the xenobiotics.

Distribution

Movement of xenobiotic molecules from circulation in to the different body organs/tissues

After absorption, xenobiotic undergoes distribution - a dynamic and complex process. Distribution is determined by the principles of transport as for any membrane. The rate of entry of a xenobiotic into a tissue is determined by the mass of the tissue and its blood supply. Distribution may be unequal in many tissues because of protein binding, regional variations in pH and characteristic permeability of various membranes. After distribution equilibrium, the concentration in the plasma reflects the concentration in tissues and extracellular fluids and vice versa.

There are basically two water compartments in the body, intracellular and extracellular. The extracellular may be divided into a plasma compartment and interstitial. The values commonly used for these compartments are as follows:

Extracellular	17% of body weight (12 liters)*
Plasma	4% of body weight (3 liters)
Interstitial	13% of body weight (9 liters)
Intracellular	41% of body weight (28.5 liters)

Total body water (58% of body weight) or (40.5 liters)/ *70 kg

Using certain reference compounds whose distribution is well known, the volume of these various compartments can be determined.

Plasma	131 I tagged albumin, Evans Blue
Extracellular	Mannitol, tagged sodium thiocyanate
Total body water	Heavy water or triturated water

Factors effecting distribution

Physiological factors

- Cardiac output
- *Regional blood flow*: the organs which are having high blood supply will get the xenobiotics in faster time after the exposure then the organs which are having less blood supply.

Physico-Chemical Properties

- Degree of ionization increases distribution decreases
- Lipid solubility increases distribution increases
- Plasma protein binding decreases distribution increases
- Binding with cellular components of tissue distribution decreases

Apparent volume of distribution : The apparent volume of distribution gives a quantitative estimate of the tissue localization of a xenobiotic. It is that volume in which a xenobiotic seem to be distributed to give the concentration in the plasma at equilibrium and following the exposure of a known quantity of the xenobiotic. This hypothetical value is calculated from the total exposure divided by the plasma concentration at zero time. This concentration is value extrapolated from the linear curve log concentration of plasma against time. This value is compared with the values obtained with the reference compounds.

Vd = Q (mg/kg) = ml/kg of body weight to Co (mg/ml)
Q = Total quantity exposed
Co = Concentration in plasma at 0 time

$$\text{Vd (liters)} = \frac{\text{total amount of xenobiotic in body (Gm)}}{\text{concentration of xenobiotic in plasma (Gm/1)}}$$

Interpretation: The lower the plasma concentration, the greater the distribution. If the Vd is greater than the total body water it is taken up by some tissue.

- For xenobiotics that are highly bound to plasma proteins –vd: 0.06lt/kg
- For xenobiotics that pass through capillary endothelium but not through cell membrane and not protein bound –vd : 0.2lt/kg corresponds to ECF
- For xenobiotics that pass through cell membrane without selectivity and evenly distributed through body water- vd:0.6lt/kg corresponding to total body water.

Sequestration of Xenobiotics

The process of accumulation of a xenobiotic in any biological organ inside the body without producing any action is called as sequestration of xenobiotics. Continous intake of xenobiotic in smaller quantities for a prolonged periods or sudden intake of large quantities of xenobiotic will enhance the possibility of sequestration of xenobiotics

- keratin - arsenic, mercury
- Nucleic acids- mepacrine (anitmalarial drug)
- Bones - tetra cyclones, lead, fluorine
- Adipose tissue : organo chlorine insecticides
- Heamopoitic tissue - phosphates
- Thyroid gland - iodine
- Lungs - tricylic antidepressants like cocaine ,impipramine
- Liver, kidneys - radio opaque xenobiotics

Distribution of Xenobiotic in Special Compartments

Blood Brain Barrier

These barriers influence the distribution of xenobiotics. The blood brain barrier is of particular significance since it is not desirable to attain lethal dose concentrations in the brain tissue of any xenobiotics. This barrier is basically anatomical but has a physiological component. The endothelial cells of the brain capillaries are tightly joined to one another. The glial connective tissue cells are closely applied to the basement membrane of the capillary endothelium. This makes for a barrier, especially for water soluble and polar substances. There is a slight difference in pH of the cerebrospinal fluid and plasma (7.3 and 7.4). These factors confer different permeability characteristics on the brain from other tissues. Lipid soluble compounds diffuse across the barrier the same as with other tissues. Certain parts of the brain do not have a barrier to the entrance of polar substance. These tissues are not really part of the brain but merely contiguous with it, in fact, the cells of these areas are not said to be non-neuronal.

Placenta Barriers

The placenta also acts as a barrier between the maternal circulation and the fetal circulation. The same principles applied here as for other membranes. Lipid soluble xenobiotics diffuse across more rapidly than polar compounds. A constant level of a xenobiotic in the maternal circulation will eventually reach equilibrium with the fetal circulation. Fortunately, this requires time. The fastest possible time is estimated to be 40 minutes.

Biotransformation of Xenobiotics

Introduction

"Biotransformation is the process whereby a substance is changed from one chemical to another (transformed) by a chemical reaction within the body. Metabolism or metabolic transformations" are terms frequently used for the biotransformation process.

Biotransformation also serves as an important defense mechanism in that toxic xenobiotics and body wastes are converted into less harmful substances and substances that can be excreted from the body.

Features of biotransformation

1. Changes activity of xenobiotics
   - Quantitative (detox or activation)
   - Qualitative (disposition and cffcct)
2. Phase I products most often more polar and less lipophilic
3. Phase II reactions most often abolish biological activity and add to polarity
4. Biotransformation requires energy or energy equivalents
5. Enzyme systems are inducible
6. Enzyme systems are saturable, frequently by depletions of cofactors
7. Systems are age, gender, and species dependent and are affected by exgogenous environmental factors

Two categories of enzyme systems are known to exist in mammals that cause chemical transformation of foreign compounds. One category consists of enzymes that normally occur in the tissues and are responsible for transformation of normal endogenous substances in tissues as well as foreign chemical e.g.,alcohol dehydrogenase. Second category consists of an enzymes system that is very important known as xenobiotic metabolizing enzymes, which are present in many tissues but are particularly in liver cells. These enzymes are located in small particles called microsomes which in turn are located in the smooth surface of endoplasmic reticulum. These microsomal enzymes are capable of catalyzing a variety of biotransformation reactions, the major ones being oxidation, reduction, and hydrolysis.

The xenobiotic metabolizing enzymes system is also called as mixed function oxidase (MFO) enzyme system for the obvious reason that is capable of catalyzing various types of reactions. The oxidase system requires the presence of a cofactor NADPH, and molecular oxygen for its activity. NADPH reduces a component of the microsomes which reacts with molecular oxygen to form an active oxygen intermediate which oxidizes the xenobiotic or the foreign chemical. The components of microsomes which is reduced by NADPH is a heme protein called cytochrome P-450.

R.T. Williams (1959) divided the biotransformation mechanism of foreign chemicals into two major types:

- Phase I/functionalisation reactions
- Phase II/biosynthetic/detoxification/conjugation reactions

PHASE I Metabolism

In phase I, a variety of enzymes acts to introduce reactive and polar groups into their substrates.

Microsomal Monooxygenation

- Enzymes bound to smooth endoplasmic reticulum
- Addition of single atom of oxygen
- NADPH - dependent

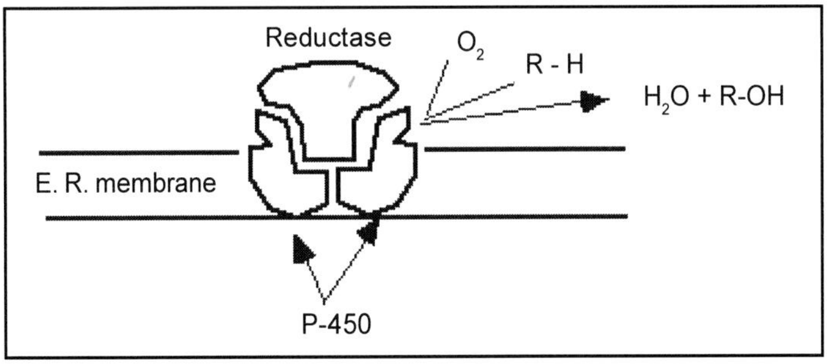

Two systems

A. FAD-containing monooxygenases
B. Cytochrome P-450s

Named for "cytochrome" (i.e. heme) functional group in enzyme

"Mixed-function oxygenases" (MFOs) – "mixed function"= 1/2 used to oxidize xenobiotic, 1/2 reduced to water.

Locations in body: Liver**, lung, brain, skin, nasal mucosa, GI tract

Microsomal (i.e., embedded in endoplasmic reticulum)

- In membrane in close association with:
  - reductase enzyme (NAD(P)H-dependent, flavoprotein)
  - phospholipid (joins two together)
- Substrate must be able to penetrate into membrane to reach active site (i.e., lipophilic)

General reaction of monooxygenase

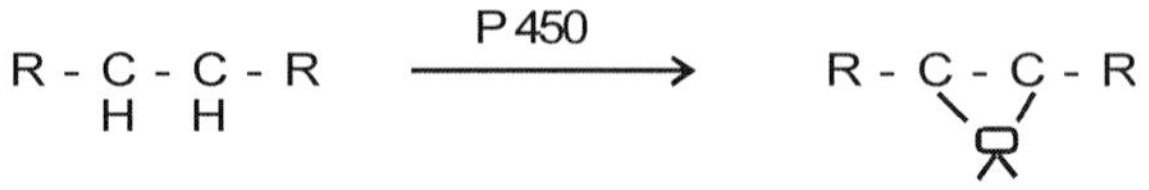

The most important phase I reactions are

- Oxidation
- Reduction
- Hydrolysis

Oxidation reactions

The following are various oxidation reactions that are taking place inside the body during the process of biotransformation

- N-dealkylation
  1. Active –inacitve : morphine – normorphine
  2. Active – active : mephobarbital – pheno barbital
  3. Inactive – active : imipramine – desimipramine
- O-dealkylation
  1. Active – inactive: codeine – morphine
  2. Inactive –active : acetaminophenetidene – acetaminophen
- Deamination
  1. Active – inactive : amphetamine
  2. Inactive – active : zoxazolamine –zoxazone
- Desulphuration
  1. Active – inactive : thiobarbiturates
  2. Inactive – active ; parathion – paraxoan

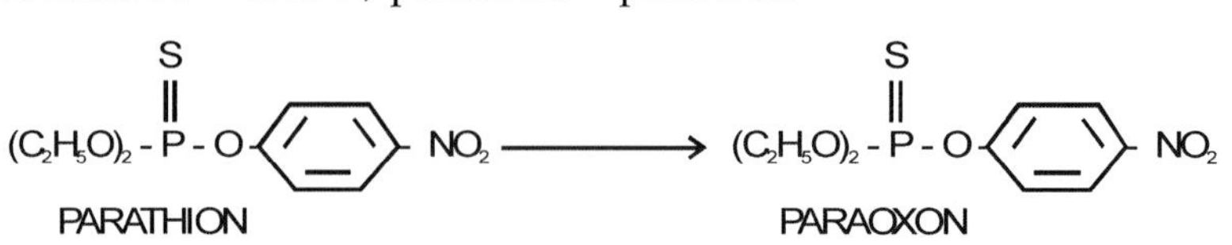

- N-oxidation
  1. Active – inactive : chlorpromazine
- Suphoxide formation
  1. active –inactive : phenothiazine derivatives
- Aromatic hydrogenation
  1. Active –active : phenobarbital –oxyphenobarbital
- Aliphatic hydrogenation
  1. Active –active : phenobarbital – hydroxy phenobarbital
- Epoxidation
  1. Inactive – active : aldrine – dieldrine

Reactions taking place outside the smooth endoplasmic reticulum in the cytoplasm of the hepatocyte through mixed function oxidases

Non-microsomal oxidations: (Enzymes of the mitochondrial or soluble fraction of cytosol).

Amine oxidation

Monoamine oxidases (MAO) - flavoproteins in the mitochondria. Primary amines are preferred:

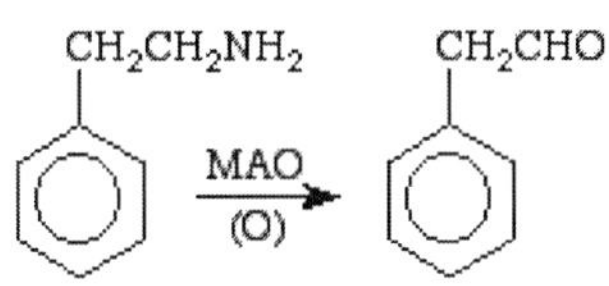

Diamine oxidases (DAO) - diamines to charectristic aldehydes

$$\underset{\text{Putrecine}}{H_2N(CH_2)_4NH_2} \xrightarrow[(O)]{DAO} H_2N(CH_2)_3\overset{H}{\overset{|}{C}}=O + NH_3$$

DAO oxidizes primary diamines only. The rate depends on the chain length, with a maximum at four carbons (putrecine) and five carbons (cadaverine), and going to 0 at nine or above.

At nine carbons and above MAO becomes active, since the separation of the amine groups is sufficient for the substrate to look like a monoamine.

Alcohol and Aldehyde Oxidation

Regardless of ethanol consumption its metabolism is important since it is endogenously produced in the large intestine by the microbial fauna to give about 0.5 mM ethanol in the hepatic portal vein! (Compare to the concentration reached after a single drink of 2-5 mM.)

Most ethanol metabolism takes place in the liver, with the primary pathway catalyzed by Alcohol Dehydrogenase (ADH) at low concentrations of ethanol since the K_M of ADH is low (approximately 1mM):

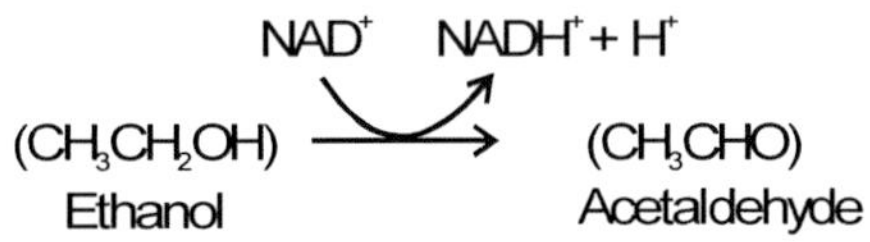

Ethanol is also oxidized by the microsomal ethanol oxidation system (MEOS), which is P_{450} based:

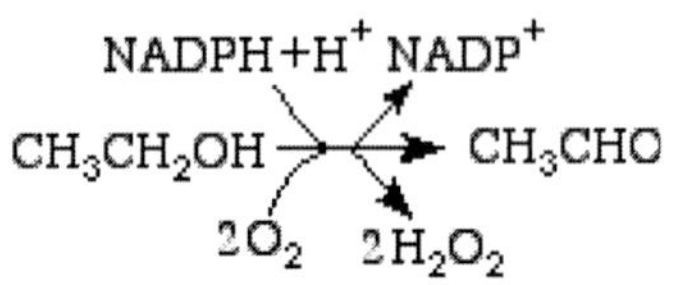

This reaction may explain ethanol's competition with drug metabolism.

- Ethanol can also be oxidized by Catalase:

$$CH_3CH_2OH + H_2O_2 \longrightarrow CH_3CHO + 2\,H_2O$$

The aldehyde produced in alcohol metabolism can be oxidized further:

$$CH_3CHO \longrightarrow CH_3COO^-$$

Aldehyde oxidation is mostly due to mitochondrial aldehyde dehydrogenase in liver (K_M = 0.01mM, cytosolic = 1 mM). The mitochodrial enzyme also has a greater capacity.

Some of the toxic effects of ethanol on the liver are due to NAD^+/NADH.

- Ethanol can lower liver NAD^+/NADH from 1000-100. Since most dehydrogenases operate at equilibrium, this can affect metabolism generally. (e.g. Glycolysis, gluconeogenesis).

- Decreased NAD^+ / NADH markedly decreases pyruvate concentrations.
- Ethanol is a potent inhibitor of gluconeogenesis, which could contribute to hypoglycemia in alcoholics and to lactic acidosis.

❒ Ethanol also decreases testosterone concentrations.

While other effects are related to acetaldehyde production.

❒ Acetaldehyde is responsible for many effects of ethanol even though its concentration in the blood is only 0.02-0.23mM.

- It can get higher concentrations if aldehyde dehydrogenase is inhibited by pyrogallol and other alliphatic aldehydes present in beverages.
- Acetaldehyde inhibits mitochondrial oxidative phosphorylation, decreasing ATP/ADP.
- Acetaldehyde reacts with biogenic amines to neurotransmitters, possibly accounting for some of alcohol's neurologic effects etc.

Reduction Reactions

Reductions take place in both the soluble and microsomal fractions under anaerobic conditions. Cytochrome P_{450} or a flavoprotein may be involved in the microsomal reactions, with NADPH as a required reductant.

Important reduction reactions may also take place in the gut by bacterial P_{450} reductases. An example is the reduction of the azo dye prontosil to give the antimicrobial drug sulfanilamide:

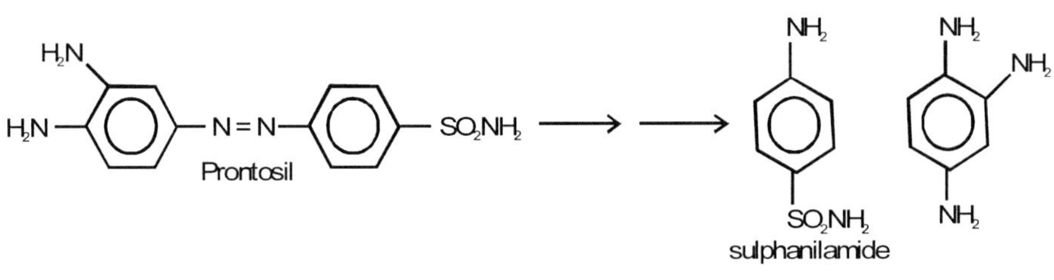

Nitrobenzene toxicity to red blood cells occurs as a result of its reduction by the microbial P_{450} / NADPH system. The nitrosobenzene and phenylhydroxylamine intermediates in this reduction are toxic to red cells.

- Nitro reduction
  1. active : inactive: chloramphenicol
- Azoreduction
  1. Inactive –active :protosil -Sulphanilamide
- Reductive dehalogenation
  Under anerobic conditions can get dehalogenation using P_{450}/NADPH. An example is the reaction of Halothane under anaerobic conditions:

  1. active –inactive : Halothane

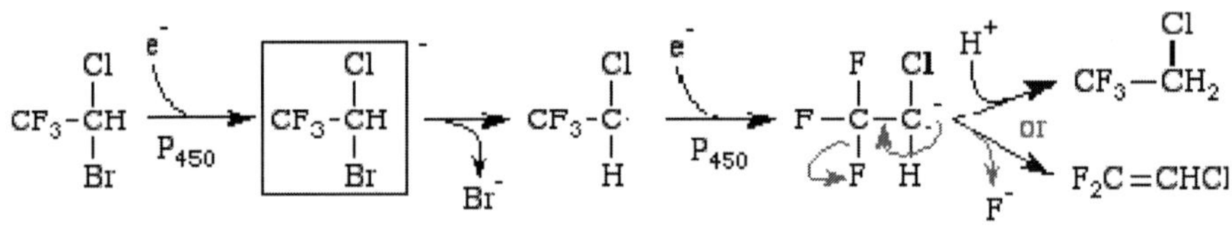

Hydrolysis Reactions

Esters and amides are commonly hydrolyzed:

$$R-\overset{O}{\overset{\|}{C}}-O-R' + H_2O \longrightarrow R-\overset{O}{\overset{\|}{C}}-OH + HOR'$$

or

$$R\text{-}\overset{O}{\overset{\|}{C}}\text{-}OR' + H_2O \longrightarrow R\text{-}\overset{O}{\overset{\|}{C}}\text{-}OH + HOR'$$

An example is the hydrolysis of the anesthetic, procaine is rapidly hydrolized by esterases in the plasma and by tissue microsomal esterases:

- Ester hydrolysis
  1. active-inactive : acetylcholine→choline + acetic acid
- Amide hydrolysis : (mitochondrial)
- Active-inactive: procainamide

The analogous amide, procainamide, is hydrolyzed more slowly by amidases in the microsomal fraction of tissue. It is not hydrolyzed at all in the plasma.

- inactive – active : nicotinamide – nicotinic acid
- Glycoside hydrolysis:

Release of HCN from ingested plant materials

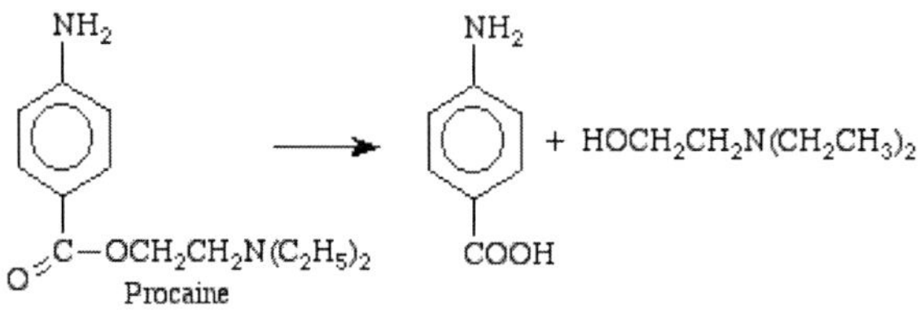

Phase II reactions

In phase II reactions, these activated xenobiotic metabolites are conjugated with charged species such as glutathione (GSH), sulfate, glycine, or glucuronic acid. These reactions are catalysed by a large group of broad-specificity transferases, which in combination can metabolise almost any hydrophobic compound that contains nucleophilic or electrophilic groups. One of the most important of these groups are the glutathione S-transferases (GSTs). The addition of large anionic groups (such as GSH) detoxifies reactive electrophiles and produces more polar metabolites that cannot diffuse across membranes, and may, therefore, be actively transported.

Conjugation of Phase I metabolite with endogenous substance.

- Most often make very water soluble
- Most often eliminates biological activity
- Energy- and/or energy equivalent-requiring reactions

S.No	Name of the conjugation	Functional groups of the xenobiotics	Conjugate donor	Enzymes involved	Remarks
1	Glucuronidation	COOh,NH_2SH,$_2$ OH	UDPGA	Glucuronyl-s-transferase	Deficient in cats
2	Acetylation	NH_2SO$_2$NH $_2$	Acetyl co A	N-acetyl transferases	Deficient in dogs
3	Methylation	SH,NH $_2$	S-methyl adenosine	Methyl transferases	
4	Sulfateester formation	OH,NH2	3′phosphoadenosine-5′phospho sulphate	Sulphate transferases	Deficient in pigs
5	Aminoacid conjugation	COOH	Glycine, glutamate serine, tuarine	-----	-----
6	Glutathione conjugation	Halides	Glutathione	Glutathione-s-transferase	

Let's look at examples for these different Phase 2 processes.

Process	*in vivo* **reactant**	**Product**
Glucuronide formation	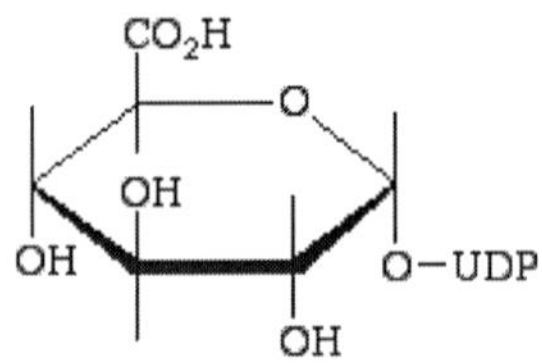 UDP-*alpha*-D-glucuronate	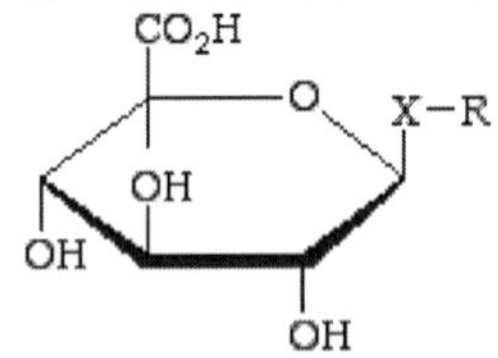 Glucuronide (X = O, N, or S)
Glutathione conjugation	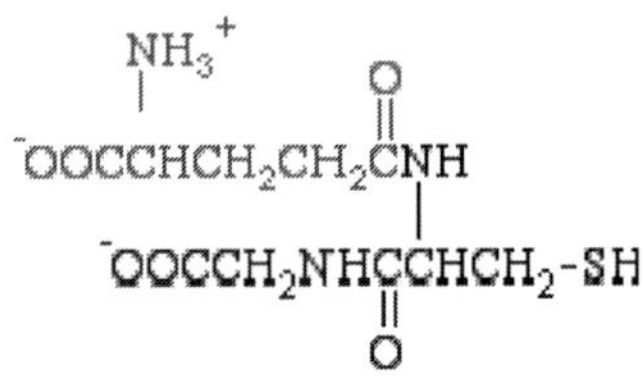 glutathione (Glu, Cys, Gly)	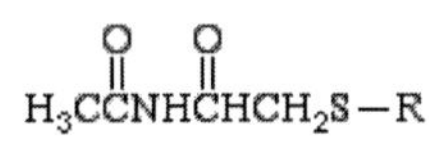 Mercapturic acid
Sulfate conjugation	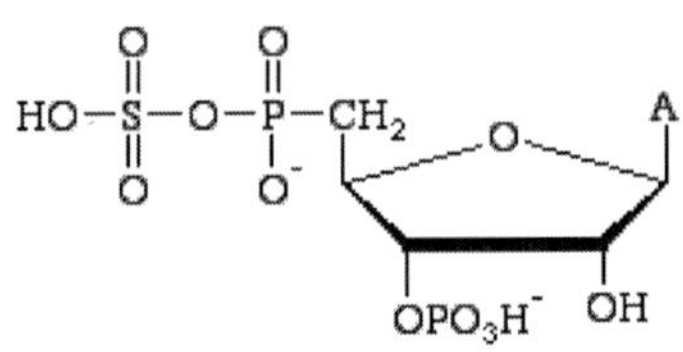 PAPS = Adenosine-3'-P-5'-Phosphosulfate	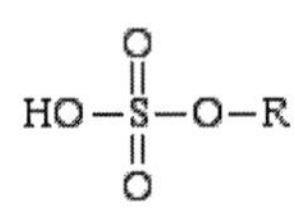 Aryl or alkyl sulfates and sulfamates
Acetylation	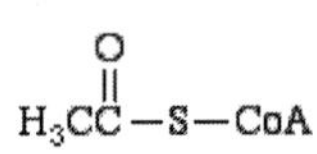 Acetyl Coenzyme A	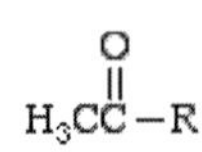 Acetylated derivatives
Amino acid conjugation	Coenzyme A, ATP & e.g. glycine	Acyl derivatives
Methylation	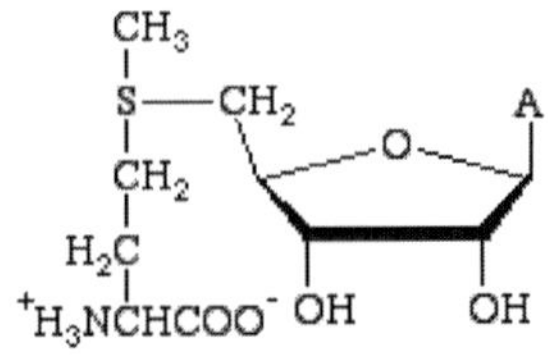 S-Adenosylmethionine	CH_3-R Methyl derivatives

Glucuronide Formation: In order to form glucuronides we must first synthesize UDP-glucuronic acid by activating and oxidizing glucose.

$$\text{Glucose} \longrightarrow \text{UDPG}$$
$$\text{Glucose} + \text{ATP} \longrightarrow \text{Glucose-6-P} + \text{ADP}$$
$$\text{G-6-P} \longrightarrow \text{G-1-P}$$
$$\text{G-1-P} + \text{UTP} \longrightarrow \text{UDPG} + \text{PP}_i$$

where PPi = inorganic pyrophosphate

PPi → 2 Pi *where* Pi = inorganic phosphate

Note that the hydrolysis of PP_i drives the reaction, since it is very favorable and the product of the previous reaction is removed. These rections take place in the cytosol.

- Conjugation by *glucuronyl transferase* now takes place on the ER, mostly via reaction with hydroxyl and carbonyl groups (but occasionally with N & S also). Generally we see S_N2 reactions, so the *alpha*-UDPG yields *beta*-glucuronides.

Example: Conjugation of phenol gives an *acetal* glucuronide, phenyl-*beta*-D-glucuronide:

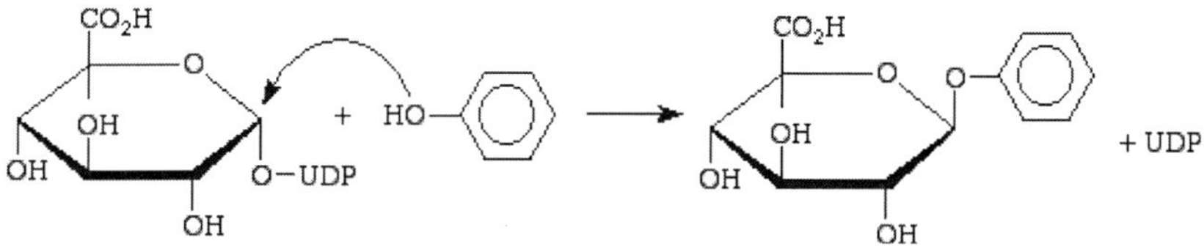

Conjugation with benzoic acid gives an ester glucuronide, benzoyl-*beta*-D-glucuronide:

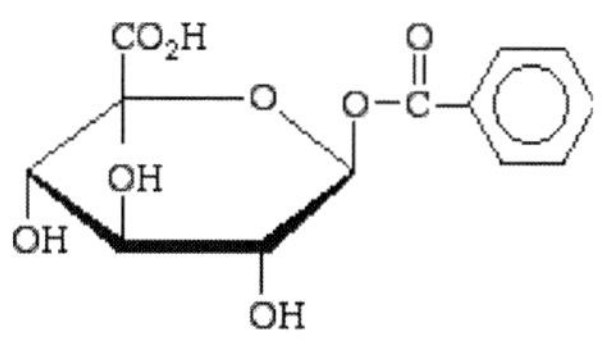

Examples with nitrogen and sulfur include the conjugation of aniline to give phenylamino-*beta*-D-glucuronide, and conjugation with 2-mercaptobenzothiazole to give the benzothiazole-2-thio-*beta*-D-glucuronide:

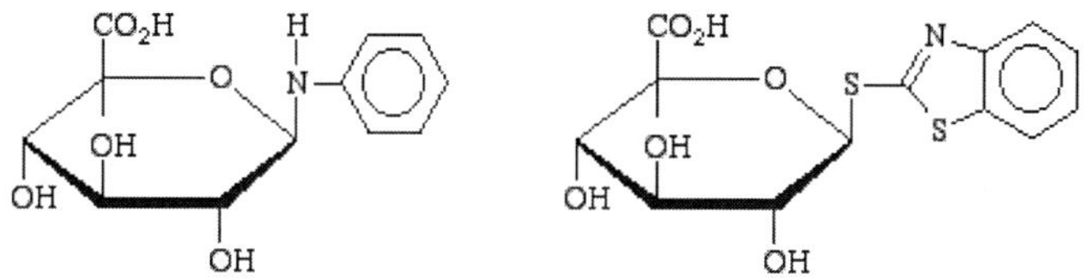

Glutathione conjugation: Glutathione is a tripeptide (*gamma*-glutamylcyteinylglycine, with the amino acid residues color coded in the structures below). It is used in cells as a recyclable anti-oxidant as well as a conjugating agent. When used in conjugation it is initially conjugated by a glutathione-S-transferase, or sometimes as a simple chemical reaction. Generally the conjugation occurs as a nucleophilic attack by the -SH group on a reactive electrophilic center. Conjugation is often followed by metabolic cleavage of the peptide to leave only the cysteinyl residue, which may then be acetylated to give a mercapturic acid.

Example

1. Glutathione S-transferase

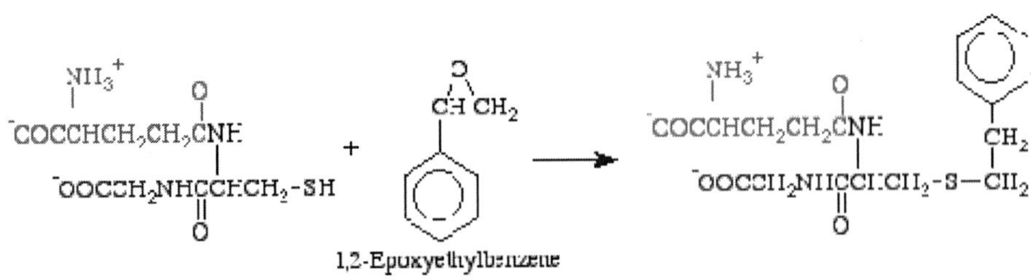

2. γ-glutamyltranspeptidase:

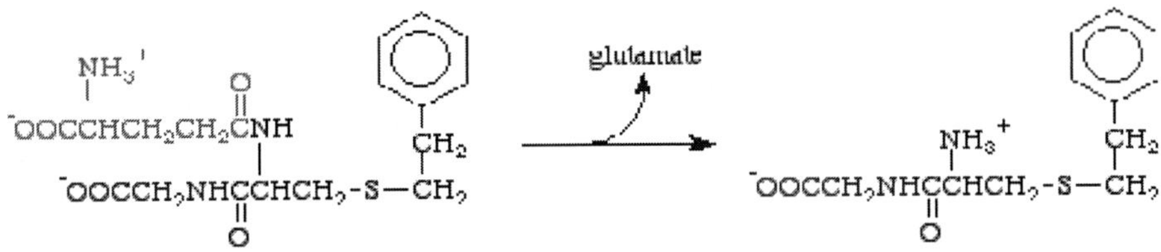

3. cysteinyl glycinase:

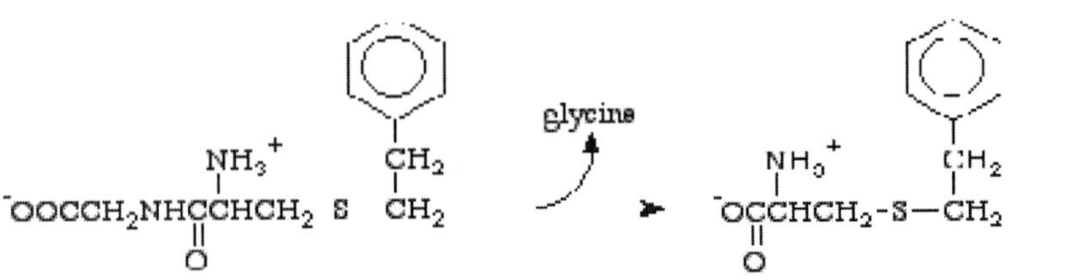

4. N-acetyl transferase:

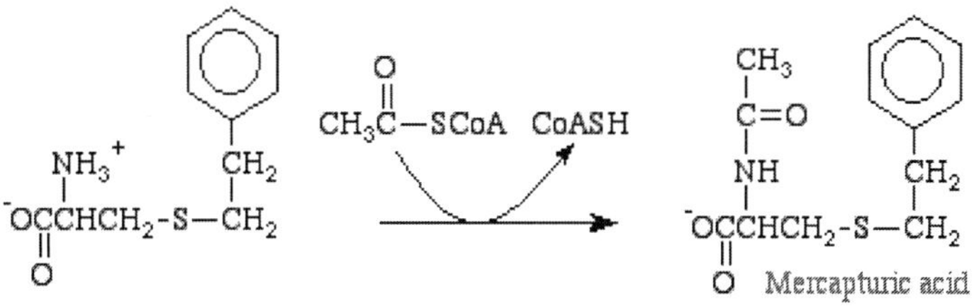

Of course not all glutathione derivatives are further metabolized, some may be excreted as is. However, if the derivative is excreted via the bile, it may be metabolized by the gut fauna and the toxin may be reabsorbed.

Sulfate Conjugation: This is the major Phase two process for a variety of hydroxyl groups and for some amines.

- The first step is to "activate" the sulfate to give "PAPS" (Adenosine-3'-P-5'-Phosphosulfate)

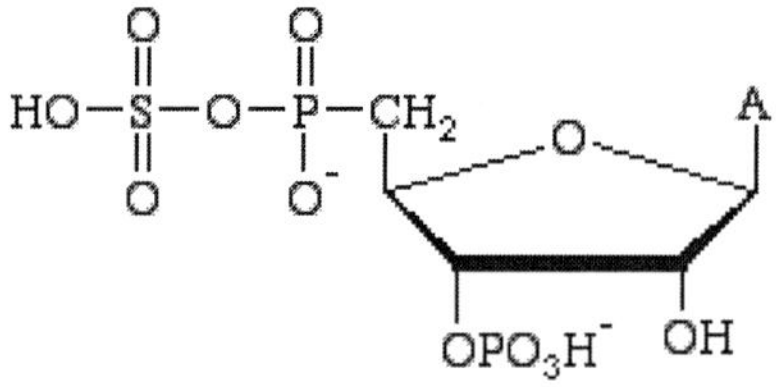

- PAPS is synthesized via Kinases:

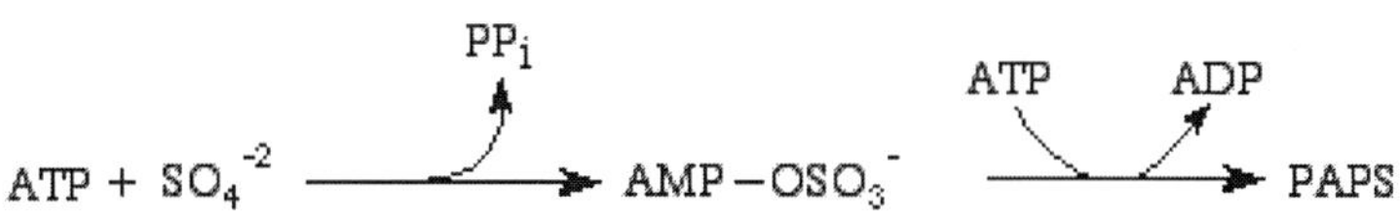

These enzymes are in the soluble fractions of a wide vriety of tissues (e.g. liver, muscle, intestine, testes, etc.).

- Can get Aryl sulfates, Alkyl sulfates, and Sulfamates via a sulfotransferase reaction.

  Example, sulfamate synthesis

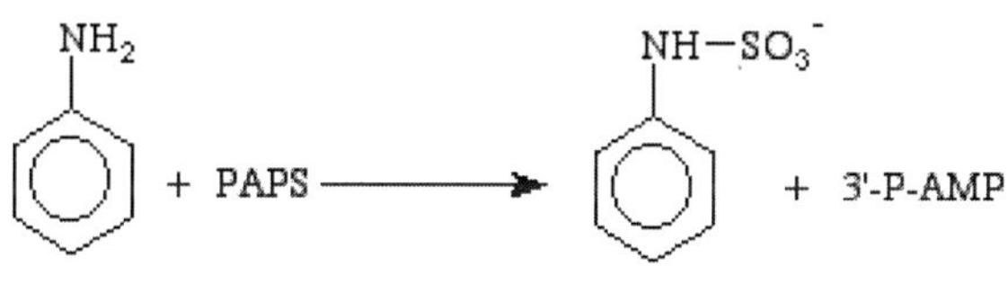

Acetylation: Acetyl transferases are found in the cytosol of hepatic endothelial cells, intestinal mucosal cells and white blood cells.

The "activated" acetyl group on acetyl CoA is used as the source of acetate, so it is readily available from normal metabolic sources. The enzyme mechanism is outlined below:

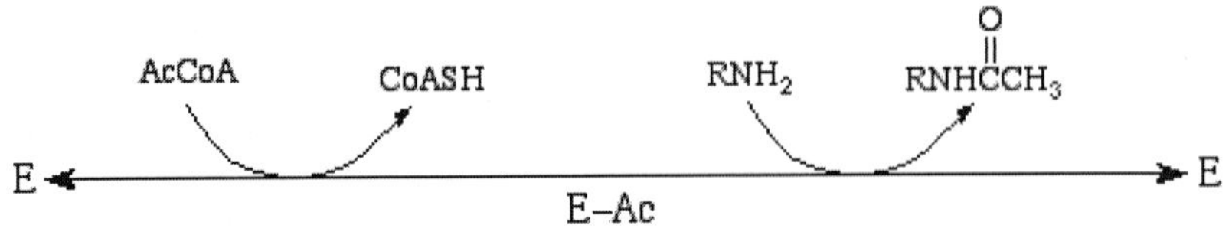

Example: acetylation of a primary aryl amine:

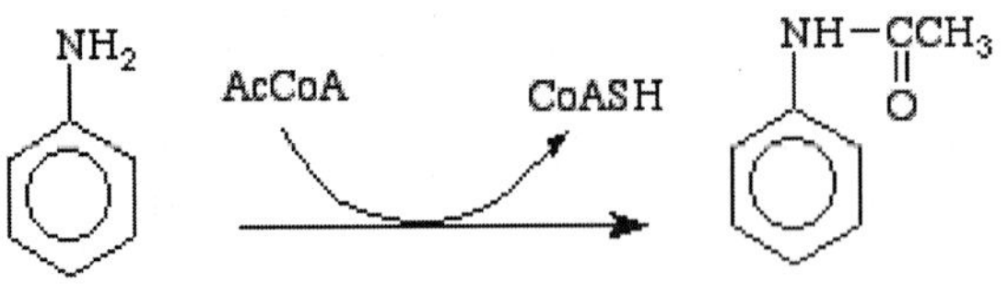

There is evidence for more than one acetylase, which provides the genetic basis for "slow" and "fast" acetylators. Apparently there is polymorphism for various acetylases.

Slow acetylators are more susceptable to xenobiotics which are inactivated by acetylation. Turns out deacetylases are also present. The two processes show dominance in different organisms, varying the importatnce of acetylation.

Acylation: Acylation is similar to acetylation in the products excreted with an amino acid (most commonly glycine, but ornithine, taurine, and glutamine are also known) substituting for acetate. However, the synthetic strategy is "reversed" in that the xenobiotic is activated by adding coenzyme A, which then reacts with the amino acid.These reactions may be catalyzed by fatty acyl CoA synthetases:

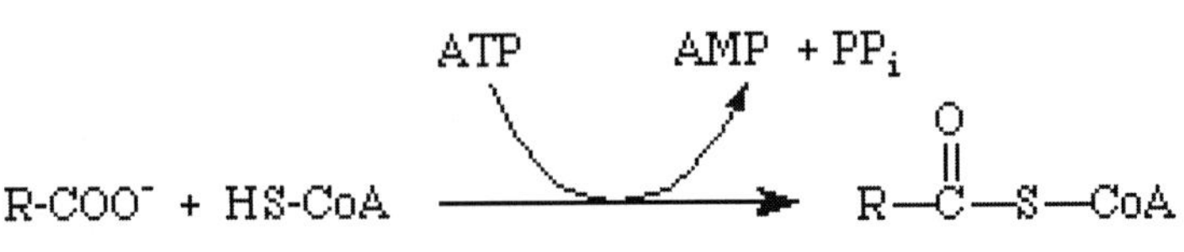

This enzyme catalyses a two part reaction:

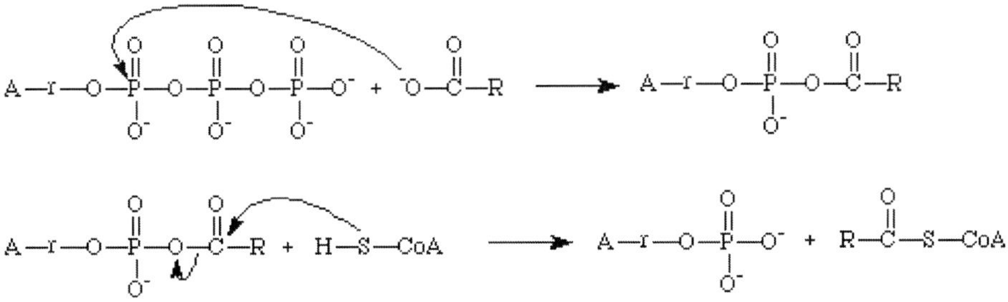

The resulting acylCoA derivative can then react with an amino acid to give the acyl excretory product.

Example: Benzoic acid is first converted to benzoyl CoA, the benzoyl CoA then reacts with glycine to give the product, Hippuric acid:

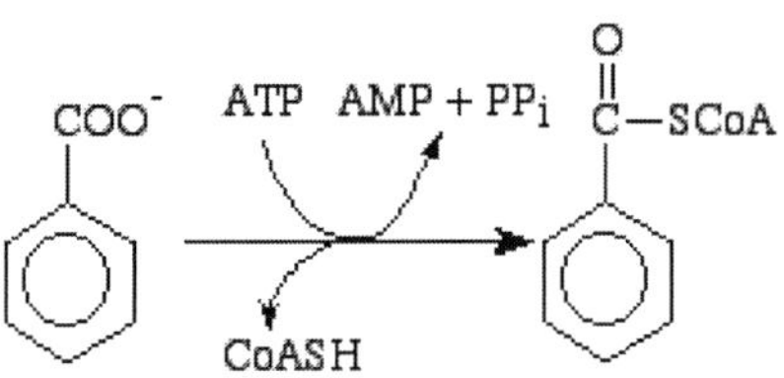

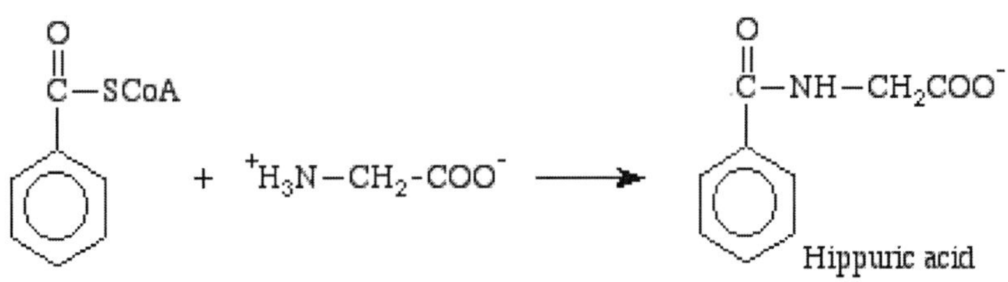

Methylation involves the transfer of an "activated" methyl group, most commonly from S-Adenosyl methionine (methyl H_4 folate and methyl Vitamin B_{12} are other possibilities). The organism can then use this system to methylate amine, hydroxyl, or sulfhydral compounds. Bacteria can also methylate heavy metals, most notoriously mercury to give dimethyl mercury.

Example : Methylation of dihydroxy benzoic acid by catechol O-methyl transferase.

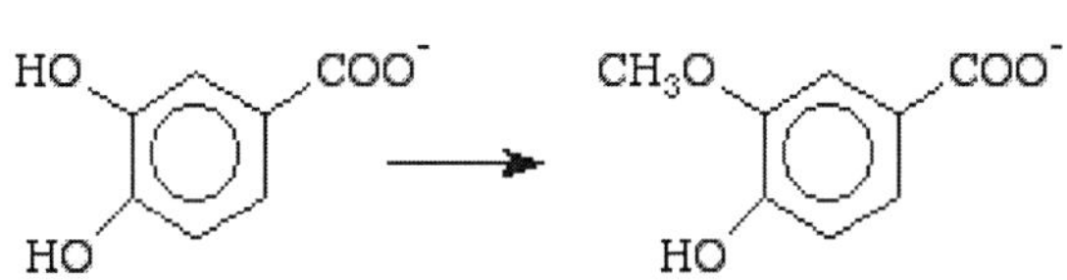

Methylation of histamine:

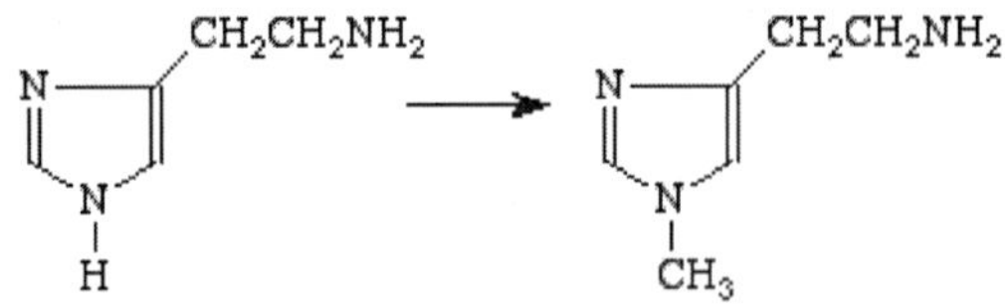

Methylation of mercaptoethanol

$$HSCH_2CH_2OH \longrightarrow CH_3\text{-}SCH_2CH_2OH$$

Factors affecting biotransformation

- *Age*: in young and old animals the biotransformation is very slow due to poor activity of liver
- *Species variation* : rabbits are resistant to atropine overdosage due to presence of atropinase enzyme cat and dogs are susceptible to certain groups of xenobiotics due to deficiency of acetyl transferases in dogs and glucuronyl transferases in cats
- *Degree of ionization* : greater the degree of ionization greater will be the biotransformation
- *Plasma protein binding* : greater the plasma protein binding lower is the biotransformation
- *Disease conditions* : diseases effecting the liver biotransformation will be low
- *Xenobiotic interactions* : Some of the xenobiotic interactions involving enzyme induction/inhibition are listed below:

Enzyme inducer	Xenobiotic affected	Remarks
Phenobarbitone	Barbiturates Chloramphenicol Progesterone; Testosterone Griseofulvin Phenytoin Phenylbutazone Cyclophosphamide	Cross tolerance can also exist between many of them due to lack of systematic specificity
Phenylbutorzone	Corticosteroids; Steroid hormones	Tolerance
Phenytoin	Steroid hormones	Hormonal imbalance
DDT	Steroid hormones	Hormonal imbalance
Griseofulvin	--	Tolerance
Diphenyl hydantoin	--	Tolerance
Inhalational anaesthetics	--	Tolerance

Enzyme Inhibitors

Chloramphenical	Barbiturates Cyclophosphamide Phenytoin Salicylates	Sleeping time enhanced Toxicity
Theophylline	Fluoroquinolones	Convulsions
Isoniazid	Phenytoin	Favour toxicity
Salicylates Chloramphenicol Phenylbutazone	Tolbutamide	Several hypoglycemic effect
Oral contraceptive	Pethidine	Respiratory depression

Excretion

The kidney is the major organ of excretion. There are, however, minor routes such as, intestines, saliva, sweat, udder milk, and lungs. The lungs become very important for volatile substances or volatile metabolites.

Xenobiotics are Eliminated by the Kidney by

a) *Passive glomerular filration*: Filtration - no xenobiotic is reabsorbed or secreted.

b) *Active tubular secretion*: Filtration and some of the xenobiotic is reabsorbed.

c) *Passive tubular reabsorption*:Filtration and some secretion.

By use of the technique of clearance studies, one can determine the process by which the kidney handles the xenobiotic .

Renal plasma clearance = UxV ml/min

U = conc. of xenobiotic in urine

Cp = conc. of xenobiotic in plasma

V = urine flow in ml/min

$$\text{Renal clearance ratio} = \frac{\text{renal plasma clearance of xenobiotic (ml/min}}{\text{GFR (ml/min)}}$$

Total Body Clearance = renal + non-renal

Interpretation

- renal clearance ratio= 1, the xenobiotic is filtered and not reabsorbed or secreted.
- renal clearance ratio=< 1, the xenobiotic is filtered and some is reabsorbed.
- renal clearance ratio= >1, then the xenobiotic is filtered and secreted.

Filtration and reabsorption are governed by the same principles already discussed under transport mechanisms and absorption. In the kidney, one may use these principles to enhance the elimination of a xenobiotic. The pH of urine may vary from 4.3 to 8 and by the use of drugs the pH can be maintained or changed to acidic or basic as desired. Acidification of the urine will hasten the elimination of basic xenobiotic. If the urine is made basic just the opposite occurs (Henderson Hasselback equation) (phenobarbital, aspirin, methamphetamine). The overall extend that pH may influence the elimination which depends on the percent of the xenobiotic cleared from the plasma by renal clearance.

Tubular Secretion: Active tubular secretion of some xenobiotic, weak organic acids and bases take place in the proximal tubule. This process is energy dependent and can be blocked by other drugs. It is specific and can be saturated. Each substance has a characteristic maximum (Tm). Anions and cations are handled by different transport systems. The anionic system generally handle metabolites conjugated with glycine, glucuronic, acid or sulfates. These various anionic compounds compete with each other transport (Probenecid-Penicillin). Similarly organic cations complete with each other but not with anionic compounds.

Following are the major ways through which xenobiotic and their metabolites are excreted.

1. Faecal excretion. Substances may find their way into faeces via bile; xenobiotic stored in the liver are slowly excreted in this way.
2. Pulmonary excretion. Volatile drugs may be mainly excreted in the expired air.The lesions found in the lungs in paraffin poisoning are probably due to irritant effect caused by pulmonary excretion.
3. Urinary excretion. This is the most important pathway of the excretion of a xenobiotic. Irritant poisons cause damage to kidney. Urine is often a convenient material for diagnostic analysis. In veterinary field it is of great importance in detecting the elimination parameters.

4. Milk and dermal excretion. Excretion can also take place through skin,e.g., arsenical compounds, and in lactating animals in milk.

Biliary Excretion: Larger, polar compounds are often preferentially excreted via the biliary system into the duodenum.

- Usually need to have a MW > 300 for this system to be effective.
- Generally active processes are specific for acids, bases or neutral compounds.
- Charged compounds will not be resorbed from the intestinal lumen and so will be lost with faces.
- Can get intestinal resorption however if the excreted conjugated compound is hydrolyzed or metabolized to give a non-polar entity by intestinal flora.

Other systems involved in excretion include the lungs (volatile substances), sweat, and milk (particularly for lipid soluble substances).

Dose-response: Relationship between the level of exposure and the magnitude of the response.

- Much of veterinary toxicology.... deals with levels of exposure that are within ranges reflected in previously generated dose-response data.
- Risk assessment (for human safety) commonly deals with extrapolation below the experimental range.
- Risk assessment (for animals in ecosystems) commonly deals with exposures in the experimental range, but *extrapolation is necessary to a range of untested and phylogenetically diverse species.*

Types of Responses - Graded as Contrasted to Quantal Responses

Graded data = varied in intensity, e.g., enzyme activity, heart rate, graphical example: egg shell thickness in eagle

Graded dose-response data can be analyzed by regression analysis, to identify linear or curvilinear relationships.

Quantal data = + or - e.g., lethality.

Quantal data (examples)

% dead vs. alive (lethal dose = LD).

% showing an increase in heart rate to 100 (a toxic dose = TD)

% showing control of seizures (effective dose = ED).

One can plot quantal responses of a group of animals vs:

Dose.

Concentration in air.

Concentration in feed.

Frequency of administration.

The steeper the dose-response curve, the more uniform the response among the test animals (i.e. more of them respond within a narrow dose range).

The flatter the dose-response curves, the greater the variation in response to the doses given. With flatter dose-response curves, it is much more difficult to predict the effects of a given toxicant dose on a given animal.

Therapeutic Index (TI) applies to pharmaceutical agents and is the ratio of the median lethal dose (LD_{50}) to that producing a desired median therapeutic response ED_{50}.

e.g. $$\frac{LD_{50}}{ED_{50}}$$

Depending on which values are used to calculate the therapeutic index the TI value will differ widely, therefore, be sure to know the basis for each therapeutic index.

Standard Safety Margin. Another useful calculation is the Standard Safety Margin, which compares the lowest lethal dose (LD1) to the highest effective dose (ED99), giving a much more conservative evaluation of safety of a product.

LD_{50}: Primary advantage is that it is generally the most reliable number (regarding the probability of a lethal effect that you can get).

- "Better than nothing" when estimating outcome of an exposure.
- Used for extrapolation.
- *Disadvantages*: Tells you nothing about shape or slope of dose response curve. Thus, you still know nothing about LD_1 or the lowest toxic dose.
- LD_{50} bears no relationship to long term toxic effects

$$M = LD1/ED99$$

If 50% died at a single dose, it could be termed the LD_{50}. However, it can be a problem to hit exactly 50% dead; and trial and error is inefficient - too many animals used, too many experience the toxicosis.

Definition: Relationships between tissue concentrations of a toxicant and time.

Differences from pharmacokinetics: In clinical toxicology cases, one deals with:

- Potential poisoning (not yet absorbed).
- Actual toxicoses (altered physiology/may alter kinetics over time).
- Residue contamination of foods such as meat, milk, or eggs.

Whether the problem relates to poisoning or residues, toxicokinetic data may be used either

- to predict "normal" rates of metabolic change (activation or detoxification) and/or elimination, or
- to choose methods to help decrease the toxicant concentration at the receptor (e.g., to limit absorption, or increase detoxification or excretion).

As compared to typical uses of therapeutic xenobiotics, in toxicoses, kinetics are more likely to be altered by

- *Saturation of enzymes* involved in metabolism (detoxification or toxification) or of enzymes employed in carrier systems necessary for elimination
- *Organ system dysfunction or failure*

e.g. toxicant-induced liver or kidney damage that alters metabolism and/or elimination of the toxicant

e.g. circulatory problems resulting in hypotension secondary to shock

e.g. acidosis due to exertion and seizures

Review of some important kinetic concepts.

Zero Order (sometimes termed as "Michaelis-Menten kinetics").

Reason Zero Order

Ab(t) = starting Ab - x t Ab

Where Ab = amount in body.

Ab(t) = amount in body at time t.

x = amount elim. per unit of time (x has no exponent, and therefore is zero order).

t = time (after dosing).

First Order Kinetics

The usual situation for most xenobiotic and other toxicant exposures.

Rate of process may be limited by blood flow through liver or kidney; e.g., if all or a fixed fraction of the compound is cleared on each pass.

Early on: Rapid fall in amount in body. Later on, rate of elimination slows as blood concentration gradually declines.

Reason first order = first order exponent

Ab(t) = Starting (e^{-kt}) Ab

Where

e = 2.72 = base of natural logs.

k = rate constant (= fraction elim. per unit of time).

Note: Kinetics may change from zero order (process saturated) to first order (no longer saturated).

More complex models may explain the disappearance of some xenobiotics, e.g., two or three compartment models.

In residue cases, one may be most interested in the terminal (elimination) phase, but ignoring the earlier phases may lead to an overestimation of the time necessary to clean up the animals.

Kinetics are influenced by the basic chemistry of the xenobiotic

Bioavailability of xenobiotics varies from 0% to 100%. The rate of absorption, metabolism and/or elimination depends on chemical size and structure, fat solubility, and ability to interact with degradative enzymes, carrier systems, and alternative binding sites.

- e.g., Ca^{++} uptake system in the gut also takes up Pb^{++}.
- e.g., Organic acids often are excreted by an active process in renal tubules (e.g., 2,4-D).
- Highly fat-soluble compounds that resist biotransformation increase in fat over time. With chronic low level exposure, biomagnification occurs (biomagnification is the redistribution to the fat in this case) (e.g., heptachlor epoxide).

Dose-Response Curves

Dose-response Curve: When lethality is plotted against log Dose the typical response is described by a sigmoidal curve.

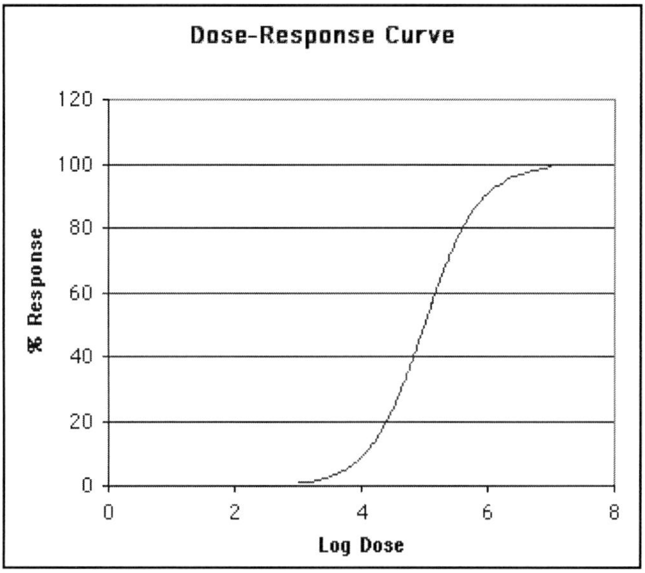

[This kind of curve shape also describes a wide range of binding phenomena, the most familiar being the pH titration curve. For the pH titration the axis are interchanged. The log is of course pH, while the % response corresponds to the % acid titrated.]

We generally consider that this relationship is based on three assumptions:

1. The toxic response is a function of the concentration of the compound at the site of action.
2. The concentration at the the site of action is related to the dose.
3. The response is causally related to the compound.

Let's look at these assumptions

- The response is a function of the concentration at the site of action:
  - The site of action may be an enzyme, a receptor site, a cell, etc.
  - The interaction at this site may be reversible or irreversible.

We generally consider that this relationship is based on three assumptions:

1. The toxic response is a function of the concentration of the compound at the site of action.
2. The concentration at the the site of action is related to the dose.
3. The response is causally related to the compound.

Let's look at these assumptions

- The response is a function of the concentration at the site of action:
  - The site of action may be an enzyme, a receptor site, a cell, etc.
  - The interaction at this site may be reversible or irreversible. For reversible phenomena

$$T + R \rightleftharpoons TR$$

  the response is proportional to [TR]

  where T = toxin, R = receptor, and TR = toxin - receptor complex

  For r = R + TR = number of receptor sites, TR/r = 1 will get the maximum response.

  K_{eq} will effect the dose-response curve, but the curve will remain sigmoidal, with:

- Strong binding giving a steep curve.
- Weak binding giving a shallow curve.

  For irreversible interactions the response may still be proportional to the concentration at the site of action, but the results may be quite different. Since the interaction is irreversible a single interaction knocks out the receptor. The response will now depend on how fast the receptors may be replaced, and if the replacement is slow, the dose may be cumulative.

- Of course for this discussion to be relevant to Dose, we must have a particular relationship between dose and concentration at the active site. Generally we **assume** tissue concentration is related to dose - but what if it isn't? What factors might affect it?
  - Absorption at the site of exposure.
  - Tissue distribution (non-polar substance deposit in fat, skin etc.)
  - Metabolism (substance may be metabolized so rapidly that it never reaches the site of action.

- Excretion (may be rapidly excreted, again active site concentration does not reflect exposure).

  Notice that the dose itself may alter any one of the above processes. For example, the substance may be actively excreted, but it "kills" the kidney, leading to a complex dose-response behavior.
- Saturation of one of the above processes.
- Saturation of a storage site, such as plasma protein, will give a curve with an initial very shallow rise, until saturation when a much steeper response curve ensues.
- Accumulation (concentration) of a compound in a particular tissue can give a higher than expected response if the tissue includes the target.

  These various processes may **prevent** a compound from reaching the site of action at low doses, particularly with irreversibly bound compounds, and thus contribute to a **threshold** phenomena. We will look in detail at some of these processes later with specific examples, demonstrating how they can drastically affect the concentration at the site of action.

3. Finally, the response **may not be** causally related to the compound.

Quantitation of Dose Response

Gaussian (Normal) Distributions: For populations often assume a Gaussian distribution, that is we assume that we in fact have a completely random distribution of values around a central value, as in the Gaussian curve below.

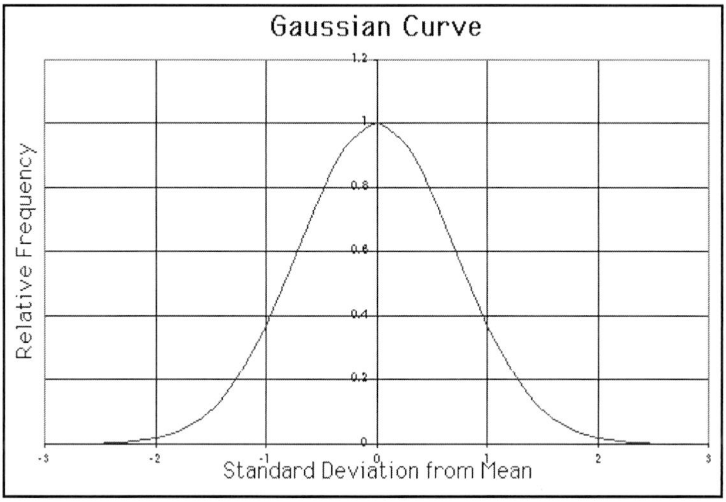

Recall that for a Gaussian distribution the the mean (arithmetic average), median (central value), and mode (most frequent value) coincide. It is also useful to note that the area under the curve between ± 1s (1 sigma) includes 68% of all values (of the population), while ± 2s (2 sigma) includes 95% and ± 3s (3 sigma) includes 99% of all values.

Of course not all distributions are randomly distributed around a central point. For example the distribution of concentrations around an average value near zero will be skewed toward high values since we cannot have concentrations below zero. This is similar to the situation we see for the speeds of gas molecules etc.

Because of the wide occurrence and common knowledge, and mathematical exactness of the Gaussian function other distributions are often transformed to get a Gaussian shape. Thus a log transformation will often convert a skewed distribution into a Gaussian. One should exercise caution however. The Gaussian is too nice, it is seductive because of its convenience etc., **but** it is not always followed. If at all in doubt one should test a distribution to be certain it is in fact Gaussian. Linear transformations are very useful in this respect. Thus one may plot data on "probability paper" or in Probit units for frequency (below) vs. log value. In each case deviation from linearity indicates a non-Gaussian distribution. This deviation in turn can be analyzed statistically etc.

Sigmoidal plot of normal distributions: If the values in a normal distribution are plotted vs. **cumulative** frequency instead of frequency, a sigmoidal plot results (Ideally the curve should intersect 0 at 50%.

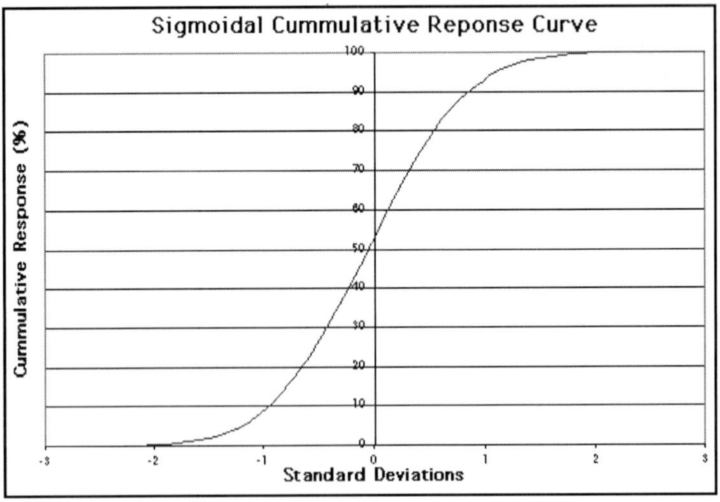

Probit Analysis gives a linear response from sigmoidal (Gaussian) Dose-response curves. For probit analysis divide data into multiples of s ("Probit units") from the mean. But **define mean = 5**. Thus -1s = 4, 1s =6 etc. The standard deviation is sometimes called NED (normal equivalent deviation). So for 50% response (mean value in Gaussian) NED = 0, for 15.9% (50 - 68.2/2) response NED = -1, for 84.1% (68.2 + 15.9) NED =1. So Probit = NED + 5.

Plotting probit units against log dose will then give a linear function for populations following a normal distribution. Plots of data in terms of probit units are very convenient. Very easy to define LD_{50} etc. can also do regression analysis, and the slope aids in judging hazards. A narrow range gives a steep slope, indicating little for warning of serious effects.

Quantitation of Dose Response

Selection of Toxic Criteria

We have looked at one of the simplest measures of toxicity, the LD_{50}. Lets define a few of these measures

- ED_{50}: effective dose. Generally used for drugs - the dose required to have a therapeutic or other effect in 50% of sample population.
- TD_{50}: toxic dose. The dose required to elicit a defined toxic effect (e.g. fatty liver, fever, etc.) in 50% of the sample population.
- LD_{50}: lethal dose. The dose required for lethality in 50% of the sample population.

Sometimes the occurrence of parallelism between the probit curves for these three measures is interpreted as indicating an equivalence in their mechanisms - not necessarily true.

Therapeutic Index

Therapeutic index is a comparison of effective versus lethal doses - an important thing to know if you are giving drugs out!

- Most commonly the median is used as the measure of centrality rather than the mean. This is because the median is generally a better measure of centrality for skewed distributions - it gives a better picture of the population, with fewer chances of error in the prediction of the behavior of individual in the population. Note that if the population does follow Gaussian statistics it makes no difference.

A safer, more reliable and thus more valuable expression for TI in drug development is thus TI = TD_1/ED_{99} or LD_1/ED_{99}. This should lead to a very safe situation.

Finally, one should keep in mind that the determination of LD_{50} etc. are not biologically constant, but in fact depend on many factors, such that we often see differences between labs and even within the same lab.

Chronic Toxicity

Chronic Toxicity can be quantified in similar ways and can reveal evidence of accumulation and therefore estimates of body $t_{1/2}$. For chronic toxicity measure TD_{50} or LD_{50} for a specific time period, such as 90 days, and compare to the same total dose delivered in a single dose. Determine the chronicity factor.

Chronicity factor: $(LD_{50})_{1\ dose}/(LD_{50})_{90\ doses}$ with units of mg/kg vs. mg/kg/day.

- Note in each case we have the same total dose top and bottom.
  - If CF = 90 then the toxin is absolutely cumulative. (e.g. for a compound with LD_{50} = 90 mg/kg, if 90 1 mg/kg doses also gave LD_{50}, then CF = 90/1 = 90)
  - If CF > 2 then relatively cumulative.
  - If CF < 2 then relatively non-cumulative.

Accumulation can be due to accumulation of the compound *in vivo* or an accumulation of effect.

Example: tri-o-cresyl phosphate (TOCP), a cholinesterase inhibitor and neurotoxin. This toxin has the same effect in chickens in one 30 mg/kg dose or in 30 1 mg/kg dose delivered daily for 30 days. Here either situation could hold, because the $t_{1/2}$ of replacement for cholinesterase is > 30 days.

Dose-Response Relationships

Dose-response relationships provide a way of quantifying toxicity. There are many ways of measuring toxicity. Toxicity is also a relative phenomena. Thus we need to understand a bit about some of the conventions used in quantifying toxicity and the types of measurements commonly used.

Criteria of Toxicity : One of the first criteria in characterizing toxicity is the lethality, generally determined in mice or rats. Usually want a minimum sample size of 50 - 100 to get good statistics and a high probability of representing the population. Probably the best known and one of the most often used measures is the LD_{50}, or the dose which is lethal for 50% of a given population. This appears to be and often is a rather gross measure unless carefully observed. Though the LD_{50} is a crude measure its value can be increased by careful observation and analysis of changes occurring during the determination of the LD_{50}. For example additional measures of toxicity which might be obtained include, in order of increasing information content (and cost):

- muscle tone, liver palpability (both are non-invasive measures)
- fatty liver (require biopsy or autopsy), serum protein changes (require blood sample)
- binding site saturation (requires isolation from tissue samples)

Each of these can provide a measurable response which will enhance the value of the toxicity test. However, much work will generally be required to get down to the detailed *biochemical mode of action*. Of course the more we know, the better we can guess and the more quickly we can assess new toxins for mode of action etc.

Interactions of Toxins: a number of terms are used to describe the interactions of toxins. It is useful to be familiar with the following:

- Additivity: the overall effect of two toxins is the direct addition of the individual toxicities of the doses given.
- *Synergism*: the toxicity of the doses of two toxins is greater than the sum of the toxicities of these two doses. Synergy gives a greater toxic effect than additive toxicities.
- *Potentiation*: similar to synergism, but the toxins have different effects. Specifically, one substance leads to a greater effect by a second toxic substance. An example is "antiabuse" in treating alcoholism - by itself at the dose given there is no effect, but when alcohol is ingested there is a toxic response to the alcohol at small doses.
- *Antagonism*: one substance reduces the toxicity of another.

Tolerance: exposure at low doses leads to a tolerance whereby subsequent exposure to toxic dose levels prove to be less toxic than normal.

Toxicodynamics

General Mechanism of Action of Poisons

I. Direct Injury

Eg: acids, alkalies, heavy metals, phenols and aldehydes

- Non-specific for any one group- anything that can cause coagulation, denaturation, a change in structure
- Action is immediate (no latent period)

II. Inhibition of Essential Enzymes

- *Reversible* Eg: carbamates- acetyl cholinesterase inhibition
- *Irreversible* Eg. Organophosphates- malathion parathion etc: irreversible acetyl cholinesterase inhibitors: due to loss of ester moiety

III. Inhibitors of Metabolism

- Uncouplers of oxidative phosphorylation Eg. Chlorophenol, dinitrophenol, arsenates (fungicides), decrease the production of ATP, increase oxygen utilization resulting in convulsions.
- Inhibitors of oxidative phosphorylation Eg: trisubstituted fungicides, decrease utilisation of oxygen and decrease ATP production resulting in weakness, fatigue and lethargy.

IV. Inhibitors of DNA and Protein Synthesis

They cause DNA alkylation and interfere with transcription Eg: aflatoxins, organomercurials, amantine (amanita phalloides, a mushroom poison).

V. Inhibitors of Release of Neurotransmitters

- Agents which alter the neurotransmitter levels. Eg: Organophosphorous compounds increase Ach levels causing paralysis. : Botulinum toxin decrease Ach levels, inhibiting cholinergic transmission, resulting in flaccid poaralysis.

  a) *Interference with receptors:* Receptors are macromolecules which are acted upon by endogenous neurotransmitter or hormones

     Eg: Curare (d- tubocurarine) is a competitive antagonist of nicotinic receptors for Ach at neuromuscular junction, results in flaccid paralysis

  b) *Interference with signal transduction :* Eg: Organochlorine compounds, synthetic pyrethroids, scorpion venom- inhibit inactivation of sodium channels resulting in excessive persistent depolarization. Tetradotoxin, saggitoxin- inhibit sodium channel and blocks axonal conduction and neurotransmission

  c) *Interference with signal termination :*

     i) Na-K- ATPase inhibition- Glutamate, excitatory neurotransmitter in brain is inhibited resulting in persistent excitation and neuronal damage.

ii) Ca ATP ase or Ca pump inhibition, accumulation of Ca in cell stimulates lysosomal membranes and liberation of degradative enzymes leading to cell death.

VI. Agents which Produce Demyelination

Eg: Lathyrus causing atrophy of hindlimb muscles, due to the active moiety diamino propionitrile.

VII. Interference with Normal Body Constituents

a) Haemoglobin- formation of carboxy haemoglobin and methaemoglobin as in carbon monoxide and nitrate/nitrite poisoning respectively which hinders the capacity to carry oxygen.

b) Vitamin K inhibition by rodenticides. Eg: warfarin; interfering with the blood clotting process

c) Fluoroacetate getting converted in to fluorocitrate, incorporating into Tricarboxylic acid (TCA) cycle.

VIII. Agents with Functional Similarity

a) Estrogenic mycotoxins Eg: zearalenone- still births and abortions: DDT, similar to estrogen, results in embryotoxicity

b) OP, Monocrotophos caused drop in number of eagles and vultures.

IX. Agents Causing Immunotoxicity

Eg: Aflatoxins, pesticides, heavy metals decrease both cell mediated and humoral immunity.

X. Agents Causing Teratogenecity

Eg: Reproduction toxicity and malformation of foetus, as caused by thalidomide. During first trimester, organ deformation and during last trimester still births were the effects noticed.

XI. Agents Causing Carcinogenesis

Initiation- directly attacking and damaging DNA

Promotion- responsible for outward expression of carcinogenicity.

XII. Agents Influencing Osmosis

Eg: In salt poisoning, Na retains iso osmotic equivalent of water, increase ECF and decrease ICF, resulting in softening and tearing of CNS (encephalomalacia).

XIII. Agents Interfering with Fat Metabolism

Decreased synthesis of lipid acceptor protein, which transports fatty acids and triglycerides from fat to tissues, resulting in fat accumulation in hepatocytes and fatty liver condition and leading to necrosis . Eg: hepatocytes, renocytes, cancerous bone marrow and GIT epithelial cells.

XIV. Agents Causing Anoxia, Hypoxia and Ischemia

Reduced oxygen supply and decreased ATP production, resulting in sodium pump failure and fluid accumulation leading to cell burst and death.

Collection and Dispatch of Specimens in Toxicological Cases

Every veterinarian will be encountered with diagnosing and treating the animals exposed to toxicant / poisoning which may be either accidental or malicious in origin. History, clinical signs and necropsy of the animals will assist in rapid tentative diagnosis which will help in the treatment of other affected animals in case of accidental poisoning. In case of malicious poisoning, which may turn up into veterolegal case, the identification of the toxin/ poison is a must to establish the cause of death. In all poisonous/toxicological cases, chemical analysis of the biological specimens is essential to know the cause of death or illness., for which proper collection and despatch of toxicological specimens to the laboratory is necessary.

History of the case is of great importance in the diagnosis of poisoning. This includes the number of animals in the farm, number of animals affected, method of feeding, regularity of feeding, recent changes in the rations or attendants, spraying of pastures with pesticides or fertilizers, rodenticides, presence of poisonous plants in the farm environment. the possibility of industrial effluents coming in contact with grazing/watering sources etc.

Postmortem

Necropsy by routine procedure is to be performed as soon as possible after the death of animal. The animal should be examined externally for the presence of any incisions (for sui poisoning, snake bite etc.,) on the skin or mucous membranes. The oral cavity is examined for corrosive lesions (acids/ alkali) or changes in colour of mucous membrane (nitrate, co, cyanide poisoning). As most of the toxins gain entry through gut, examination of gut mucosa, the contents, their smell, colour and pH (acids, alkali, urea) is a valuable guide in diagnosing toxicoses. Poisoning by salts of heavy metals results in significant post mortem lesions but poisoning by alkaloids like strychnine produces very feeble lesions.

The natural orifices, sub-cutaneous fat tissue, muscles, bones and teeth (in fluorine poisoning), body cavities, and internal organs should be examined. The stomach should be punctured rather than cut open for examination to note the character of smell. Puncture ensures greater accuracy and a longer time smell. Some of the poisons emit characteristic smell like bitter almond in hydrogen cyanide poisoning, garlic odour in phosphorus poisoning, rotten garlic or horse radish smell in selenium, tobacco odour in nicotine, acetylene odour in zinc phosphide and ammoniacal odour in urea poiosoning.

The colour of stomach contents also to be examined as copper salts impart a greenish blue colour whereas picric and nitric acid impart yellow colour to the contents.

The contents of the stomach, small intestine and large intestine vary from traces to flakes of paints or lead objects, grains or baits, seeds etc. Blood should be examined for its colour and clotting characters. Cyanide poisoning imparts cherry red colour, arsenic imparts rose red colour and nitrate poisoning turns the blood to brown colour.

Examination of other visceral organs should be done in relation to their size, colour etc. Spleen size is decreased and colour is changed to dark brown or black in copper poisoning and spleen size is increased in mycotoxicoses. The description of morphological changes should be noted clearly and absence of changes should be notified.

Submission of Specimens

A complete set of tissues collected from PM examination should include the brain, eyeball, thymus, thyroid, heart, lung, spleen, kidney, liver, urinary bladder, pancreas, lymphnodes, various sections of the gastrointestinal tract, ovaries, placenta, testes etc. In case of many animal being affected, sample from more than one animal should be used.

The following specimen samples are preferred to be sent for different suspected poisoning/ toxicant diagnosis in the laboratory.

Suspected poison	Preferred specimens in order of importance
1. Antimony	Liver, thyroid, kidney, urine, stomach contents.
2. Arsenic (acute)	Liver, kidneys, gastrointestinal contents, urine, feed.

Contd...

Table Contd...

3.	Arsenic (chronic)	Hair, liver, urine, spleen, altered organs.
4.	Alkaloids	Liver, urine, brain, stomach contents.
5.	Ammonia	Whole blood or serum, urine gastro-intestinal contents.
6.	Alpha napthyl thiourea	gastrointestinal contents.
7.	Barbiturates	Blood, brain, liver, adipose tissue.
8.	Cadmium	Kidney, liver, hair
9.	Carbon monoxide	Blood (refrigerated).
10.	Copper	Liver, blood, kidney, feces, and urine
11.	Cyanide	Gastrointestinal contents, liver,muscles,
12.	Oxalated blood, brain, suspected feed	
13.	Fluorides	Altered parts of bone, teeth, urine,
14.	Stomach contents, liver, kidney,	
15.	Feed and / or drinking water.	
16.	Organochlorines	Body Fat, liver, gastrointestinal contents, brain
17.	Only glass containers	
18.	Organophosphates	Heparinised blood, whole blood, liver, Stomach contents.urine
19.	Lead (acute)	Kidneys, liver, urine, whole blood.
20.	Lead (chronic)	Hair, liver, kidneys, bone, feces,
21.	Mercury	Liver, kidneys, intestinalcontents, stomach contents
22.	Muscle, brain, feces	
23.	Molybdenum	Feed, liver, kidneys, alteredorgans (bone), hair
24.	Mycotoxin	feed
25.	Nitrate and nitrite	Water, Stomach contents whole blood, Urine, suspected feed, forage, silage
26.	Oxalates	Fresh forage, kidneys
27.	Pesticides	Blood, liver, gastrointestinal contents
28.	Phenol and cresol	Liver, gastrointestinal contents, kidneys
29.	Phosphide	gastrointestinal contents, suspected material (Grain, flour etc.)

Contd...

Table Contd...

30.	Phosphorus	Gastrointestinal contents, liver, oxalated blood, Altered organs (lung), vomitus, faeces.
31.	Rodenticides	Gastrointestinal contents, liver, urine
32.	Selenium	Suspected feed, altered organs,whole blood, liver, hair
33.	Sodium chloride	Oxalated and whole blood,brain
34.	Sodium fluoroacetate	Gastrointestinal contents, liver, kidney, urine
35.	Strychnine	Gastrointestinal contents,urine, liver, kidney and brain.
36.	Urea	Feed, stomach contents
37.	Warfarin (other anticoagulants)	Whole blood, liver, feed
38.	Zinc	Liver, kidney, pancreas, feces, bone (humerus)
39.	Zinc phosphide	Liver, gastrointestinal contents, feed.

Quantity of the Sample

The following table indicates the minimum quantity of the samples need to be sent to the laboratory for the analysis

Kind of sample	Quantity
• Whole blood (EDTA/ Heparinised)	10-20 ml
• Serum	5ml
• Body fluids	10-20ml
• Cerebrospinal fluid	1ml
• Water	1L
• Cardiac blood clot in dead animal	
• Epidermal tissues (nail, hair, feathers)	20-30g
• Liver	100-250g
• Stomach/Ruminal contents	0.5-1kg
• Kidney	100g / whole kidney
• Bone	100g/one long bone
• Brain	50%, sagital section
• Fat	Supra renal-100g

Contd...

Table Contd...

• Brain	entire or a section
• Serum	10-20 ml
• Urine	50-100 ml
• Pancreas	100g
• Faeces	50 g
• Small species (poultty small dogs, gamebirds, rabbits)	as many of the carcasses as possible
• Dry Feed (granules, powder)	1kg
• Fresh feed (grass, forage)	2kg in ordinary paper
• Silage, pulp	2kg in plastic sack not to be filled completely after squeezing all the air out
• Straw, Hay	0.5 kg
• Fresh plant material	Whole fresh plant if it is small Leafy branch with flowers in case of large plants and trees Uncrushed bulky parts-root, fruits in a plastic bag
• Dried plant material	In a rigid cardboard box taking care not to break branches/detach leaves

Packing

Samples submitted to the laboratory should be individually packed and labelled so as to avoid any confusion about specimen identification. Sample should be -wrapped in foil to protect light sensitive compounds from degrading or frozen to prevent volatile compounds from escaping. All specimens should be double bagged and submitted in appropriate shipping containers to prevent leaking.

Following points to be taken in to consideration during packing the sample to be sent for the investigation.

- Samples must be placed in strong waterproof plastic bags or wide mouthed glass container without adding any preservatives/fixative to the sample.

- The container tightly stoppered, properly sealed with paraffin sealing wax should be kept in a larger wooden box which is sealed in cloth.
- All the specimens are to be taken in separate containers (polythene jars/ covers), securely tied, properly labelled with particulars of date, case number, organs collected, species, name of preservative used etc.
- A sample of the preservative used, brief history of the case along with treatment given particulars should be sent.
- Details of the addresses of the sender and the address of the laboratory is written on outside the box which can be sent either through a messenger or by post.
- The sample should not come in direct contact with any absorbent material like cotton wool, gauze which will dry out the sample.
- Empty used medicinal bottles, plastic mineral water bottles should not be used.
- Glass containers if used, must be well protected to prevent breakage in transit, by packing with sufficient absorbent material like sawdust, newspaper etc.
- The containers should never be filled completely as fermentation may occur particularly with stomach/ ruminal contents.
- The samples transported at ambient temperature or higher must be provided heat seal, screw caps must be reinforced with tape.
- In case of the samples being transported in refrigerated or frozen state using ice pack/ waterproof frozen sachets, screw caps should not be used.
- Rumen contents/vomitus is preferred to be sent to establish that the toxin has been ingested.
- Liver, spleen and blood are preferred to establish toxin/ poison absorption.
- Kidney, urine and milk are preferred and be sent for detecting toxin excretion.
- A sample of preservative in a separate sealed container to be sent particularly in veterolegal cases.
- The container with indelible pen / marker labelling must be sealed properly to ensure that the original contents are not being tampered or so as to to provide proof for being tampered especially in vetero legal cases.

In case of small animals (poultry, small dogs, lab animals) the cadavers are sent as it is, in case of large animals the gastrointestinal contents are collected from the vicinity of changes in the gastric/intestinal mucosa. If there are no changes, a representative sample is collected, but in medium sized animals the stomach tied at oesophageal and duodenal end, intestine tied at both ends and bladder with tied ends is sent separately.

- It is always preferable to send the specimens through a special messenger.
- In medico legal cases, the specimens should be sealed in the presence of a witness
- A sample of the preservative used should be sent.

It is always better to have a duplicate sample stored properly in a refrigerator for future reference.

Preservatives

- For visceral organs like pieces of liver, kidney, stomach, intestine, contents of a stomach and intestine saturated solution of sodium chloride can be used.
- Suspected plants or food can be sent to the laboratory without adding any preservative
- Ice pack/ waterproof frozen sachets, are used in case of the samples being transported in refrigerated or frozen state
- Rectified spirit (95% ethyl alcohol) 1 ml/ g of tissue is the ideal preservative for toxicological specimens. (except in alcohol, phosphorous and carbolic acid poisoning conditions)
- Formaline should never be used for toxicological analysis of specimen samples as it hardens the tissue without giving scope for scraping and interferes in with the analysis by making the extraction of poison much more difficult. Blood, urine and serum should be refrigerated and never be frozen.
- The materials for histopathological examination can be kept in a fixative preferably 10 percent formalin in a wide mouthed glass container with proper labelling and well protected by cotton padding/covering.

Labelling Information

The samples being sent to the laboratory must be accompanied by proper protected labelling with all the details regarding the case, including the following information.

1. Name and address of the doctor and the owner of the animal
2. Animal identification characteristics-species, colour, age, sex, breed etc.
3. Number of animals affected and number of animals dead
4. Date of onset of symptoms and the death
5. Clinical signs recorded by the doctor and symptoms noticed by the owner
6. Type and the quantity of samples sending
7. Postmortem findings
8. Suspected poison/toxicant
9. Any other circumstantial fact or information which may assist the laboratory in identifying the causative agent.

In veterolegal cases, the label containing the details is placed inside the specimen container and another label is pasted on the wooden box/cloth covering the container. The sample is then sent to the forensic laboratory, with the forwarding letter, a copy of request letter from the police and a copy of the postmortem report.

Diagnosis of Poisoning Conditions

Antemortem Diagnosis

The diagnosis of toxicological diseases on the basis of signs alone is not only very often difficult or impossible but may be dangerous as well. Each body system can react in a limited number of ways, producing clinical signs, and there are thousands of toxic agents that may affect these systems. In addition, when a clinician observes an animal with signs of illness or poisoning he may see only one phase of the syndrome. Toxicological diseases may be acute or chronic, and the clinical presentation will vary depending upon the route, extent, and frequency of exposure; the species involved; the time elapsed since the most recent exposure; and many other factors. A confirmed toxicological diagnosis often rests upon appropriate findings, including:

a) exposure history
b) clinical signs
c) time of onset
d) duration of effects that are compatible to the toxic potential of the agent involved, as well as
e) detection of the toxicant in the animal to confirm exposure (e.g., blood Pb), and in some cases

f) specific evidence of pathophysiologic derangement (e.g., acetylcholinesteraseinhibition). Even when an individual animal may no longer benefit from laboratory confirmation, positive or negative laboratory results may ultimately protect other animals or humans from toxic substances or missed diagnoses. Many specific antidotes have inherent toxicity, and their use in unconfirmed cases of poisoning can sometimes be hazardous. Also, clinical signs alone are not considered determinative evidence when presented in court.

The 5 basic routes of exposure to poisoning are: ingestion, cutaneous (topical), inhalation, injection (or envenomation), and ocular. Most toxicoses result from the oral ingestion of a toxicant, but some chemicals including many insecticides, phenols, and other lipophilic substances may also be efficiently absorbed through intact skin. Abraded skin may absorb some substances that otherwise might not reach toxic concentrations following dermal exposure. Of course, many volatile, aerosolized, or even solid particulate agents may be absorbed from the respiratory tract. For most agents, the rate of absorption is injection > respiratory > oral > topical. The route of exposure often influences the choice of specimens for confirmation. In addition to toxicosis due to systemic absorption of a compound, many compounds (e.g., corrosives) may result in direct tissue damage.

Identifying the Source

When poisoning is suspected, efforts should be made to determine the possibility and likelihood of exposure. Encourage the client to look in all places to which the animals have access. Be persistent and have them contact you after the search. If on a house or farm call, look with the client. If suspected toxicants are found, they should be saved for laboratory submission. When containers are found, read the ingredients list and any antidotal procedures (bearing in mind that some labels are out of date with regard to treatment recommendations). When toxic plants are suspected and there is evidence of significant consumption, be sure to get specimens for identification. Plants may be wrapped in wet newspapers and placed in a plastic bag prior to shipment (preferably with cold packs) to the laboratory or to a local botanist for identification.

Specimens from Animals

Care to avoid cross contamination of any sample by a potential toxicant is absolutely essential. It is therefore advisable to obtain specimens from animals before handling suspected source materials. If at all possible, before treatment is begun, refrigerate specimens of whole blood (10 - 20 ml with calcium EDTA as the anticoagulant) and freeze samples of serum (10 - 20 ml). Smaller specimens may be sufficient for certain tests. Volumes obtained may be reduced in particularly small species/individuals. In addition, save liberal portions of vomitus, urine, and faces for laboratory analysis. If vomitus cannot be collected and if gastric lavage is indicated, the initial lavage washings (using water only), should be submitted. The vomitus or lavage washings should be frozen in a tightly sealed jar. If topical exposure is suspected, hair may be frozen in a sealed container and submitted for analysis.

Feed and Water

When feed contamination is suspected, representative specimens of the material being consumed immediately prior to the onset of apparent toxicosis must be obtained. Delays in securing such samples may result in continued exposure to the toxicant and the subsequent absence of remaining feed for toxicologic analysis. For dry concentrate feedstuffs, obtain 2-kg samples of a composite from several areas of the incriminated feed. If moisture concentration is 13% or less, such feed can generally be shipped with no special method of preservation. Higher moisture feeds and forages should be kept frozen prior to and during shipment to the laboratory. When volatile substances are suspected as feed contaminants, however, the feed should be placed in clean glass jars and tightly capped and frozen. Water specimens may be similarly preserved and, if not filled more than 2/3 full, usually tolerate being frozen (in a tilted position) prior to shipment. In attempting to determine an antemortem diagnosis, one must remember that only a few toxicological tests can be done on a "stat" basis by most laboratories, e.g., blood lead, acetylcholinesterase. Due to the difficulties in chemical analysis for many toxicants, delays in receiving results of days to weeks must be anticipated. Serum chemistry, serum electrolytes, and other clinical diagnostic tests may rapidly contribute to a specific diagnosis (e.g., hypercalcemia in cholecalciferol toxicosis).

Postmortem Diagnosis

At necropsy it is essential to obtain a complete set(s) of specimens for chemical analysis and a complete set(s) of tissues for histopathology and other (e.g., bacterial and/or viral) studies. Many toxicologic diagnosis rely not only on residues of the toxicant but also on compatible lesions and/or the absence of evidence of other diseases capable of causing similar clinical effects. Specimens for analysis should be individually frozen and double bagged (with a paper label marked in pencil between 2 tightly sealed Whirl-Pack bags). The following specimens should be routinely collected: stomach or rumen contents, intestinal contents, faces, 1/2 of the brain, liver (without the gall bladder or bile contamination), kidney, body fat, and urine. Specimens should be large (i.e., up to 250 grams of stomach or intestinal contents, parenchymal organs, or body fat). In case of dermal exposure contaminated skin should be bagged, frozen, and submitted. In such cases, specimens of internal organs must not be contaminated from contact with the skin. Repeated cleaning or changing of instruments and gloves may be desirable after the skin has been reflected from the animal. Similar concerns exist when higher concentrations of toxicants may be present in the gastrointestinal tract than in organs for analysis.

General Line of Treatment of Poisoning in Animals

For the majority of cases of poisoning treatment with an antidote is not possible, instead prompt medical intervention to improve the condition of the animal can ensure its survival. These practices focus on promoting the removal of the poison or neutralizing it, whilst maintaining the vital functions of the animal.

Removal of the poison

Decontamination of the Skin

Some substance (hydrocarbons, acids, alkalis, agrochemicals, etc.) may, as a result of an accident or a spillage, contaminate the feathers or fur of animals. In general it is important that in such circumstances the following are undertaken:

- Epidermal structures (wings, nails, claws, feathers, fur) should all be cleaned with the greatest care, paying particular attention to areas such as the ears, between toes, etc. The cleaning should be undertaken quickly to avoid licking and ingestion of the poison, and to limit cutaneous absorption.
- Use soapy water (preferably a soap with a low pH), rinsing with copious tap water; repeat as often as necessary
- Dry carefully and thoroughly (e.g. with a hair dryer)
- The following must never be used: organic solvents (alcohol, white spirit, etc.) or oily substances which may actually increase percutaneous absorption of the toxin.
- Do not rub the area vigorously; cleaning and drying must be gentle but thorough

- The animal could well be in a state of shock and must be handled accordingly
- Move to a quiet place with additional heating (e.g. a heat pad, if necessary).

Gastric Emptying

Emetics

Use emetics if ingestion has taken place within the preceding 2-3 hours. Never induce vomiting in following circumstances:

- If caustics or hydrocarbons have been ingested
- If the condition of the animal does not allow such treatment, specifically if the patient is presenting with convulsions (unless controlled), coma or severe respiratory difficulties; this avoids any secondary complications due to aspiration.
- In pregnancy? And ingestion of slow releasing drug formulations.

Recommended emetics for use in dogs and cats (if necessary, in pigs)

- *Apomorphine for dogs*: Prompt effect, thorough, but does have a central depressive effect and the possibility of cardio-toxicity (arrhythmias)

  Dogs: 0.05-0.1 mg/kg s.c or im; contraindicated in cats or pigs
- *Xylazine, for dogs and cats*: Acts within 10-20 minutes; 0.25-0.5 ml of a 2% sol.,s.c.
- *Ipecachuana (10% syrup) for dogs and cats*: Acts in 20-30 minutes; orally, 10-20 ml for a dog, 2-5 ml for a cat administered in a phased manner

If none of the above compounds are available, possible alternatives include

- Sodium chloride (salt), p.o, 1-3 teaspoons in warm water
- Hydrogen peroxide, by mouth, 1 ml/kg
- Copper sulphate is not recommended as it is an irritant and facilitates the absorption of poisons. Preferred in pigs (4% solution, max: 60ml,p.o)

Gastric lavage

Currently used in dogs. It is indicated:

- If ingestion has taken place in the preceding 2-4 hours
- On anaesthetized animals with endotracheal intubation

Use 10 ml/kg of an isotonic solution of sodium chloride (occasionally sodium bicarbonate); repeat the procedure until the washout fluids are clear.

Manual gastric emptying is used in ruminants. Emergency gastrotomy with manual emptying may be necessary in some cases of plant poisoning or for indigestible materials (such as plastic, polyurethane foam).

Purgatives

- Never use irritant purgatives and
- Oil-based purgatives as they facilitate absorption

Recommended purgatives

Sodium sulphate, magnesium sulphate, by mouth or as enema, using solutions of various strengths (make up to 20%):

- Small animals : 2-25 g, Large animals: 100-200 g (max: 300 – 400g)
- Liquid paraffin (mineral oil), by mouth:Dogs: 5-15ml, Cats: 2-6ml

Diuretics

- Increase glomerular filtration by instituting a forced diuresis or osmotic diuresis
  - 5% glucose solution, by slow intravenous infusion
    Large animals: 2-5 ml/kg per 24h, Small animals: 5-20 ml/kg per 24hr
  - 10% glucose solution, by slow intravenous infusion
    Large animals: 0.5-1 ml/kg per 24 h, Small animals: 1-2 ml/kg per 24 hr
  - 10% mannitol solution, by intravenous infusion
    Large animals: 1-2 ml/kg per 24 h, Small animals: 2 ml/kg per 24 hr
- With diuretics (Note: strong diuretics are contraindicated)
  - Frusemide (im or iv), Large animals: 0.5-1 mg/kg, Small animals: 2.5-5 mg/kg
- Reduce tubular reabsorption by modifying urinary pH

  Forced acid diuresis to eliminate weak bases can be done by
  - Ammonium chloride, PO
    Large animals: 20-40 g, Small animals: 2-5 g
  - Arginine chloride, im, or iv
    Large animals: 7-10 g, Small animals: 0.1-0.2 g/kg

- Ascorbic acid, iv, all species: 40 mg/kg

  Forced alkaline diuresis to eliminate weak acids

  Sodium bicarbonate, 1.4%w/v, iv infusion, Large animals: 2-4 ml/kg per 24 hr

  Small animals: by regular monitoring of the acid - base balance (number of ml to perfuse = base deficit (in mmol) x 0.6 x body weight in (kg)
- Ringer's lactate, by iv infusion: all species: 5-10 ml/kg per hr
- Trometamol, 3.66% solution by iv infusion

  Dogs: 1-4 ml/kg per 24 hr
- Use a diuretic such as acetazolamide

Dialysis

In cats and dogs peritoneal dialysis with an appropriate dialysate* 20-25 ml/kg is suggested. Repeat the procedure several Times as necessary. Very effective in case of renal failure/renotoxicity.* Commercial preparations meant for human use can be employed.

Neutralization of Poisons with in the Gastrointestinal Tract

Adsorbents

Activated vegetable charcoal (fine medicinal charcoal or BCK granules). These are the most effective and most highly polyvalent adsorbents. They can be administered preferably as a suspension in water, several minutes to 24 hours after ingestion, if possible before any emetic.

- Large animals: 250-500 g, Small animals: 5-50 g

  Other adsorbents: All other adsorbents are less effective than activated charcoal and are of academic interest only
- Magnesium oxide (magnesia), Kaolin, Universal antidote (vegetable charcoal 10g+ magnesia 5g + kaolin 5g + tannin 5g with water added up to 200 ml).

General Chemical Antidotes

Substances which form a complex or insoluble precipitate with poisons and neutralize them in the gastrointestinal tract. The effects are often limited and debatable. This category includes:

- Water-containing albumens (proteins which are capable of forming insoluble complexes with heavy metals and which neutralize acids and bases).
- Tannins (these precipitate heavy metals aluminum, lead, silver and some alkaloids)

  Less useful against copper, mercury and nicotine), Lugol's iodine can partially precipitate heavy metals like Pb, Hg, Ag and Strychnine.
- Ferric hydrate (action as above).

Milk is commonly believed to act as the best general antidote; in fact, milk promotes the absorption of liposoluble poisons. A cardinal rule, therefore, is *"never administer milk"*.

Specific antidotes: See antidotes list

Additional treatment measures

These vary widely according to the symptoms observed, but one of the main preoccupations of the practitioner will be to support vital functions (respiration and circulation). The most frequently used agents are:

- *Doxapram*: A respiratory stimulant, Dog/Cat: 2 mg/kg, iv, repeat as required
- *Caffeine and theophylline*: Cardiovascular and respiratory stimulants, which also have a diuretic action. Dosage: 100-250 mg iv, im, hypodermally or as required
- *Nikethamide*: A respiratory stimulant. Dog: 22-44 mg/kg, im, iv,
- *Heptaminol*: A cardiac stimulant.

Rational Use of Charcoal

Activated charcoal is useful in following circumstance. Charcoal is ineffective against cyanide. It can also adsorb vitamins/minerals and therefore continued use may prove to be harmful.

Aconite	Antimony	Antipyrene	Parathion
Alcohol	Arsenic	Atropine	Nicotine
Camphor	Iodine	Barbiturates	Phenolpthaline
Cocaine	Oxalates	Morphine	Phenothiazine
Digitalis	Selenium	Mercuric chloride	Sulfonamides
Glutethimide	Silver	Strychnine	Penicillin
Methylene blue	Phosphorus	Salicylates	Ethylene glycol
Copper sulphate	Stramonium	Muscarine	Ipecacuana
		Quinine	Penicillin

Note: This is not an exhaustive list

Method of administration

Make slurry of the activated charcoal using lukewarm water. The rate of 2-8 g/kg should be given in a concentration of 1g/5-10ml water. Administration can be done by a stomach tube using either a funnel or a large syringe. Administer a cathartic (sodium sulphate or magnesium sulphate) 30 minutes after the administration of charcoal.

In pet animals this technique can be modified if the charcoal is used in conjunction with an emetic or gastric lavage (Normal saline: 10 ml/kg) with endotracheal intubation.

Systemic antidotes-Dosage and method of treatment (Large Animals)

Poisoning	Antidote/ treatment	Dosage and method of treatment
Hydrocyanic acid/Cyanide	Sodium nitrite followed by Sodium thiosulfate	Administer 1% sodium nitrite @ 15-25mg/kg,i.v followed by 25% sodium thiosulphate @ 1.25g,i.v **In emergency:** **Na nitrite + Na thiosulfate** Cattle: 20%, 10ml + 20% ,50 ml Horse: 20%, 10ml + 20%,50ml Sheep: 10%,10ml + 10%,20ml • Administer 4L of vinegar in 10 - 20Lcold water; give a large dose of vitamin B_{12} • Administer anticonvulsants if necessary

Contd...

Table Contd...

Nitrate/nitrite	Methylene blue	1% methylene blue @ 8.8mg/kg, i.v
	or Ascorbic acid	Administer 8-10L cold water and saline purgatives; Broad spectrum antibiotics intra-ruminally
Heavy metals *(Arsenic, antimony mercury, etc.)*	British anti-Lewisite (BAL)	*BAL*: 3mg/kg as 5% mixture of 10% benzyl benzoate in mineral oil. Give deep i.m injection every 4hr.on first two days, every 6 hr on third day and then *b.i.d* for next 10 days.
	or	• In cattle and horse sodium thiosulfate can also be used @ 8 - 10gram in the form of 10 - 20%solution (i.v) or 20 -30gram per-orally in 300ml water. • Fluid therapy and other supportive treatment as required
Arsenic poisoning	d-penicillamine (Expensive)	Administer @ 30-40mg ,i..v + 60-80mg/kg ,p.o, *b.i.d* or *t.i.d* for 3-4 days
Urea	Reduce the rumen pH	Administer 20-30L cold water and drench 4-6L of 5 % acetic acid
Strychnine *(Strychnous- nux -vomica)*	Phenobarbital sodium	@ 30mg/kg,i.v **or**
	or Chloral hydrate	5g/45 kg body weight, i.v • Drench tannic acid and then cathartic • Anticonvulsants, Leave the animal in calm, noise free and dark room
Lead	Calcium disodium EDTA	Make 6% solution and administer @ 73 mg/kg,i.v(repeat, if required). After two days gap start therapy again for next 5days
Copper	Ammonium tetra molybdate	• Anticonvulsants 1.7 mg/kg,i.v drip daily for 3-5 days.Allow 2days gap and then start therapy for next5days
	or Ammonium molybdate + Sodium thiosulphate **or**	Give ammonium molybdate 50-500mg p.o, *s.i.d* and sodium thiosulfate 300-1000mg,p.o,*s.i.d* for three weeks
	d-penicillamine (Expensive)	• Supportive treatment • 26mg/kg,p.o,*b.i.d* for 6 days
Warfarine	Vitamin K_1	300-500mg,*s.c*,every 4-6hour • Blood transfusion and supportive care
Ethylene glycol	Ethyl alcohol	20% ethanol @ 5ml/kg for every 4-8 hours interval

Contd...

Table Contd...

Carbamate insecticides	Atropine sulphate	0.25mg-0.5mg/kg,give ¼ intravenously and remaining ¾ by intramuscular or subcutaneous route. • *See general line of treatment for poisoning*
Organophos-phates	Atropine sulphate + 2-PAM	*Atropinization*: 0.25mg-0.5mg/kg,give ¼ i.v,remaining ¾ by i.m or s.c for every 3-6 hours. Observe for papillary dilatation and recovery symptoms and continue treatment as required . *2-PAM*: 20%solution @ 25-50mg/kg,i.v • Fluid therapy and supportive care • *See general line of treatment for poisoning*
Organochorines	Pentobarbitone sodium	30mg/kg,i.v and supportive care
(D.D.T;, B.H.C & endosulphan etc.,)	**or** Chloral hydrate	5g/45 kg, i.v and supportive care • *See general line of treatment for poisoning*
Dinitro-compounds (Herbicides like DNOC, dinitrophenol)	*In ruminants only:* Treat for methaemoglobinemia with methylene blue or ascorbic acid	*Methylene blue*: 2-4%,8-10mg/kg,i.v every 8hr. **or** *Ascorbic acid*: 5-10mg/kg, i.v every 8hr. for first 24-48hr. • *Do not give antipyretics to control hyperthermia. Use cold water or ice packs. Administer saline purgatives. Fluid therapy with dextrose saline*

Systemic antidotes-Dosage and method of treatment (Small Animals)

Toxic agent	Systemic antidote	Dosage and method of treatment
Acetaminophen	N-acetylcysteine	150 mg/kg loading dose PO or IV, then 50 mg/kg q 4h for 17-20 additional doses.
Amphetamines	Chlorpromazine	1 mg/kg IM or IV: administer only half dosage if barbiturates have been given; blocks excitation.
Arsenic, mercury and other heavy metals except cadmium, lead silver, selenium and thallium.	Dimercaprol (BAL) [Knoll Pharma]	10% solution in oil:give small animals 2.5-5.0 mg/kg IM q6h for 2 days then q12h for the next 10 days or until recovery (Note: With severe acute poisoning, 5 mg/kg should be given only on the first day).

Contd...

Table Contd...

	D-penicillamine (Artamin)® - VHB (Cilamin)® - IVIL	Developed for chronic mercury poisoning and now seems most promising drug. No reports on dosage in animals but give 3-4 mg/kg q6h.
Atropine, belladonna alkaloids	Physostigmine salicylate	0.1-0.6 mg/kg (do not use neostigmine)
Barbiturates	Doxapram	2% solution: give small animals 3-5 mg/kg, IV only (0.14-0.25 ml/kg). Repeat as necessary. (Note: The above is reliable only when depression is mild; in animals with deeper levels of depression ventilatory support (and oxygen) is preferable).
Bromides	Chlorides (sodium or ammonium salts)	0.5-1.0g PO daily for several days to hasten excretion
Carbon monoxide	Oxygen	Pure oxygen at normal or high pressure artificial respiration, blood transfusion
Cholecalciferol	Calcitonin	4 IU/kg SC or IM q8h-q12h
Cholinergic agents	Atropine sulfate	0.02-0.04 mg/kg as needed
Cholinesterase inhibitors	Atropine sulfate	0.2 mg/kg repeated as needed for atropinization. Treat cyanosis (if present) first. Blocks only muscarinic effects, atropine in oil may be injected for prolonged effect. Avoid atropine intoxication
Cholinergic agents and cholinesterase inhibitors Organophosphates, some Carbamates but not carbaryl, dimethan or carbam piloxime)	Pralidoxime chloride (2-PAM)	5% solution 20-50 mg/kg IM or by slow IV (0.2-1.0 mg/kg) injection (maximum dose is 500 mg per minute). Repeat as needed. 2-PAM alleviates nicotinic effect and regenerates cholinesterase. Morphine, succinylcholine and phenothiazine tranquilizers are contraindicated.

Contd...

Table Contd...

Copper	d-penicilamine (Artamin)	*See arsenic*
Coumarin-derivative anticoagulants.	Vitamin K (K_1) 1% emulsion or capsule	Give 3-5 mg/kg SC or PO per day with canned food. Treat 7 days for warfarin-type. Treat 21-30 days for second generation anticoagulant rodenticides, oral therapy is more effective than parenteral route
	Fresh whole blood. Fresh plasma or fresh frozen plasma	Blood transfusion 10-25 ml/kg; as required.
Curare	Neostigmine methylsulfate	Solution 1:5000 or 1:2000 (1ml = 0.2 or 0.5 mg/ml. Give 0.005 mg/5 kg SC; Follow with IV injection of atropine (0.04 mg/kg)
	Edrophonium chloride Ventilatory support	1% solution give 0.05-1.0 mg/kg IV.
Cyanide	Methemoglobin (sodium nitrite is used to form methemoglobin) and	1% solution of sodium nitrite, dosage is 16 mg/kg IV (1.6 ml/kg)
	Sodium thiosulfate	Follow with 20% solution of sodium thiosulfate at dosage of 30-40 mg/kg (0.15-0.2 ml/kg) IV. If treatment is repeated, use only sodium thiosulfate (Note: both of the above may be given simultaneously as follows:- 0.5 ml/kg of combination consisting of 10g sodium nitrite and 15 g sodium thiosulfate in distrilled water QS. to 250 ml. Dosage may be repeated once and if further treatment is required give only 20% solution thiosulfate at 0.2 ml/kg.)
Digitalis glycosides Oleander and Bufo toads	Potassium chloride	Dogs : 0.5-2.0 g PO in divided doses or in serious cases as diluted solution given IV by slow drip (ECG monitoring is essential)

Contd...

Table Contd...

	Diphenylthydantoin	25 mg per minute IV, until ventricular arrhythmias are controlled.
	Propranolol (β-Blocker)	0.5-1.0 mg/kg IV or IM. Give as needed to control cardiac arrhythmias (ECG monitoring is essential)
	Atropine sulfate	0.02-0.04 mg/kg as needed for cholinergic and arrhythmia control.
Fluoride	Calcium borogluconate	3-10 ml of 5-10% solution.
Fluoroacetate	Glyceryl monoacetin (Sigma)	0.1-0.5 mg/kg IM hourly for several hours (total 2-4 mg/kg) or diluted (0.5-1.0% solution IV: danger of hemolysis). Monoacetin is available only from chemical supply houses.
	Pentobarbital	May protect against lethal dose (experimental) (Note: all treatments are generally unrewarding).
Hallucinogens (LSD; phencyclidine hydrochloride.	Diazepam (Valium®, Roche)	As needed-avoid respiratory depression (2-5 mg/kg)
Heparin	Protamine sulfate	1% solution give 1.0-1.5 mg by slow IV injection to antagonize each 1 mg of heparin. Reduce dose as time increases between heparin injection and start of treatment (after 30 minutes give only 0.5 mg)
Iron salts (Iron tonics)	Deferoxamine mesylate (Desferal, Ciba)	Dosage for animals not yet established. Dosage for humans is 5 g of 5% solution PO, then 20 mg/kg IM q4h-q6h. In case of shock, the dosage is 40 mg/kg by IV drip over 4-hour period. May be repeated in 6 hours then 15 mg/kg by drip q8h.

Contd...

Table Contd...

Lead	Calcium disodium EDTA (CaEDTA)	Maximum safe dosage is 75 mg/kg per 24 hours (only for severe case); EDTA is available in 20% solution for IV drip, dilute in 5% glucose to 0.5%; For IM, add procaine to 20% solution to give 0.5% concentration of procaine.
	EDTA and BAL	BAL is given as 10% solution in oil. (a) In severe cases (CNS involvement with > 100 μg lead per 100 μg whole blood) give 4 mg/kg BAL only as initial dose: follow after 4 hours and q4h for 3-4 days with BAL and EDTA (12.5 mg/kg) at separate IM sites: skip 2 to 3 days and then treat again for 3-4 days: (b) In subacute cases with < 100 g lead per 100 μg whole blood give only 50 mg EDTA/kg per 24 hours for 3-5 days:
	Penicillamine (Cuprimine, Merck, Artamin® VHB)	(c) May use after either treatment (a) or (b) with 100 mg/kg per day PO for 1-4 weeks.
	Thiamine hydrochloride	Experimental to treat CNS signs: 5 mg/kg IV q12h for 1-2 weeks: give slowly and watch for untoward reactions.
Metaldehyde	Diazepam (Valium®)	2-5 mg/kg IV to control tremors
	Triflupromaize	0.2-2.0 mg/kg IV.
	Pentobarbital	
Methanol	Ethanol	Give 1.1 g/kg (4.4 ml/kg) of 25% solution IV: then give 0.5 g/kg (2.0 ml/kg) q4h for 4 days. Prevent or correct acidosis with sodium bicarbonate 0.4 g/kg IV. Activated charcoal, 5 g/kg PO if within 4 hours of ingestion.

Contd...

Table Contd...

Methemoglobinemi a- producing agents (nitrites, chlorates)	Methylene blue (not recommended for cats)	1% solution (maximum concentration) give by slow IV injection 8.8 mg/kg (0.9 ml/kg), and repeat if necessary. To prevent fall in blood pressure in cases of nitrite poisoning, use a sympathomimetic drug (ephedrine or epineprine)
Morphine and related drugs	Naloxone hydrochloride	0.1 mg/kg IV: do not repeat if respiration is not satisfactory.
	Levallorphan tartrate (Lorfan®, Roche)	Give IV 0.1-0.5 ml of solution containing 1 mg/ml (*Note: use* either of the antidotes only in *acute poisoning. Ventilatory support may be indicated. Activated charcoal is also indicated*).
Oxalates	Calcium	10% solution of calcium gluconate IV; give 3-20 ml (to control hypocalcemia)
Phenothiazine	Methamphetamine hydrochloride	0.1-0.2 mg/kg. Treatment for hypovolemic shock may be required.
	Diphenhydramine hydrochloride	For CNS depression, 2.5 mg/kg IV to treat extrapyramidal sings.
Phytotoxins and botulin	Antitoxins not available commercially (attempt to obtain through National poison information center)	As indicated for specific antitoxins, examples of phytotoxins: ricin, abrin, robin, crotin.
Spider bite	Antivenin (Merck)	Caution: equine origin; administer IV undiluted.
Black widow	Dantroiene sodium	For neurologic sings. 1 mg/kg IV. followed by 1 mg/kg PO q4h
Strychnine and brucine (Nux-vomica)	Pentobarbital	Give IV to effect: higher dose is usually required than that required for anesthesia. Place animal in warm and quiet room.

Contd...

Table Contd...

	Amobarbital	Give slowly IV to effect: duration of sedation is usually 4-6 hours.
	Thiobarbiturates	Dog/cat : 60-70 mg/kg IP.
	Glyceryl guaiacolate	110 mg/kg IV 5% solution; repeat as necessary
	Diazepam (Valium®, Roche)	2.5 mg/kg; controls convulsions
Thallium	Diphenylthiocarbazone	Dogs: 70 mg/kg PO q8h for 6 days: hastens elimination but is partially toxic.
	Prussian blue	0.2 mg/kg PO in 3 divided doses daily.
	Potassium chloride	Give simultaneously with thiocarbazone or Prussian blue; 2-6 g PO daily in divided doses.

Toxicity Testing Methods

Acute Toxicity Testing

- These tests assess the potential of a toxicant to cause adverse effects after a single dose or multiple doses during a 24-hour or shorter period.

Subchronic Toxicity Testing

- These assess the potential to cause effects after 30 to 90 days of repeated or continuous exposure.

Chronic Toxicity Testing

- These assess the potential to cause effects after prolonged exposure:
  - 1.5 years in mice.
  - 2 years in rats.
  - 3 or more years in dogs.
  - Included are tests for carcinogenicity.

Reproductive Toxicity Testing

- Evaluate the effects of the toxicant on:
- Ovulation, conception, implantation.
- Embryo and fetal development, length of gestation.

- Parturition.
- Lactation.
- Early postnatal growth.
- *Usually 2 or 3 successive generation (rat) studies are done.*
- Males and females are exposed from 60 days before breeding until the end of gestation and lactation.
- The offspring are dosed from weaning through their complete reproductive cycle, including lactation.
- Embryotoxic Vs. Fetotoxic Agents: If an agent produces a stillbirth or *in utero* death, the correct term is *embryotoxic* if it occurs *in the embryonic period*, and *fetotoxic* if it occurs *during the fetal period.*

Teratogenicity Testing

- Teratogen: An agent which, when administered during gestation, produced *nonlethal structural or functional changes* in the embryo or fetus.
- Teratogenicity testing is usually separated from chronic reproductive toxicity tests.
- Goal is to administer the toxicant *during the period of* differentiation *of fetal organs and tissues*: e.g., mice exposed during days 6 to 15 of gestation; rats during days 6 to 18.

Mutagenicity Testing

- Mutagenesis: *Induction of changes in DNA*. This may include observable structural changes in the chromosomes, such as breaks, etc.
- But, changes in DNA are more often evident only at the biochemical level with no obvious structural alterations in the chromosomes. Most such changes are harmless change due to DNA repair, which is a common event.
- Note: Mutations are of concern because they can result in misreading the genetic code.
- Genetic changes may be harmless (new peptide sequence works as well as the original version) or even beneficial (trial and error process —> evolution of the more successful).
- However, evolution has already lead to considerable refinement; and mutagenesis is therefore generally undesirable. The primary concerns are that it may result in carcinogenesis or hereditary defects.

- Four Types of Mutagenicity Tests (commonly used for testing of chemicals).
- *Dominant lethal test*: Males are treated with the test compound and females are examined for an increase in pre- and post-implantation losses.
- *Cytological test*: Animals exposed to test compound - examine mutation susceptible cells (i.e., rapidly dividing cells of bone marrow, germ cells, etc.) for chromosomal aberrations.
- *Ames Test*: Expose a mutant Salmonella bacterium that requires histidine for growth. If "back mutation" occurs, the organism grows in histidine-free media.Test compounds are often metabolically activated to a reactive form through exposure to liver cells, liver extracts, or hepatic enzymes.
- *Host-mediated assay*: Animal is given both the *test agent* and the mutant *Salmonella* ip. Host may metabolically activate the compound which then causes the "back-mutation" in the *Salmonella* so that it propagates in histidine-free media.
- "Special Studies"
- *Hemolysis tests*
- *Irritation tests*: Well-founded controversy over tests done with known irritants which are nevertheless applied at high concentrations. Tests *in vitro* are coming on line to lessen the need to test commercial products for irritancy. Generally these can result in elimination of toxic components so that they do not need to be tested in animals. Final products are either formulated from ingredients already thoroughly evaluated in animal studies or are tested with animal irritations tests before manufacture and sale in quantity.
- *Draize eye irritation test*
- *Draize skin irritation tests*
- *Other irritation tests*

Chapter 3

HEAVY METAL TOXICOLOGY

Arsenic

General Information

1. Exists in elemental form (-3), trivalent As+3 and pentavalent As+5 oxidation states
2. Arsenic is an essential element for rats, chicks, mini-pigs and goats
3. The second most important pollutant for livestock.

Source

- Inorganic form is used in paints.
- Pasture near smelters may be contaminated.
- Industrial effluents released into nearby water body.
- Insecticides (arsenic trioxide, lead arsenate).

- Herbicides (Sodium arsenite, lead arsenate)
- Rodenticides (arsenic trioxide) all can kill non-target species. (As arsenic is poisonous, all such products are being replaced with safer substances).
- Milk from affected dams poisons the calves.
- Arsenical preparations (Sodium thiacetarsamide for blood parasites, acetylarsan as a skin tonic) cause toxicity.
- Arsenic is used as a growth promoter in pigs and poultry. This form causes peripheral nerve demyelination that differs from inorganic arsenic toxicity.

  Ex: Roxarsone in poultry, Arsanilic acid in pigs.

Factors Affecting Toxicity

1. *Species* : all species are effected

   Ruminants, horses, dog, cat - inorganic arsenic

   Swine, poultry -organic arsenic
2. *Toxicology rating*: $RAs\text{-}X < As^{+5} < As^{+3} < AsH_3$ (Arsine, gas)
3. *Physical state* : finely divided granules readily absorbed than coarsely divided.

Toxicokinetics: Delivery - Absorption, Distribution and Excretion

1. Variable absorption - $As^{5+} > As^{3+}$
2. *Distribution*: liver and kidney, hair and nails - As binds to SH groups
3. Readily bypass placenta
4. Excretion- Excreted in faeces, bile, milk, saliva and sweat

   a) Arsenite in feces and arsenate in urine

   b) Pentavalent - rapid excretion, trivalent - slow excretion

Toxicodynamics: Arsenic compounds are directly toxic to body systems

Arsenic irrespective of route of absorption affects tissues rich in oxidative enzymes like intestine, liver and kidney. It crosses the placental barrier but does not seem to cross BBB.

At cellular level Arsenic mainly causes relaxation of capillaries and increases capillary permeability. Increased capillary permeability causes oedema in gastric sub mucosa and overlying mucosa is dishelmed.

Capillary endothelial cells of GIT, skin, liver, kidney
↓
Induce vasodilatation
↓
Haemorrhages
↓
Sub mucosal edema of GIT
↓
Blood pressure
↓
Colloidal osmotic pressure
↓
Shock
↓
Weakness, trembling, collapse

At molecular level inhibits SH group of enzymes of lipoic acid, which is essential for glycolysis and citric acid cycle.

Arsenicals are uncouplers of mitochondrial phophorylation
↓
interact with dihydrolipoic acid cofactor
↓
inhibits activities of succicinic and pyruvate dehydrogenase
↓
inhibits energy linked reduction of NAD
↓
competes with inorganic phosphate
↓
stimulates ATPase activity
↓
Causes decrease in ATP production and increase in H_2O_2
↓
Induces oxidative stress and generation of ROS (reactive oxygen species)
↓
Production of major stress proteins + oxidative stress
↓
Causes DNA damage and induces carcinogenesis

At local level Arsenic causes corrosion of the gastro intestinal mucosa.

Corrosive → GIT → epithelium → necrosis → colic

Particularly in the trivalent (As3+) form, they are able to bind to sulphydryl (-SH) groups of enzymes in the pyruvate dehydrogenase system.

They are also able to bind to enzymes in the Kreb's (Tricarboxylic acid, TCA) cycle and they therefore can interfere with oxidative phosphorylation in cells.

In the pentavalent (As+5) form, they can also exert their toxicity by competitively substituting their ions for the body's phosphate ions. This can lead to the breaking down by hydrolysis of high energy bonds in compounds such as ATP.

Organic arsenicals (pentavalent) causes myelin degeneration of peripheral nerves. This leads to atrophy of weight bearing animals ex-swine moves on hocks.

Clinical Signs

Toxicology Effects – 3 D's of Arsenic: Diarrhea, Dementia and Dermatitis

1. Circulation - increase permeability of capillary
2. Gastrointestinal - bad diarrhea "rice and water" stools
3. Kidney - glomerular capillaries
4. Skin - "mild and rose" complexion
5. CNS - peripheral neuritis, encephalopathy
6. Blood - cause decrease in Red blood Cell and other cells
7. Liver - fatty infiltration and necrosis
8. Metabolic effects - not a tonic
9. Carcinogenesis human carcinogen - skin and lung, bladder and liver

Per acute cases – animal found dead *or* sudden and severe colic, staggering, collapse, paralysis and death are seen.

Acute cases - Severe colic, staggering, weakness, trembling, salivation, vomiting, thirst, projectile watery diarrhoea (rice water stools in humans), dysentery, rapid and weak pulse, prostration, normal or sub-normal temperature, death in 1-3 days.

Sub-acute cases - Same as acute toxicity except for partial paralysis of hind limbs, cold extremities, stupor, hematuria and convulsions.

Chronic cases - rare as the metalloid is excreted very fast. The symptoms could be wasting, poor condition, haemorrhagic dermatitis in buffaloes and humans as arsenic accumulates in skin, nails and hair. (tissues rich in thiol groups). Polyuria and anuria, haematuria, weak irregular pulse, brick red m.m (Mucous Membrane).

Lesions : are quite prominent except in per acute cases

1. Congestion and haemorrhages in abomasal or duodenal mucosa and sub mucosal oedema resulting in sloughing of the duodenal mucosa or perforation of gut wall.
2. The intestinal contents are fluid; foul smelling, bloody with shreds of intestinal mucosa.
3. Liver soft and yellow.
4. Lungs oedematous and congested.
5. Haemorahages on heart, peritoneum, kidneys and liver.
6. Heamorrhagic dermatitis.

- In *humans arsenic accumulates in nails known as - meres lines*

Swine: Inflamed and oedematous fauces, which extends to larynx and trachea causing asphyxia.

Poultry: Intense inflammation of proventriculus and gizzard, horny lining of gizzard may slough because of underlying gelatinous exudates. Duodenal mucosa is congested.

Diagnosis

Based on

1. Case history
2. Clinical Signs
3. Lesions
4. Tissue analysis - Reinch's test
5. Laboratory examination of Samples

Liver, kidney	100g
Whole blood	15ml
Urine	50ml
Ingesta	100g
Feed	1-2kg

Differential Diagnosis: Pesticides, urea and lead show colic and other GI signs but watery diarrhoea with blood and mucous and foul smell, severity and the sudden onset, is only seen in arsenic.

Irritant plants, certain insects that harbour on plants too cause severe diarrhoea.

Treatment

Arsenic binds to dithiol groups in the body; hence BAL (dimercaprol) is the drug of choice to revive inhibited enzyme activity. But caution is to be exercised and the treatment schedule be maintained strictly as **BAL itself is toxic.**

Large Animals

1) BAL 3 mg/kg I/M 5% solution (in 10% of benzyl benzoate in peanut oil).

   Repeat every 2 hours for first 2 days, every 6 hours 3rd day, 12 hours for the next 10 days till recovery.

2) Sodium thiosulfate

   20-30 gm in 300 ml water orally. Also 8-10 gm. In 10-20% solution I/V.

   Or

   30-40 mg/kg. I/V 2-3 times a day until recovery.

   60-80 mg/kg orally.

Small Animals

1. BAL 2.5-5 mg/kg. 10% solution in arachis oil. Deep intramuscular.

   Dosage intervals same as for large animals. Use 5 mg/kg on the first day in acute cases only.

2. Sodium thiosulfate 5-6 gm in 60 ml water orally,

   2-2.5 gm in 10-20 % solution I/V.

Disadvantages of BAL

- Overdose can kill the animal
- Ineffective incase of delayed poisoning
- Should be administered before the start of clinical signs.

Symptomatic Therapy

I/V fluids and electrolytes. Antibiotics, analgesics and demulcents.

Contraindicated: emetics and parasympathomimetics

Mercury

General Information

Major Species effected: All species, especially swine, cats

Usual Duration (if survives): Mercury is a growing concern in the environment. Mercury may be encountered as:

- Elemental mercury (Hg^o ; in the form of metallic mercury or Hg^ovapor).
- Mercury salts (also called inorganic mercury) such as mercuric chloride, mercuric oxide, etc.
- Organomercurial compounds (includes alkyl forms such as ethyl, methyl, propyl, dimethyl, etc., and aryl forms of mercury, such as phenylmercuric acetate).

Sources

- Mercury metal Hg^o. Elemental mercury - mercury vapor
  - Electrical equipment
  - Mercury circulates in the environment. Because of its volatility the earth continuously "degasses" mercury.
  - Paints
  - Thermometers
  - Dental amalgum used for fillings.
  - Chlor-alkali plants
  - Barometers.
  - A major source of mercury in the biosphere is mercury vapor produced by burning coal (and to a much lesser extent, other fossil fuels).
  - Metallic mercury is sometimes used in crude gold mining techniques directly contaminates the local streams and the atmosphere.
- Mercury in manufactured formulations (several compounds; inorganic and organic). As compared to aryl organic mercury compounds, alkyl organics such as methyl or ethyl mercury tend to be more toxic, especially after repeated exposure. Inorganic mercury salts include monovalent mercurous compounds and divalent mercuric compounds.
  - Mildew proof or antifouling paints such as some types used on boat bottoms.

- Batteries (some small batteries are high in mercury).
- Fungicides (some are inorganic, many are organic compounds).
- Fungicide treated seed grains used in feeds.
- Highly toxic mercurial fungicides have been largely replaced by far less toxic nonmercurial or phenylmercurial fungicides.

❐ Mercury-containing medications.

- Mercurial diuretics are similar in toxicity to mercury salts and are no longer used appreciably.
- Phenylmercuric acetate—sometimes used in dermatology—topical application.

❐ Sewage sludge may be very high in mercury in some instances.

❐ Mercury in living organisms.

- Methyl mercury and, to a lesser extent, ethyl mercury are primary concerns with regard to environmental forms of mercury. All forms of mercury are converted to these by anaerobic bacteria. Methyl mercury is the principle tissue residue form in eggs, regardless of the mercury compound ingested by a bird.

  a) Aquatic organisms accumulate methyl mercury from polluted watersheds, bays, etc. In fish - biomethylation

     i. Minamata Bay, Japan

     ii. Tuna and swordfish in U.S.

- Methyl mercury can accumulate in eggs and animal tissues.
- Dimethyl mercury is also produced in sediments. Like metallic mercury, dimethyl mercury is somewhat volatile and may therefore leave the aquatic ecosystem.

Toxicokinetics

❐ Elemental Mercury

- Orally - nontoxic
- Lung - readily absorbed, oxidized by Red Blood Cell to divalent mercuric cation (Hg^{2+})
- Distribution - because mercury vapor crosses membranes more readily, a significant amount of mercury enters brain before it is oxidized

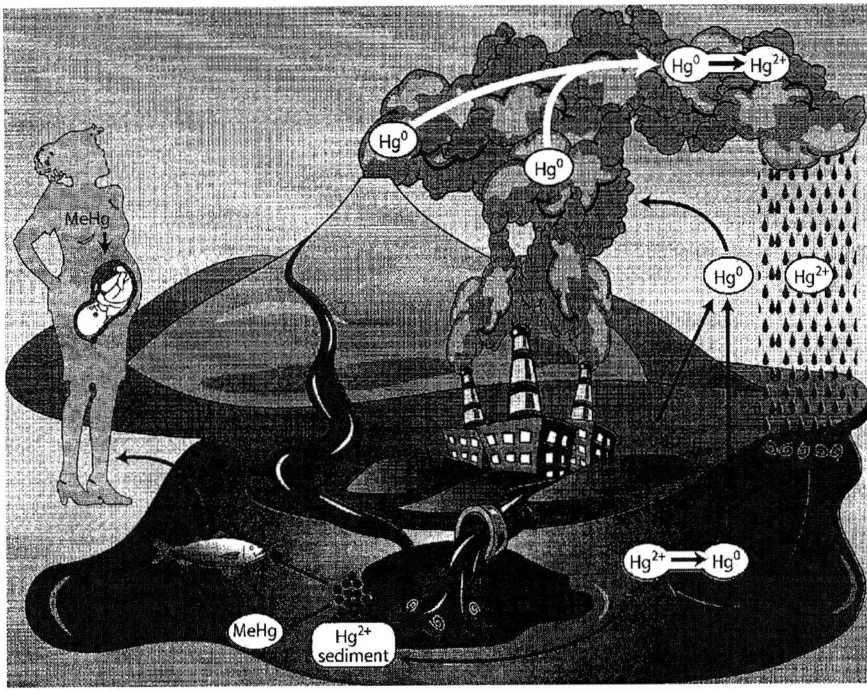

Picture showing the bioaccumulation of mercurial compounds

- Inorganic Mercury Salts
  - About 10% absorbed from G.I tract
  - Concentration in Red Blood Cell and plasma are similar - not like lead (which concentrates in RBC)
  - In ionized form, so doesn't readily pass blood-brain barrier or placenta
  - High concentration in kidney
  - Fecal excretion - in bile
  - Half-life - 65 days
- Organic Mercurials
  - About 90% absorbed from G.I. tract
  - More lipid soluble - more evenly distributed and enters brain and passes placenta
  - 5 times higher concentrated in Red Blood Cells than in plasma
  - Half-life - 65 days

- *Elimination* - Inorganic Hg is eliminated primarily via the urine; organic mercury is eliminated mainly via the bile and feces, less than 10% appears in the urine.
- if eliminated through sweat causes dermatitis
- if eliminated through saliva causes ginigivitis and has metallic taste

Note: Marine mammals and some other marine organisms may have extraordinarily high mercury concentrations. This is possible primarily because of formation of insoluble, 1:1 complexes of mercury and selenium intracellularly.

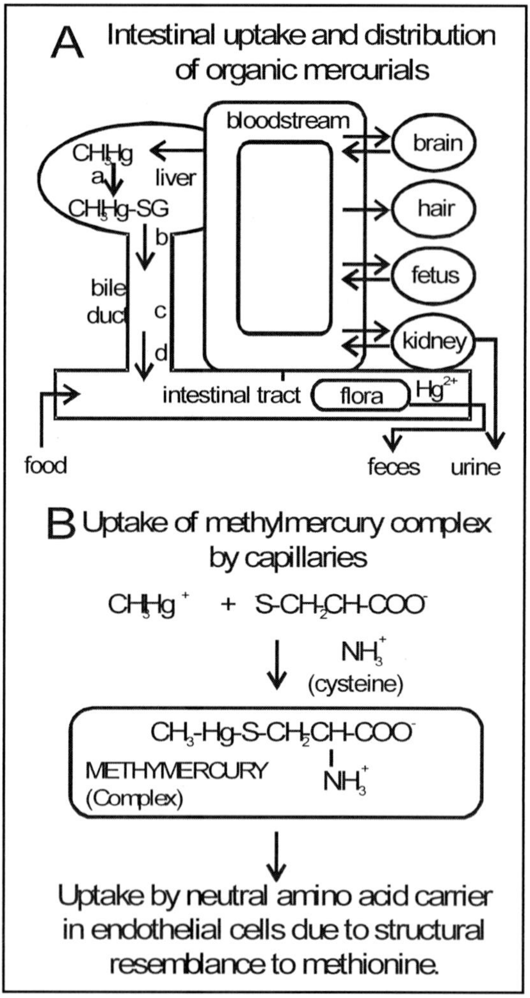

Toxicodynamics

- Sulfhydryl groups of enzymes and other proteins are affected (bound to mercury). Hg readily forms covalent bonds with sulfur. Hg replaces H2 (Note: 2 atoms) to form mercaptides: X-Hg-SR and Hg(SR)2 (where R = a protein and S = an electronegative radical).
- Associated epithelial & neuron damage may explain some of the problems.
- Gastrointestinal mucosal damage.
- Skin lesions.
- Renal tubular damage (especially with inorganic mercury).
- Vascular and neuronal damage in the brain (especially with methyl mercury).
- Blood-brain barrier can be disrupted with less than 1.0 ppm Hg ions in the brain.

Elemental form
↓
Blood RBC (stored)
↓
Oxidized by catalase
↓
Haemolysis
↓
Anaemia

- Both methyl mercury and Hg^{++} can disrupt ion exchange across both voltage-gated and ligand-gated channels.
- Mercury may irreversibly inhibit voltage-gated K^+ outcurrent in the early developing nervous system. This may explain neurologic teratogenicity.
- Methyl mercury-induced neurotoxicity is believed to be the result of an increase in reactive oxygen species caused by a disruption of the mitochondrial electron transport chain. This increase in free radicals in turn depletes glutathione and mediates neuronal injury.
- Methyl mercury also inhibits ATP production and release of Ca^{++} from mitochondria, resulting in increased intracellular Ca^{++} concentration, which leads to spontaneous depolarization and release of acetylcholine.
- Methyl mercury decreases uptake of choline by nerve terminals, so there is decreased synthesis of acetylcholine.
- *In vitro*, methyl mercury has been shown to disrupt microtubule assembly and cellular migration.

Organic form

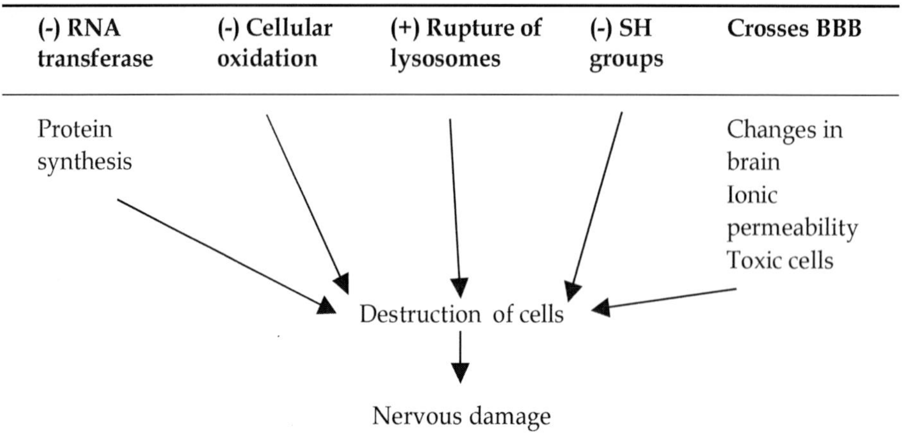

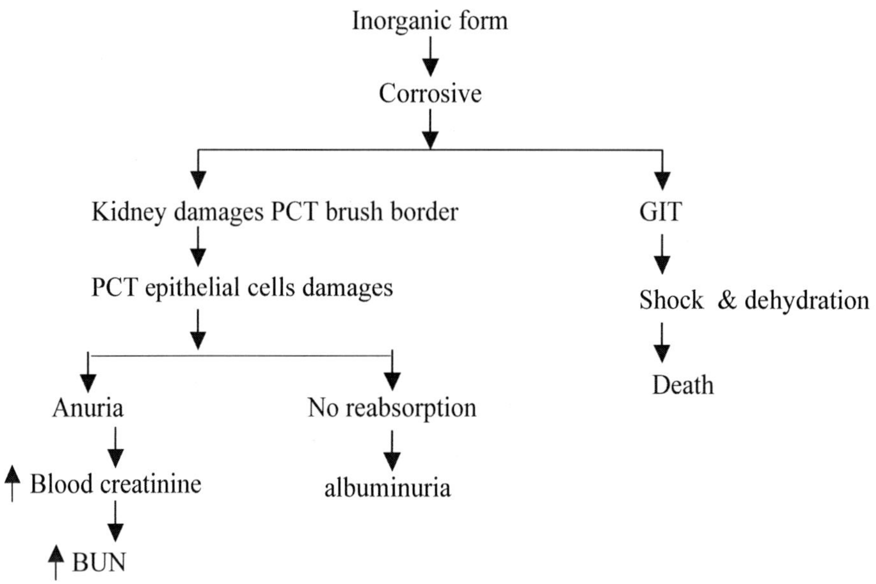

Clinical Signs

Acute Mercury Poisoning

- Local effects
  - G.I. tract effects – pain, vomiting, diarrhea
  - Inhalation – pneumonitis, coughing, etc.
  - Systemic effects

- Metallic taste, sore gums, excessive salivation
- CNS - lethargy, excitation, hyperreflexia and tremor
- Kidney injury
- Central neural effects.

Chronic Mercury Poisoning

- Mercury vapor - largely neuropsychiatric: depression, irritability, shyness, insomnia, emotional instability, forgetfulness, confusion, excessive perspiration, uncontrolled blushing (erethism) and tremors
  - Mad Hatter
- Methylmercury - organic mercury
  - Paresthesia (abnormal spontaneous sensation such as tingling)
  - Visual changes - constriction of visual field
  - Hearing defects
  - Dysarthria (disturbance of articulation)
  - Ataxia
  - Fetus is extremely susceptible - so methylmercury is a teratogen
  - Elemental mercury - shyness, irritability, spontaneous fits of laughing and crying, intellectual deterioration.

Kidney – Target Organ of Inorganic Mercury Toxicity

- Other Effects
  - Mouth - gingivitis, stomatitis and excessive salivation
  - Mercurialentis - colored reflex from lens.

Species Wise Clinical Signs

- Cattle
  - Stomatitis, salivation, loose teeth, gastroenteritis.
  - Nasal discharge, bronchopneumonia, dyspnea.
  - Dermatitis, pustules, skin ulceration, depilation, hyperkeratinization.
  - Weakness, anorexia, emaciation, prostration, low total protein, low globulin, proteinuria (in severely affected).
  - CNS depression, ataxia, stumbling, hyperesthesia, convulsions (rare).
  - Epistaxis, hematuria, bloody feces, non-regenerative anemia.
  - High fever, severe skin lesions, hemorrhage all give poor prognosis.

- Swine - more commonly poisoned with Hg.
  - Anorexia, weight loss, constipation, poor growth.
  - Weakness, flaccid abdominal muscles.
  - Gagging, vomiting.
  - Fever.
  - Thickened, scaly skin.
  - Cyanosis.
  - Blindness.
  - Abnormal posture, staggering, stiffness, disorientation.
  - Depression, tremors, paresis, paddling, coma.
  - Excitation, chewing, but without prehension of food.
  - Death often within 2 - 3 days of onset of major neurologic signs.
  - At high doses: Gastrointestinal upset, tachycardia, CNS depression, cyanosis, hypothermia, dyspnea, coma and death within 1 day.
- Feline
  - Sensitive to environmental mercury (especially methyl mercury in seafood); entry of environmental/food contamination for humans.
  - Paresis, rear leg rigidity, knuckling over at the carpus and/or tarsus, hypermetria, cerebellar ataxia, tremors, hypersalivation, sensory impairment, tonic-clonic, convulsions.
  - Blindness, persistent vocalizing, paddling, coma, hyperthermia.
  - Weakness, lateral recumbency.
  - Vomiting, diarrhea.
  - Skin pustules.
  - Death.
  - Cerebellar hypoplasia (mimics panleukopenia) and other teratogenic effects in kittens, deaths prior to 3 months of age.
- Birds
  - Reduced hatchability, eggs without shells.
- General
  - Pulmonary damage and associated clinical signs may predominate in cases of inhalation of toxic amounts of Hg^{o}.

- Lesions
  - Renal: pale swollen kidneys; renal tubular damage especially affecting the proximal tubular epithelium, glomerulonephritis is possible with chronic exposure due to the antigen-antibody complex deposition.
  - Hepatic: liver is pale and reduced in size; microscopic examination may reveal hydropic change.
  - Digestive tract: possible necrotic pharyngitis, focal erosive or ulcerative gastritis; necrotic enteritis and typhlitis.
  - Lungs : degenerative changes.

Organic mercurials : Brain: no grossly evident brain lesions.

  - Cerebral precapillary arterioles exhibit fibrinoid degeneration especially in swine and cattle.
  - Cerebral laminar necrosis and myelin loss.
- Peripheral nerves: myelin and axonal damage.
- Inhalation of mercury vapor may produce an acute, corrosive bronchitis and interstitial pneumonia.

Diagnosis

Based on

- Case history
- Clinical signs
- Postmortem lesions
- Kidney (especially cortex) Hg usually 10 - 15 ppm or more. With time, Hg may decrease to a few ppm. Submit cortex and medulla.
- Liver and brain are also worth analyzing for mercury (in addition to kidney).
- Gross and histologic lesions (send fixed specimens also).
- Test blood, plasma and urine antemortem, though false negatives are possible in urine as excretion is concentration and time dependent.
- Based on laboratory test- reinch's test
- Samples to be submitted for analysis

Kidney	100g	Heparinised, do not use EDTA
Whole blood	10ml	
Liver	100g	
Urine	15ml	

Differential diagnosis : lead, thallium, phenylarsonic feed additive, and ethylene glycol toxicosis, encephalitis, polioencephalomalacia, hog cholera, and erysipelas.

Treatment

- Neurologic damage may be permanent (give appropriate prognosis before owner decides to treat).
- Keep in mind that meat from livestock can be a **hazardous** source of mercury for humans.
- Acute oral exposures
    - Feed egg then use an emetic if not contraindicated.
    - Activated charcoal and saline cathartic.
    - Sodium thiosulfate orally also safe to bind Hg.
    - Cattle 30 grams orally in a 10% solution.
    - Scarlet Drench Powder, 10% sodium thiosulfate solution.
- Seizures
    - Diazepam (0.2 - 2.0 mg/kg, I/V, to effect) (dogs) or barbiturates (e.g., phenobarbital or, if it fails, pentobarbital) (most species).
    - Fluids and electrolytes for corrosive GI syndrome.
    - Support renal function.
- Any acute mercury toxicosis.

Chelation therapy in general is not very effective with the organic Hg compounds as only a small fraction is in the plasma and available for excretion.

Dimercaprol (British Anti Lewisite or BAL, is 2, 3-dimercaptopropanol

- Can't be given orally
- Unable to reduce brain Hg level
- Most effective for protection of kidney injury from inorganic mercury salts

- Is not very effective after chronic exposure to organic mercurial compounds. BAL British Antilewisite dimercaprol. It is contraindicated with organic mercurials as it will increase the brain concentration. BAL also contraindicated with preexistent liver or kidney damage.
- BAL (in oil) injections may still be recommended for more acutely poisoned small animals (with inorganic mercury sources) although its efficacy is not well documented.

- BAL - reportedly not highly effective in large animals or humans.
- Nevertheless, the recommended dose for cattle is 3 mg/kg QID for 3 days, then BID for 10 days; for horses, 3 mg/kg every 4 hours for the first two days, QID on third day, BID for next 10 days (until recovery is complete).
- When using BAL, it is recommended that one should alkalinize the urine - helps maintain BAL mercury complex which may otherwise dissociate in acid urine and thereby damage renal tubules.
- **DMSA and DMPS**. Mesodimercaptosuccinic acid (DMSA) and dimercaptopropane sulfonate (DMSA) are water-soluble analogs of BAL which are less toxic and have greater water solubility than BAL but have limited lipid solubility. They are effective when given orally. DMSA is preferred.
  - DMSA (e.g., Succimer®) was 4 times more effective than N-acetylpenicillamine in increasing urinary excretion of MeHg.
  - With inorganic mercurials, DMSA > BAL > DMPS at increasing urinary excretion.
  - D-penicillamine (15 - 50 mg/kg) orally, but only after gut is free of significant ingested mercury and only if renal function is present, otherwise is dangerous.

Polythiol resins for methylmercury

Oral administration of polythiol resins are useful as they bind mercury in the G.I. tract, which helps to prevent absorption into the body.

Copper

General Information

- Major Species effected: Sheep, cattle, certain breeds of dogs
- Usual Time of Onset Hours to chronic.

Susceptibility

- The most common and serious problem is copper toxicosis-molybdenum deficiency in **sheep**
- **Cattle** are sensitive to an **excessively low dietary copper to molybdenum ratio**
- **Goats** are 3 - 4 times more tolerant of copper than sheep.

- Genetic defects in some dog breeds (**Bedlington terriers**) cause excessive storage of copper in the liver eventually resulting in liver damage.
- All species are sensitive to excessive copper intake and are potentially affected by acute or subacute copper toxicosis.

Sources of Copper-Containing Compounds

- Anthelmintics Copper sulfate used as an anthelmintic or in solutions to treat infectious pododermatitis in ruminants can be a source of toxic levels of copper
- Foot baths used for livestock (see below)
- Pesticides including fungicides and algicides
- Copper is routinely added to livestock mineral supplements and is a GRAS (generally recognized as safe) feed additive
- Molybdenum is not recognized as an essential and safe element and its addition to feeds is thereby prohibited
- Feeding to sheep of complete feeds intended for cattle or poultry can provide copper levels toxic to sheep
  - Cattle can tolerate somewhat excessive copper and low molybdenum ratios, but sheep cannot
- When a vitamin-mineral supplement is added to a ration, the copper concentration may be increased to 30 ppm or more
- Natural molybdenum concentrations in rations are often 2 ppm or less
- Consumption of forage plants naturally low in molybdenum and high in copper or confinement of sheep without green forage containing adequate molybdenum will skew the copper: molybdenum ratio
- Consumption of plants contaminated by copper in pesticides such as bordeaux mixture (contains 1 - 3% copper sulfate) which is sometimes used in orchards
- Water from ponds treated with copper containing algicides can cause toxicosis
- Soils and vegetation contaminated from mining or smelting operations
- Grazing on pastures amended by poultry or swine waste from animals fed copper-containing growth promotants.

Factors Affecting Toxicity

- Age : young and old are effected due to ill developed detoxification mechanisms.

- Species: sheep and dogs are worst effected ex: Doberman, bedlington terrier, west land terrier due to presence of autosomal recessive gene.
- Sheep are deficient glucose-6-phosphate enzyme this is essential for pentose phosphate pathway. This forms essential component of RBC metabolism. So heamolysis seen.
- Malnutrition, improperly compounded feeds especially Zn, S, Mo enhance the toxicity.
- The proper dietary ratio for sheep is 6 parts copper to 1 part molybdenum. Ratios in excess of 10:1 often result in clinical copper toxicosis in sheep.
- Copper sulfate is somewhat less toxic than many other copper salts, perhaps because of a sulfate-enhanced excretion of copper.
- Copper in dry forages may be more available than copper from green forages.
- Toxicosis is often brought on by **stress**,fasting and excess physical activity.

Toxicokinetics

Absorption

Copper absorption is poorly understood, but it is thought that a complex of copper with a protein, and another organic compound or another metal may be formed.Copper absorption takes place in the small intestine and, in sheep, considerable absorption also occurs in the large intestine. Most of the ingested copper is not absorbed and is therefore passed in the faeces. Zinc and copper may compete for the same carrier protein for transport across the intestinal mucosa into the blood. Once absorbed, about 90% of the copper is firmly bound to a serum protein called ceruloplasmin and is loosely bound to albumin and amino acids. Copper bound to ceruloplasmin is not as readily available for exchange or transfer as is free copper. Copper in red blood cells exists primarily in 2 forms: 60% is in a superoxide dismutase enzyme called erythrocuprein and the remainder is loosely bound to other proteins. When copper reaches the liver, it is largely incorporated into the mitochondria, endoplasmic reticulum, nuclei, and cytosol of hepatocytes. The copper-molybdenum complex reduces copper accumulation in the liver.in hepatocytes Cu combines with metallotheionin and chelatin and stimulates their sysnthesis. Cu crosses placental barrier but no reports of crossing Blood brain barrier hence effected animals does not exhibit neuronal symptoms.

Elimination

- Fecal excretion is the primary route of elimination

- Small amounts of copper are also excreted in the urine. Increased dietary concentrations of molybdenum and sulfate increase urinary and biliary excretion of copper.

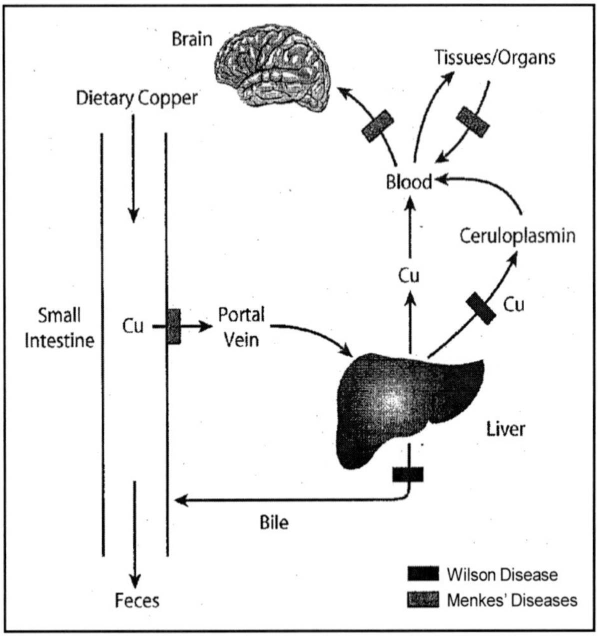

Figure showing the toxicokinetics of Copper inside the body

- Sulphur converted into sulphate, sulphite and sulphide forms CuS_2 and get excreted out through bile and faeces Plants or other toxicants that cause hepatic necrosis may impair the metabolism and excretion of otherwise tolerable amounts of copper.

Toxicodynamics

After copper builds up to about 150 ppm or more in the liver, copper toxicosis is initiated by the sudden release of copper from the liver into the blood. This may occur spontaneously, but it often seems to occur after some stress such as reduced feed intake, handling, or vigorous exercise. Generally, a sudden hemolytic crisis occurs. Associated with the hemolysis is a marked reduction in red blood cell glutathione concentrations and an increase in methemoglobin, indicating that copper may, in some way, promote oxidative reactions that result in red blood cell destruction.Because of hemolysis, death may result from hemoglobin-induced renal damage and anemia.

Copper buildup in liver from excess copper intake
(low molybdenum and low sulfate increase copper buildup)

(A)

Liver damage

+

Usually some stress factor

↓

Sudden release of copper

↓

Inhibits SH group of enzymes

↓

Detoxification

↓

Necrosis of hepatocytes

↓

Releases Cu in lysosomes

↓

Cu enters blood

↓

RBC (Hb in Fe^{+2} form)

↓

Cu+Hb(Fe^{+2})

↓

Methemoglobinimea (pays way for the formation of
Heinz bodies attach to RBC membrane → Hemolysis

↓

oxygen carrying capacity of RBC lowered

↓

Dyspnoea and anoxia, hemoglobinemia, hemoglobinuria

↓

Collapse and death in 24 - 48 hours

Copper also acts on the vascular smooth muscle and produces edema of the surrounding tissue due to transudation of plasma which increases colloidal osmotic pressure causing shrinkage in the RBC and also causes extensive heamorrhages in the body cavities.

(B)

Binds with SH groups of glutathione (GSH)
↓
Increased radical oxygen species (ROS)
↓
Increased lipid peroxidation
↓
Decreased cell membrane integrity
↓
Increased fragility of RBC
↓
Rupture of RBC
↓
Heamolytic crisis with heamaturia
↓
Heamolytic debris clogs glomerular filter
↓
Necrosis of kidneys
↓
Renal failure (tubular epithelial cells are effected)
↓
Anuria and uremia
↓
Effects brain (squeal to RBC heamolysis)
↓
Death

Clinical Signs

Acute Toxicosis

An acute syndrome of copper toxicosis results from ingestion or administration of copper containing formulations at a highly toxic dose. Frequently a period of stress precedes the onset of signs. Sudden onset of weakness, trembling, anorexia, hyperventilation, hemoglobinuria (red or coffee-colored urine), and icterus are usually present. Low morbidity generally (usually less than 5%), but mortality in affected animals is high (usually over 75%). If the syndrome progresses to death, the course generally lasts only 24-48 hours after the initial signs.

- Vomiting
- Hypersalivation
- Signs referable to abdominal pain
- Diarrhea, often greenish tinged
- Collapse and death sometimes occurs within 2 days

Chronic Toxicosis

Three syndromes occur

- Young dogs, 6 years of age and less may exhibit :
  - Anorexia
  - Vamition
  - Weakness
  - Lethargy
  - Dehydration
- These effects are believed to be due to active liver disease
- Older dogs, 6 - 12 years of age, may exhibit a chronic syndrome characterized by
  - Anorexia, weight loss
  - Occasional vomiting, diarrhea
  - Jaundice
  - Ascites
  - Hepatic encephalopathy, death
- The third form is comparatively rare and consists of sudden, severe, hemolytic crisis and anemia.

Non-Ruminants

Stage – I

- lasts for 2-3 months reduced ruminal fermentation and ruminal stasis

Stage – II

- lasts for 14-25 days
  - Anorexia
  - Loss of apetite
  - Diarrhoea

Stage – III

- Lasts for 2-5 days
- Generalised jaundice
- Hb in urine

In terminal stages animal dies due to

- Hepatic failure
- Renal failure
- Brain failure

Lesions

- Before the hemolytic crisis, liver biopsies may show swelling and necrosis of isolated hepatocytes with swollen Kupffer's cells, rich in acid-phosphatase and containing PAS-positive, diastase-resistant material, and copper.
- After the death of affected sheep, gross lesions usually include:
  - Generalized icterus.
  - Greatly enlarged gun-metal colored kidneys that sometimes are mottled with hemorrhage.
  - Slightly enlarged, friable, yellowish liver (or small, firm, pale liver).
  - Gallbladder distension with thick, greenish bile.
  - Splenic enlargement with a blackberry jam consistency and brown to black color in the parenchyma.
- Histologic changes include:
  - Cytoplasmic vacuolation and necrosis.
  - All liver lobules may contain clusters of necrotic cells.
  - Portal fibrosis begins early.
  - Renal tubules are clogged with hemoglobin with degeneration and necrosis of both tubular and glomerular cells.
  - The spleen is crowded with fragmented RBCs.
  - Status spongiosis in the white matter of the central nervous system.

Diagnosis

- Based on Appropriate clinical history, signs, and lesions.
- Normal concentrations of copper in the blood range from 0.75-1.35 ppm. Concentrations above this range are often associated with copper poisoning. Normal liver copper concentrations in sheep range from 10-50 ppm (wet weight basis). Liver copper concentrations associated with copper toxicosis are usually greater than 150 ppm on a wet weight basis, whereas kidney concentrations are generally greater than 15.0 ppm.
- Complete sheep rations containing 25 ppm or greater with 2 ppm or less molybdenum may produce copper toxicosis. As noted under **Toxicity**, lesser amounts of copper may also be associated with toxicosis.
- Based on laboratory examination of suspected samples.

Kidney, Liver	100g
Serum	2-5ml
Whole blood	10ml
Feed	1-2kg
Faeces	100g

I. Liver enzymes such as SGOT, LDH, sorbitol dehydrogenase, arginase, and glutamic dehydrogenase may be increased for 6 - 8 weeks before the hemolytic crisis. The serum activities of these enzymes often return to near normal values 1 - 2 weeks before the hemolytic crisis, but increase to very high values shortly before or during the crisis.

II. The enzyme activities do **not** correlate with copper concentrations in the blood.

III. An increase in methemoglobin concentration may be seen.

IV. Hemoglobinemia, hemoglobinuria.

V. Increased plasma bilirubin.

VI. Reduced PCV.

VII. Increased WBC, normal platelet counts.

Treatment

- Eliminate the source
- Free access to salt licks be prevented for 2-3 days
- The prognosis for animals in the hemolytic phase of the disease is often poor. Usually the most benefit is derived via efforts to alleviate copper buildup in the rest of the flock.
- Urinary copper excretion is increased 10 - 20 times by the chelation agent, D-penicillamine, at 52 (40-100mg/kg/day) mg/kg/day for 6 days, although it may be expensive for treating on a flock basis.
- Individual animals may benefit from alkalinization of the urine to decrease renal damage from hemoglobin. Animals may also improve in response to blood transfusions if serious anemia is present.
- Intravenous ammonium tetrathiomolybdate at 100 mg 2 times per week has been used to treat or prevent hemolytic crisis, minimize tissue damage, and decrease liver copper deposition.
- Ammonium molybdate at 50 mg(50-500mg) per head per day with 0.3 - 1 gram of thiosulfate orally daily for 3 weeks may help to prevent chronic copper toxicosis.

- Molybdenized superphosphate (ammoniumtetra thio molybdate) (at 2ppm molybdenum per acre) increases molybdenum content of pastures and reduces copper retention.
- Alternatively, molybdenized licks comprised of 190 lb salt, 140 lb finely ground gypsum, and 1 lb sodium molybdate may be used.
- Zinc may play a preventative role since supplementation of the ration with 250 ppm zinc as zinc oxide reduce liver copper buildup The effect was synergistic with that of added sodium molybdate.

Supportive therapy

- Glucocorticoids for lysosomal stabilization in acute disease.
- Ascorbic acid, 500-1,000 mg/day, to enhance urinary excretion of copper

Lead (Plumbism)

General Information

- *Major Species effected*: Most species, especially dogs, horses, cattle, waterfowl. Swine resistant
- *Usual Time of Onset*: Hours to months.

Sources

Large Animals

Acccidental grazing or licking of

- Batteries in pastures, broken in feed mixers, etc.
- Roofing coat
- Motor oil from engines that burn regular leaded petrol
- Grease if it contains lead
- Lead paint (licked from the walls, in paint cans, etc.)
- Lead smelters-effluent onto forage; also, some uptake by plants
- Lead mine tailings
- lead arsenate pesticides
- *Note: With lead arsenate pesticides; signs and lesions of poisoning relate much more to arsenic than to lead*
- News paper print contains lead chromate
- Milk from lead poisoned animals (98% absorbed through milk)
- Cosmetics PbO or lead tetraoxide.

Small Animals

Accidental ingestion or licking of

- Lead paint, especially paint chips
- Lead objects Toys, drapery weights, sinkers, solder, caps from glass bottles especially a concern for dogs
- Plumbing materials.
- Improperly glazed bowls.
- Leaded petrol (contains tetraethyl lead, which is highly absorbed by all routes). Also burning of tetraethyl lead produces particulate lead in the exhaust of engines burning regular leaded petrol.

Toxic Levels In Animals

- Cattle-intakes of greater then 6-mg/kg-body weight can lead to chronic poisoning and intakes greater than 10 mg/kg BW may cause acute lead poisoning.
- Sheep-generally occurs only in lambs and symptoms of poisoning appear at intakes greater than 4.5 mg/kg BW.
- Pigs, Goats and Rabbits-more resistant than sheep or cows. Very minor signs of poisoning occur at intakes of 60 mg/kg BW. This is equal to blood concentrations of 130 micrograms per dl.
- Horses-respiratory "roaring" occurs at intakes of 6.4 mg/kg BW. Signs of anemia occur at intakes of 7.4 mg/kg.
- Birds-poultry can withstand dietary intakes of 100-mg/kg feed with no symptoms. Levels of 500 mg/kg induce serious poisoning.

Dogs and cats-nervous symptoms of poisoning appear at intakes of 5 mg/kg BW/day.

Factors affecting toxicity

- Susceptibility
    - Young more susceptible: absorb greater fraction than adults.
    - Dogs, horses, cattle, and waterfowl are all poisoned comparatively more.
    - Horses may be even more sensitive than cattle.
    - Swine, goats, and chickens are comparatively tolerant.
    - Rare in cats

- *General health* : debilitated animals are more susceptible,pregnant animals are more susceptible
- *Route of entry* : oral route is the most common route can also enter through skin. inorganic cannot cross skin. Lead bullet shots in skeletal muscles dissolution slow compared to stomach where it is fast due to acidic pH
- *Rate of ingestion* : large dose over a short period causes death where as small quantity over a prolonged period of time does not produce death
- *Physical form* : solid form poor absorption low toxicity where as pure form more absorption high toxicity
- *Condition of the GIT* : presence of ingesta delays absorption
- *Dietary factors*: Low selenium concentration enhances Pb toxicity.

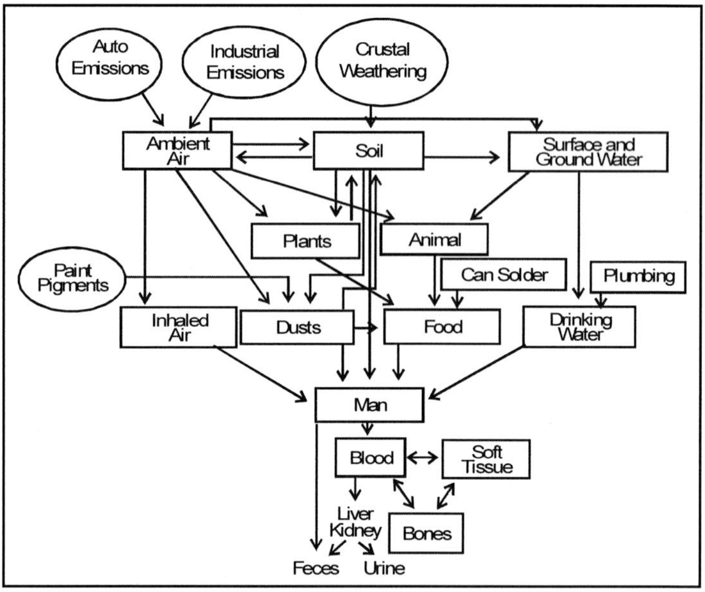

Figure 1. Pathways of lead from the environment to man & animals, and body disposition of lead (EPA, 1986).

Toxicokinetics

Most common route of exposure is oral ingestion. However, inhaled lead particles are cleared by mucociliary action and then swallowed. A greater degree of absorption occurs in the young, especially when low Fe and calcium are deficient in diet. 10% ingested absorbed in adults and 50% in young ones. Bone is the sink for lead (hence an x-ray picture shows lead lines in bone).

This is considered to be a protective mechanism of the body. Other two protective mechanisms are the sequestration of lead in liver and kidney. Lead crosses the placenta and can enter milk. Doesn't readily enter CNS, except in youn ones - their blood-brain barrier not fully developed. Initial distribution in liver and kidney, redistribution is 95% in bone (detected by X-ray). Half-life is one month. Excretion is limited and is excreted predominately via the bile. Enterohepatic circulation not known. Urine excretion is minimal unless chelation therapy is administered.

Toxicodynamics

Acts as surrogate for Ca^{2+} which results in subtle disruption of essential functions-

↓

Inhibits uptake of Ca^{2+} through membrane channels/ Na+-K+ ATPase

↓

Substitutes for Ca^{2+} in Ca^{2+}-Na+ ATP pump

↓

Blocks entry of Ca^{2+} into nerve terminals

↓

effects generation of action potential/signal transduction

↓

Interferes signalling processes at the post and presynaptic junctions

↓

Interferes with two intracellular Ca^{2+} receptors i) calmodulin and ii) protein kinase C (Protein kinase C: cell division, proliferation, cell-to-cell communication & organisation of cytoskeleton)

↓

Activation of PK C in microvessels alters normally tight BBB

↓

Also alters activity of tyrosine hydroxylase, phenyl-ethanolamine-N-methyltransferase and choline acetyltransferase causing alteration in the concentration of NA, DA & ACh in brain and nerve terminals

a. *In developing brain*: impairs timed programming of cell-to-cell connections (modify neuronal circuitry) and induces precocious differentiation of the glia (affect migration)

b. Interferes with metabolism of Vit D

c. Depresses functioning of adrenal and thyroid gland

Lead Inhibits Biosynthesis of Haeme

Succinyl Co-A + glycine

↓ X δ-ALA synthase

d-aminolevulinate (δ-ALA)

↓ X X δ-ALA dehydratase

porphobilinogen

↓ Isomerase deaminase

Uroporphyrinogen III

↓ Urogen decarboxylase

Coproporphyrinogen III

↓ X coproporphyrinogen oxidase

Coproporphyrin III

↓ coproporphyringenase

Protporphyrinogen

↓ progen oxidase

Protoporphyrin IX+Fe^{2+}

↓ X ferrochelatase + Fe^{2+}

Haeme

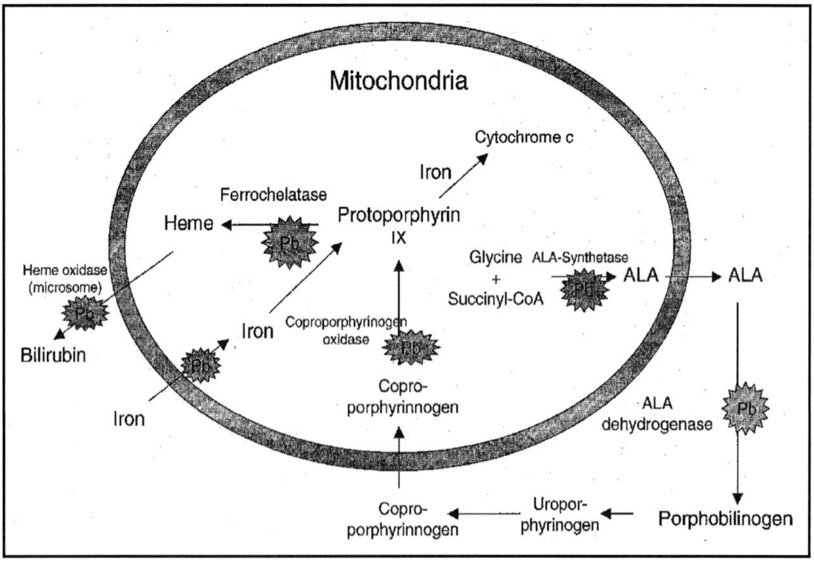

Diagrammatic representation of theame synthesis inhibition by lead

Other Effects

- Interferes with thiol (-SH containing) enzymes.
- Lead may replace zinc in some enzymes.
- Cerebral edema and neuronal damage centrally, demyelination and reduced nerve conduction velocity peripherally
- At very high concentrations inhibits inhibitory interneurons of GABA
- Inhibition of the enzyme nucleotidase is responsible for basophilic stippling and increased fragility of RBCs. Basophilic stippling can be normal in ruminants and is therefore not considered to be a diagnostic feature where as in dogs it is pathological importance
- Failure of heme synthetase to insert iron atoms leaves protoporphyrin free to chelate endogenous zinc atoms.

Clincal Signs

- Neurologic Effects
  - Nervous system signs often predominate.
  - Blindness. Swelling of optic disk. Iridocyclitis.
  - Hysteria, chomping, seizures, muscle spasms, opisthotonus.
  - Circling.
  - Pushing against objects (head pressing).
  - Ataxia.
  - Cattle - rhythmic bobbing of the head, twitching of the ears, exaggerated blinking, fine muscle tremors, marked excitement or seizures (bad prognostic sign).
- Horse
  - Paresis of lower lip, *recurrent laryngeal paresis* **(stertorous sounds),** pharyngeal paresis, and rectal sphincter paresis.
  - Regurgitation of water from nose during drinking.
- Gastrointestinal Tract
  - Mucosal damage, abdominal distress, tucked abdomen.
  - Anorexia, vamition.
  - Constipation, then diarrhea, colic.
  - Cattle - rumen motility reduced or abolished, grinding of teeth.

- Reproductive
  - Crosses placenta causes abortion, resorption, and sterility.

Other Signs

- Behavioral signs - anxiety, hyper excitability, bellowing, rolling eyes, pressing of head against a wall or post, attempts to climb walls, rolling of eyes, jumping into the air, frenzied or maniacal behaviour. Lead disrupts learning and memory in young ones directly or through mother's milk.
- Nervous signs – depression (specially in sheep and horses), muscle spasms, paralysis of pharynx and larynx (roaring in horses) blindness, torticollis, convulsions etc.,
- Autonomic signs- salivation (due to inability to swallow), lacrimation, colic (tucked abdomen, tooth gnashing, groaning) constipation or diarrhoea, atony of rumen, urinary incontinence and vomiting even in cattle.
- Locomotor disturbances- stiff gait, ataxia, inco-ordination, muscle weakness to compulsive hyper motility (circling, pacing, running).

Lesions

- Lead objects, paint, or used motor oil in the gastrointestinal tract in some cases.
- Mild gastritis or enteritis.
- Esophageal dilatation in some dogs.
- Pale liver, acid-fast intranuclear inclusions in hepatocytes.
- Muscle may also be pale.
- Kidneys Degeneration and necrotic changes, acutely hyperemic or hemorrhagic. acid-fast intranuclear inclusions may occur in the renal tubular epithelial cells
- Oedema, swelling, increased prominence of vessels in the brain.
- Capillary damage in the CNS. Collapse of small arterioles.

Diagnosis

- Antemortem
  - Base on Case history, clinical signs
  - Blood lead (whole blood: heparinized or EDTA tubes).

- 0.6 ppm or greater is diagnostic
- Blood lead concentrations are a valuable indicator of exposure but they do not indicate the length of exposure or total amount of lead deposited in the body.
- Nucleated RBCs or basophilic stippling (in dogs, cat, horse) is suggestive
- X-ray abdomen or reticulum of ruminants when possible.
- X-ray epiphyseal plate.
- Serum ALA dehydratase inhibition and erythrocyte protoporphyrin assays are highly sensitive tests for indication of a possible effect of lead.
- Urine increase in delta ALA.
- *Hair*: shedding in animals decreases the value of lead analysis and hair is not as good an indicator of chronic exposure as in man.
- *Fecal lead*: 35 ppm is suspect.
- Samples for laboratory examination.

Kidney	100g	Heparinized,
Whole blood	10ml	do not use EDTA
Liver	100g	
Urine	15ml	

- Postmortem
  - Liver and kidney. Renal cortex more reliable to assay than liver because kidney stores more lead.1 - 10 ppm;
  - Characteristic lesions.

Differential Diagnosis

- Dog, cat: rabies, distemper, hepatitis, other heavy metal toxicoses.

Ruminants	major DDx	rabies, poliencephalomalacia, TEME, listeriosis.
	minor DDX	hypomagnesemic tetany, nervous ketosis, hypovitaminosis A, nervous coccidiosis, mercury poisoning, meningitis, encephalitis, hepatoencephalopathy, organic insecticide poisoning.

OC - body temperature is increased, marked neuromuscular signs, abnormal posturing and severe convulsive activity with postictal depression, and absence of blindness.

Urea - no blindness, diarrhoea is not prominent. Strychnine like convulsions with post ictal rigidity.

OP & carbamates have parasympathetic activity that can be treated with atropine.

Other substances that show the same signs - salt, strychnine, nicotine, fluoroacetate, arsenic, mercury and hypovitaminosis-A. In dogs the symptoms may mislead the vet. to diagnose it as either CD or Rabies.

Treatment

- Eliminate the source and prevent further exposure.
- Remove remaining lead from digestive tract.
    - Saline cathartic.
    - Sodium sulfate or magnesium sulfate (0.5 mg/kg in a 10% solution in water PO or by stomach tube),Promotes evacuation, plus insoluble (poorly absorbable) lead sulfate is formed.
    - Gastric lavage (infrequently needed).
    - Surgery to remove large objects, particularly those not progressing through the GI tract.
- Surgical removal of lead shot from tissue after gunshot, but if it is delayed case than not needed
- Flush and siphon lead pellets from gizzard or feed large amount of grit to expel pellets.
- Feeding peanut butter in baby cereal to provide lubrication to aid in passage of lead foreign bodies in avian species.
- Chelation therapy.
    - Orally administered chelation agents may enhance absorption of metals when present at elevated concentrations in the GI tract. They are, therefore, used (by this route) only after the metal has left the digestive tract.
    - CaEDTA = Ca disodium EDTA = Ca disodium ethylene diamine tetraacetate = Ca disodium versenate. (Na EDTA chelates calcium and can cause hypocalcemia).

- Horse/cattle - CaEDTA (6.6% solution) at 73 mg CaEDTA/kg using slow I/V administration in divided doses 2-3 times per day for 3-5 days. If necessary to treat more than 5 days (based on clinical signs, urine lead), a 2-day rest period is provided before the second 5-day course of therapy.
- Dog - CaEDTA at 100 mg/kg for 2-5 days. The daily dose is divided into four portions, administered SC after dilution to a concentration of 10 mg CaEDTA/ml of a 5% dextrose solution. Clinical improvement can occur in 24-48 hours. Do not exceed 5 days of continuous therapy or 2 grams as a single day's total dose because of potential nephrotoxicosis.
- Psittacine birds - CaEDTA at 35 - 40 mg/kg undiluted IM twice daily for 5 days. Do not exceed 5 days of continuous therapy. Second course of therapy, if needed, is given after a 5-7 day waiting period. Seizures controlled with diazepam 0.5 - 1 mg/kg IM BID to TID as needed.

  *Zinc supplementation may reduce the gastrointestinal upset associated with CaEDTA therapy.
- BAL removes lead directly from parenchymatous organs.
- BAL increases Pb excretion in urine, and removes Pb from red blood cells.
- DMPS (2,3-dimercapto-1-propanesulfonic acid sodium salt) and DMSA (Mesodimercapto- succinic acid - Succimer®) a structural analog of BAL, show considerable efficacy as a chelation agent. DMSA is available as a human product in 30 mg capsules. It is used in pet birds at 25 - 35 mg/kg PO BID 5 days a week for 3 - 5 weeks. DMSA appears to be a more rapid and effective chelator of lead, than Ca EDTA and is also less toxic.
- Penicillamine is given at 10 - 15 mg/kg BID up to 55 mg/kg BID for 1 week or for 2 weeks (separated by 1 week interval) given orally on an empty stomach. To minimize side effects give in divided doses TID to QID. It is contraindicated when lead is still present in the gastrointestinal tract.

Cattle and Calves

1. $CaNa_2$ EDTA

(1-2% W/V solution in 5% glucose @ 110 mg/kg b.i.d/2 days I/P or S/C).

Skip the next 2 days, rpt. after 2 days.

(This interruption allows time for redistribution of lead from soft tissue into bone, the site where chelator acts). Ca. Na_2 EDTA is not free from side effects; hence it has to be used very cautiously.

Dogs

$CaNa_2$ EDTA 1% w/v solution in 5% glucose @25 mg/kg 4 times a day/ 5days.

D-penicillamine orally as a follow up to $CaNa_2$ EDTA.

Dose- 35-110 mg/kg. Divided into 3or 4 daily doses for 1 wk. on 1wk. off.

D-penicillamine is contraindicated in animals with penicillin allergies.

DMSA(meso-2,3 dimercaptosuccinic acid)is the current drug of choice and is more specific than $CaNa_2$ EDTA against lead, mercury and arsenic.

Dose-10mg/kg every 8hrs.orally for 10days.

Symptomatic Therapy

- Thiamine HCl
  - Cattle 250 - 1000 mg (total dose) BID for 5 days. Dogs 100-300 mg/ kg. S/C or I/ M
- Seizure control
  - Cattle - phenobarbital 30 mg/kg I.V. or chloral hydrate 50 - 70 mg/ kg I/V as a 5 - 7% solution.
- Cerebral edema
  - Dexamethasone (cattle, horse, 0.1 mg/kg I/V, SC, or IM; dog, 1 - 2 mg/kg SC, IM, or I/V)
  - Mannitol (20% solution, 1 - 2 gm/kg slowly I/V)
- Broad-spectrum antibiotics to control secondary bacterial infections.

Prevention

- Avoiding exposure is essential.
- Adding organic material in soil tends to increase its ability to bind metals, including lead. The increase in binding capacity is limited because the organic material will tend to be degraded over time in the environment.
- Altering the pH (alkalinizing) is another method being studied in efforts to immobilize lead in soil.

Selenium

General Information

- Most domestic animals require selenium in their diet. For food-producing species, a level of 0.3 ppm in the total diet is often recommended.

  Available in 3 oxidation states
  - +6 Selenate
  - +4 Selenite : most toxic
  - -2 Selenide

Source

- Shampoos and fungicides containing Se
- Errors in feed formulation but rare
- Mine wastes, especially from copper, silver and high sulfide ores
- Iatrogenic administration of excessive doses of selenium intended as therapy or prevention of musculoskeletal disorders
- Selenium levels are highest in low rainfall areas with alkaline soil
- Leaching of selenium from the soil as a result of irrigation and transport downstream to evaporation basins has resulted in widespread teratogenesis
- Plants growing in high selenium soils are classified into three forms based on their ability to accumulate selenium
- *Obligate indicator plants /Selenium indicators* - require Se in large amounts for growth. Therefore their presence indicates the presence of high selenium. These plants concentrate 15000ppm Se
  - Examples include
  - *Xylorrhiza* = woody aster
  - *Oonopsis* = goldenweed
  - *Stanleya* = prince's plume
  - *Astragalus* = locoweed
- *Facultative indicator plants* - absorb Se if present in high concentrations, but do not require large amounts for growth. These are, therefore, found in both seleniferous and non-seleniferous soils. If not seleniferous soils, they may concentrate 1500 ppm of Se
  - Examples include
  - Other asters

- *Atriplex* = saltbrush
- *Sideranthus*
- *Machaeranthera*

- Non-accumulator plants / Passive accumulators - such as crop plants when grown on seleniferous soils may also accumulate 150 ppm Se as part of their protein make-up in integral proteins (i.e., seleno-cystine, selenocysteine, selenomethionine and selenocystathionine) in a water insoluble form.
  - Examples include
  - Wheat
  - Oats
  - Barley
  - Grasses
- Susceptible Species

  All species are susceptible

Toxicity

Acute Selenosis

- Due to ingestion of obligate indicator plants or iatrogenic toxicosis after parenteral administration
- 1 to 5 mg Se/kg BW orally is acutely toxic.
- Parentarally 0.2 mg Se/kg BW is acutely toxic.
- LD_{50} in sheep of intramuscularly administered Selenium 0.7 mg Se/kg BW.
- Oral LD_{50} of sodium selenite in Horse 3.3 mg/kg, Cattle 10 mg/kg, Swine 17 mg/kg. and 25 ppm (of selenium) in the diet causes subacute poisoning.

Chronic Selenosis

- Alkali disease (chronic selenosis) in livestock is due to the ingestion of nonaccumulator plants grown on seleniferous soils (150 ppm selenium) over a period of weeks or months.
- Primarily seen in cattle and horses.

Mechanism of Action

- Se^{+4} replaces sulphur from aminoacids (Cystien & Methionine) and forms abnormal structural protein.
- Se^{+4} causes glutathione depletion and secondary lipid peroxidation.
- Se^{+4} interfers with metabolism of vitamin A & C and hampers the availability of vitamin C.
- Se^{+4}combines with hemeprotein and inhibits cell oxidation.
- Se^{+4} reduces GSH concentration in the body of the effected animal which decreases the scavengingof free redicals resulting the oxidative free radical damage of various cell membranes

6Se+2GSH $\rightarrow$ formation of Se GSH complex Se binds with oxidized GSH inhibits the regeneration of GSH resulting in decreased concentration.

Clinical Signs

Acute Selenosis

- Onset of clinical signs within 1-2 hours
- Lethargy, nonresponsiveness.
- Dyspnoea blood tinged fluid oozes from nostrils with fluid sounds in lungs cyanosis and nasal discharge
- Teeth grinding
- Anorexia
- Prostration
- Mydriasis
- Elevated temperature
- Incoordination
- Uncertian gait "rooted to one spot" animals stands at on spot with head and ears lowered
- Bloody watery diarrhoea
- Polyuria
- Bloat

Lesions

- Edematous lungs, hydrothorax, pale heart.

Subchronic Selenosis/Blind Staggers

It occurs in 3 stages

System	Stage I	Stage II	Stage III
GI	Partial anorexia	Complete	Colic ,emaciation
CNS	Wanders aimlessly	Depression incordination foreleg weakness animal goes down on knees due to arthritis	Swelling & inflammation of eyelids → cloudy cornea → blindness
Respiration	Normal	Normal	Dyspnoea and tachypnoea
Temperature	Normal	Normal	Subnormal

Chronic Selenosis /Alkali disease

Sloughing and cracking of old hoof and onset of new hoof

↓

Fusion of old and new hoof

↓

Formation of long hoof (rocker shaped hoof)

↓

Deformities of the legs

↓

Lameness

↓

Results in emaciation and anorexia

Signs

- Decreased vitality
- Anemia
- Joint stiffness
- Lameness
- Rough hair coat
- Hair loss (tail and mane in horses).
- Horn and hoof deformities (circular break in hoof below coronary band).
- Horizontal hoof-wall cracks is the characteristic sign.

- Paresis
- Peripheral circulatory insufficiency
- Partial blindness.

Lesions

- Carcass emaciated
- Congestion, haemorrhages and oedema in all vital organs
- Cardiomyopathy and liver cirrhosis
- Degenerative changes in liver and kidney
- Hydropericardium and hydrothorax.

Teratogenesis in Poultry

- Missing or underdeveloped, legs, lower or upper beak, eyes.

Diagnosis

Based on

- Case history
- Clinical signs
- Presence of rotten garlic smell or horse radish smell in the stomach contents
- Postmortem lesions gross and histopathologic lesions
- Laboratory diagnosis of whole blood selenium (acute 25ppm and chronic 4ppm) and kidneys and liver 4-25 ppm acute) hair 5-10ppm chronic.
- Samples to be submitted for analysis

Kidney	100g
Liver	100g
Urine	15ml
Feed	10g

Differential Diagnosis

- *Acute selenosis /blind staggers:* Pneumonia, Anthrax, Infectious hepatitis, Enterotoxaemia, Pasteurellosis
- *Chronic Selenosis/Alkali disease:* ergotism,fluorosis,molybdenosis and laminitis.

Treatment

- Eliminate the source and minimize absorption
- Symptomatic and supportive treatment no specific antidote
- Symptomatic therapy (diuretics)
- Bromobenzene increases elimination of urine
- To replenish the glutathione levels Acetylcysteine: loading dose 140 mg/kg I/V followed by 70 mg/kg I/V QID
- Supplementation of Cysteine and Methoinine
- Increase protein content of ration (SH groups).
- Increase linseed meal content of ration
- Vitamin E contraindicated (synergistic with Se) Vitamin A & C can be supplemented)
- Low level feeding of Hg,Cu,Cd,Ag etc

Adding organic arsenic to diet to increase biliary excretion has been suggested for poultry, cattle, and pigs(not recommended for horses)

Molybdenum

General information

- Major Species effected: Ruminants
- Usual Time of Onset: Days to week
- The critical copper to molybdenum ratio in cattle feeds is 2:1.
- Usually a concomitant copper deficiency is also present.

Sources

- Animals grazing in the contaminated soils and forages in the vicinity of certain mining or smelting operations in which molybdenum containing ores are heated to high temperatures.
- Industrial contamination of farmland near metal alloy production plants.
- Contamination of soils with molybdenum containing fertilizers.
- In areas of excessive molybdenum and/or deficient copper in soils and associated forages and grain may result in problems in cattle and sheep.
- Molybdenum is added to fertilizers to increase nitrogen fixation in legumes.

- The molybdenum concentration of forage can be unusually high when:
  - There is a naturally high content of Mo in the soil
  - Industrial contamination of pastures occurs in the vicinity of mining or metal alloy production plants.

Factors Affecting Toxicity

- Cattle are more susceptible than sheep and young animals are more susceptible than old.
- Water soluble molybdenum in growing herbage is most toxic
- Young animals are more susceptible than adults
- Accumulation of molybdenum in plants is starts more in summer (spring) and is maximum in early winter (september-october)
- When the ratio of copper to molybdenum in feed drops below 2:1, molybdenum toxicosis can be expected in cattle.However, the 2:1 ratio is not absolute even in cattle because increasing the copper concentration of the diet even 5 ppm above normal to 13 - 16 ppm will protect cattle against 150 ppm molybdenum.
- Morbidity averages about 80% of the herd.
- When copper concentrations in feeds and forages are in the normal (8 - 11 ppm) range, cattle may be poisoned by molybdenum concentrations above 5 - 6 ppm, and sheep may be poisoned when molybdenum concentrations are greater than 10 - 12 ppm.
- Calves may be poisoned by milk from cows on high molybdenum diets.
- High dietary sulfate concentrations exacerbate the condition.

Toxicokinetics

- Molybdenum excretion is enhanced by increasing dietary inorganic sulfate.
- Increase in dietary molybdenum and sulfate increase urinary excretion of copper.
- Urine is the major route of elimination of molybdenum

Toxicodynamics

The major damage of molybdenum in the body is due to the creation of Copper deficient condition. copper is an important metal component (often at a catalytic site) in many enzymes including: tyrosinase, lactase, ascorbic acid oxidase, uricase, monoamine oxidase, deltaaminolevalenic acid dehydratase, dopamine-beta-hydroxylase, and cytochrome oxidase. Deficiency of copper may reduce certain enzyme activities.

- Reduction in the activity of a copper containing enzyme, amine oxidase, in the aorta resulting in reduced deamination of lysine in elastin, which may result in less conversion of lysine to desmosine, a cross-linkage group of lysine. In turn, this may result in lessened elasticity of the aorta and other major blood vessels. The tensile strength of the aorta is apparently markedly reduced, and there are spontaneous ruptures of the major blood vessels. The myocardium becomes friable
- Progressive atrophy of the myocardium with replacement by fibrous tissue and resultant sudden deaths, usually after excitement or exercise, has been associated with molybdenum toxicosis (falling disease) of cattle
- Complex formation with catechol compounds like phenols in the GI tract causes diminishing bacteriostatic activity resulting in liquid diarrhea full of gas bubbles
- In ruminants, osteoporosis and spontaneous fractures have been documented with excess dietary molybdenum due to excess displacement of phosphorus from the bony tissue
- Disrupts the maintenance and function of myelin, and nerve damage and demyelination causing "enzootic ataxia" and "sway-back" (usually in lambs).

Clinical Signs

- Anemia (microcytic, hypochromic)
- Emaciation
- Liquid diarrhea (peart scours)(full of gas bubbles) which may begin 8 - 10 days after being placed on a high molybdenum diet
- Depressed growth
- Osteoporosis, spontaneous fractures, beaded ribs (pacing gait)
- Depigmentation of hair (spectacled appearance)
- Gastrointestinal disturbances
- Vascular damage

- Achromotrichia
- Heart failure
- Impaired reproductive performance
- Swollen genitalia
- Prolonged purgation may result in poor weight gains and even death
- Neonatal ataxia
- Loss of libido and general unthriftiness
- Rough hair coat
- Drop in milk production
- Sudden deaths.

Sheep

- Depigmentation of wool
- Abnormal wool growth, loss of crimp and quality of wool, stringy wool and anemia in ewes condition is called as "enzootic ataxia" (Australia) and "Sway-back" (United Kingdom)
- Enzootic ataxia and swayback are noted in lambs less than 1 month old. The lambs are severely uncoordinated, ataxic, and usually blind
- Death results from starvation, exposure, or pneumonia.

Lesions

- Coarse, stringy, poorly pigmented hair or wool
- Emaciation
- Hemosiderosis
- In prolonged cases, osteoporosis and bone fractures are common
- In lambs with "enzootic ataxia" or "swayback", there is lysis of the white matter of the cerebrum and degeneration of the motor tracts of the spinal cord. The damage in the white matter varies from microscopic foci to massive subcortical destruction. There is often neuronal degeneration and demyelination.

Diagnosis

Based on

- Case history,clinical signs and lesions.
- Copper and molybdenum concentrations in feeds and forages.

- Response to the administration of copper.
- Copper and molybdenum concentrations in tissues.
  - Liver-copper concentrations of less than 10-30 ppm on a wet weight basis and molybdenum concentrations of greater than 5 ppm are significant. Normal liver-copper concentrations range from 30-140 ppm on a wet-weight basis, and liver molybdenum is normally below 3-4 ppm.
  - Blood:Whole blood copper concentrations of less than 0.6 ppm and molybdenum concentrations above 0.1 ppm are usually present in molybdenum toxicosis-copper deficiency. Normal blood copper concentrations range from 0.7 - 1.3 ppm, while a normal molybdenum level is around 0.05 ppm.
  - Based on laboratory examination of suspected samples.

Treatment

- Providing copper orally or parenterally; good response usually. Use with caution in sheep.

Methods

- Copper sulfate added to salt-mineral mixture at 1 - 5% depending on molybdenum levels in the feed.
  - Provide 1 gram of copper sulfate/adult cow. Alternative methods include:
  - 37.5mg/1 ltr $CuSO_4$/250 gal of water
  - 450mg of $CuSO_4$ to 45.35kg of salt
  - 45.35kg of protein concentrate, 45.35kg of salt, and 1.14kg of $CuSO_4$ (feed at rate of 77mg/hd/day).
- Copper glycinate inj. (S/c) at 60 mg for calves and 120 mg for mature cattle. May need to be repeated during a season.
- In areas where molybdenum content of forage is <5%ppm the use of 1% copper sulphate has provided effective control and with higher levels upto 5% has been used.

Cadmium

General Information

- Cadmium is a metal which has become an environmental contaminant as a result of effluents from plants smelting zinc, copper and lead, as well as from industries using cadmium in batteries, alloys and paints.

Sources

Accidental ingestion or licking of substances

- Associated with lead and especially zinc
- During use in electroplating
- Cadmium-Nickel battery
- Coal and fossil fuels
- Paints
- Cadmium-containing fungicides
- Cadmium (and lead) are often components of municipal sewage sludge in many communities in which the appropriate industries are located. Commercial sludge may contain up to 1500 mg of cadmium per kg dry material.

Toxicokinetics

- Low levels of dietary protein, calcium, iron, or zinc causes increased cadmium absorption
- Young absorb more than adults
- 1-5% absorbed from G.I. tract
- 10-40% absorbed from lung
- Distribute to kidney and liver - binds to Metallothionein
- Half-life: 10-30 years
- Excretion: bile.

Toxicodynamics

- Cadmium inhibits enzymes associated with zinc and displaces it from metalloenzymes
- Inhibits zinc uptake by the male reproductive tract
- Chronic cadmium toxicosis causes increased copper and iron deficiencies
- Blocks renal synthesis of the active form of vitamin D, resulting in anemia, poor bone mineralization and growth inhibition.

Clincal Signs

Acute Cadmium Poisoning

- Acute oral exposure to high concentrations may cause excessive salivation, persistent vomiting, diarrhea, abdominal pain, ataxia, loss of consciousness, severe gastroenteritis, subdural hemorrhage and testicular necrosis.

- Inhalation of cadmium is generally characterized by dyspnoea, cough, fever, and pulmonary edema.

Chronic Cadmium Poisoning

- *Kidney* : Most cadmium sensitive organ injury when 200 μg Cd/g Quantitate by β2-microglobulin in urine

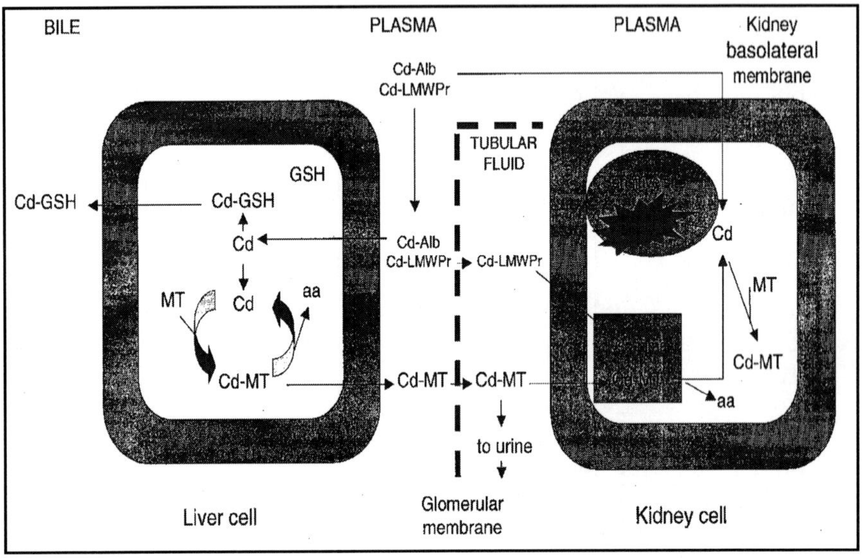

Diagrammatic representation of Cd damage of liver and kidney

- Lungs
  - a) After inhalation
  - b) Emphysema
    - i. Loss of ventilatory capacity and increase in lung volume
- Cardio vascular: hypertension
- Bone
- Testes - sensitive after acute, not after chronic

Diagnosis

Based on

- Case history
- Clinical signs

- Postmortem lesions gross and histologic changes in the kidneys, bone, gut, etc.
- Laboratory examination of Liver, kidney, and/or blood calcium
- Horses tend to have much higher cadmium (in normal animals) than with other domestic species
- Appropriate history, clinical signs.

Treatment

- Eliminate the source
- For acute toxicoses, BAL and calcium EDTA decrease mortality, but for chronic toxicoses are generally ineffective and may increase cadmium concentrations in the kidney, BAL is considered contraindicated after chronic exposure due to increased risk of nephrotoxicity
- Efforts to remove cadmium from the digestive tract should be employed in recent exposures
- In cases of chronic exposure, supplementation with zinc, copper and iron in more than normally adequate amounts are significantly protective. Vitamins C and D, cysteine and selenium also aid in protection. Naturally, steps to terminate exposure should be instituted.

Comment

Cadmium is rarely recognized as a toxicant in veterinary practice.

Iron

General Information

- Major Species Dogs, piglets, other species
- Usual Time of Onset Minutes to Hours
- Usual Duration (if survives) chronic permanent damage to acute death most common in piglets

Sources

Iron toxicosis usually results when too much iron is injected or less often when too much is given orally. Any of the iron complexes and iron salts may be involved. Baby pigs are most often involved, however, all species are potentially susceptible.

Iron From	Percent (%) Elemental Iron
Ferric phosphate	37
Ferric pyrophosphate	12
Ferrocholinate	12
Ferrous gluconate	12
Ferrous fumarate	33
Ferrous sulfate (hydrate)	20
Ferrous sulfate (dried)	37
Ferrous carbonate (anhydrous)	48
Ferroglycine sulfate	16
Peptonized iron	17

Toxicity

- Ingestion of 20 to 40 mg elemental iron/kg may result in toxicosis.
- > 60 mg elemental iron/kg is potentially serious.
- > 200 to 300 mg/kg is lethal dose.

Factors affecting toxicity

- Animals with enough iron are more susceptible than those actually needing iron.
- Pigs born to vitamin-E/Selenium deficient sows are more susceptible to
- Massive doses break down the mechanism controlling Gastrointestinal absorption causing toxicosis.

Toxicokinetics

In gastric and intestinal mucosal cells, iron is metabolized to the ferric state and is then transported across the cell membrane into the blood where it is bound to a α-glycoprotein (transferrin) transport protein. In an acute iron overdose, the transferrin can become saturated, allowing total serum iron to exceed iron-binding capacity, increasing free circulatory iron. Absorption is enhanced in the presence of acid. Peak absorption may occur between 1 and 6 hours after ingestion.

Toxicodynamics

- Direct (caustic) irritant effect on gastrointestinal tract.

- Presumably interferes with sulfhydryl groups of enzymes and other proteins.
- Enhances free radical damage by superoxide radical.
- precipitation of phosphates in the gut as a complex with iron causing stunted growth and rickets
- Enters the mitochondria where it acts as a mitochondrial poison, interfering with cellular respiration and resulting in metabolic acidosis.
- Two main syndromes are involved:
  - Per acute syndrome comprised of an anaphylactoid reaction causing Sudden death within a few minutes to hours after an iron injection.
  - Sub acute syndrome causing death accompanied by severe depression and coma.

Signs

- *Per acute condition*: anaphylactic shock reaction, vascular collapse followed by rapid death.
- *Sub acute condition*: animal may be drowsy, may exhibit vomiting and diarrhea, may be bloody, cardiovascular collapse and death occur.
- In small animals, early signs from the corrosive effect on the gut with vomiting and diarrhea develop in 0 to 6 hours post ingestion. Apparent recovery may occur 6 to 24 hours post ingestion followed by shock, CNS depression, GI hemorrhage, acidosis, and liver failure.
- Oliguria, anuria. Secondary to shock-induced acute renal failure.

Lesions

- Yellowish-brown discoloration and edema of the tissues, especially near the injection site.
- The nearby lymph nodes, and the liver and kidneys may all be dark in colour.
- Gastric ulceration and edema
- Histologically is characterized as Periportal necrosis.

Diagnosis

- Based on case history, clinical signs and lesions
- Samples should be taken at 3, 6, 9, and 12 hours
- Abdominal radiographs for the presence of metallic foreign bodies.

Treatment

- Anaphylactoid reaction
  - Antihistamines, epinephrine, oxygen
- Subacute
- Desferrioxamine (Desferal ®) effective as a chelation agent given at 40 mg/kg, I/M, q 4 to 8 hours, slowly in an IV drip (< 15 mg/kg/hour). or more often as deferoxamine is to enhance the excretion of iron. One hundred mg of deferoxamine will bind approximately 9 mg of iron. Its highest affinity for iron in the ferric (+3) state causes a "vin rose" (reddish-brown) appearance to the urine
  - Ascorbic acid in large oral doses doubles or triples the iron excretion after defesrrioxamine. However, ascorbic acid should be used only after the gut is thoroughly cleared of iron sources. recommended when serum iron values in dogs greater than 350 ˈg/100 ml are present
- Oral exposure
  - Early, eggs, water, milk and emetic are indicated
  - The milk of magnesia (MgOH) complexes with iron to form FeOH which precipitates and is therefore not as effectively absorbed. MgOH may be of limited value in dogs
  - I/V fluids and appropriate supportive measures.

Prognosis

Iron toxicosis usually carries a poor prognosis.

Zinc

Sources

- Ingestion of coins
- Drinking water (especially when it's acidic) from galvanized tanks.
- Ingestion of acidic food or beverages from galvanized containers.
- Birds may ingest zinc from "welded wire" fencing.
- In dogs as a result of ingestion of zinc nuts from hardware used on transport cages or those in veterinary facilities or from repeatedly licking off zinc oxide ointment used to treat skin lesions.

Susceptible Species

Dogs, cats, ferrets, mink, sheep, horses, cattle, caged birds.

Toxicity

- Cattle and sheep have decreased feed consumption when the diet exceeds 1,000 ppm zinc
- Rats, pigs, and poultry tolerate dietary levels of 1,000 to 2,000 ppm without adverse effect
- An acute oral LD_{50} for zinc chloride was 96 mg/kg in the guinea pig.

Toxicokinetics

- Approximately 2/3 of the zinc in serum or plasma is loosely bound to protein and the remainder is tightly bound
- Zinc is excreted primarily via the bile and pancreas.

Clinical Signs

- The most common clinical signs in small animals include: vomiting, depression, anorexia, hemoglobinuria, diarrhea, weakness, icterus. Can also see clinical signs (e.g., oral ulcers) associated with acute renal failure
- Cattle may present with anorexia, depression, polydipsia, polyphagia, decreased milk yield, chemosis, exopthalmia, convulsions, and death
- Subacute or chronic zinc toxicosis primarily affects the renal, hepatic, and hematopoietic tissues
- Mucosal irritation can result from ingestion of certain zinc salts (e.g., zinc oxide)
- Single ingestions of zinc oxide ointment are characterized mainly by Vamition
- Regenerative anemia; hemolytic anemia with hemoglobinemia and hemoglobinuria possible.

Clinical Pathology

- Increased serum alkaline phosphatase, bilirubinemia
- Hypophosphatemia, isosthenuria or hyposthenuria, proteinuria, hematuria, azotemia, and renal casts all consistent with acute renal failure.

Lesions

- Hemorrhagic gastritis.

- Proximal renal tubular epithelial necrosis
- Centrilobular hepatocyte vacuolization, necrosis of individual cells occurs. Bile casts in bile canaliculi.

Diagnosis

- Elevated serum, tissue (kidney, liver), and urine zinc concentration. Note: Special tubes for elemental analysis (Royal blue top) are recommended. In addition, syringes used in collecting blood should contain no rubber gromets (i.e., all glass or all plastic). This is necessary because certain blood tubes and syringes have zinc stearate present in the lubricant which can contribute up to 5-6 ppm extraneous zinc.
- Radiograph of abdomen for presence of zinc hardware.

Treatment

- Symptomatic and supportive therapy.
- Slow I/V fluid and bicarbonate for acute renal failure.
- Emetics
- If zinc foreign bodies are present Gastrotomy or enterotomy is required.
- Chelation therapy : CaEDTA or penicillamine
- If hemolysis is a problem blood transfusions is indicated.
- Chronic zinc toxicosis interferes with absorption and utilization of iron and copper.

Chapter 4

NON METAL TOXICOLOGY

Nitrate – Nitrite Poisoning

Sources

Accidental ingestion/grazing of

- Plants which are Nitrate accumulators

Species of Plants

Sudan Grass (*Sorghum* spp.)*	Sweet Clover (*Melilotus*)
Johnson Grass (*Sorghum* spp.)*	Flax, linseed (*Linum*)
Sorghum (*Sorghum* spp.)*	Pigweed (*Amaranthus*)
Beets (*Beta*)*	Jimson weed (*Datura*)
Rape (*Brassica*)*	Wild Sunflower (*Helianthus*)
Corn (*Zea*)*	Cheeseweed (*Malva*)
Rye (*Secale cereale*)	Smartweed (*Polygonum*)
Wheat (*Triticum*)	Dock (*Rumex*)
Oats (*Arena*)	Nightshades (*Solanum*)
Fescue (*Festuca*)	Soyabeans (*Glycine*)
Alfalfa (*Medicaqo*)	

* Indicates plants of greatest risk.

Factors Increasing Nitrate Concentrations in Plants

- Heavy fertilization
- Factors that tend to reduce plant nitrate reductase activity
  - Drought or rainy period after drought
  - Decreased light (cloudy weather, early in the day before exposure to much sunshine). For these reasons, it is wise to cut hay or green chop relatively late on a sunny day to minimize concentrations of nitrate
  - Decreased temperature

Accidental drinking of water

- Run-off from fertilized fields
- Run-off from decaying manure in fields
- Nitrates or nitrites may leach through soil to deep and especially shallow, poorly cased wells.
- Concentrations are less likely to be excessive in ponds with abundant algal blooms
- Concentrations may be highest after high surface run-off (heavy rains) especially when recently applied fertilizer washes into small ponds or very small streams

Accidental ingestion or licking of

Fertilizers

- Large animals (sodium, potassium, or ammonium nitrate) since it is salty in taste
- May be eaten directly from bags, spilled, unevenly spread, or washed into water
- Fertilizer is the primary source of nitrate for small animals
- Some nitrogen fertilizers are high in urea.

Factors Affecting Toxicity

- Species
  - Ruminants are much more susceptible to nitrates than monogastric animals
  - Rumen microorganisms reduce nitrate (NO_3) ion to nitrite (NO_2) ion

- Age
  - Fetuses and neonates are more susceptible than are the older young or the adults.

- Time
  - Concentrations in plants are generally highest just prior to flowering and rapidly drop after pollination and grains or fruits set on.
  - Post harvest reduction of nitrate to nitrite in feedstuffs such as moist hay and silage, a factor which could increase toxicity with completion of the ensiling process, nitrate-containing feeds often become less hazardous with conversion of the nitrite to ammonia and dissipation.

- Diet
  - Vitamin A deficiency may be an effect of nitrate toxicosis and contribute to the occurrence of abortion (but this is only a theory, it has not been substantiated)
  - Urea toxicity
  - Availability of Mo,Cu,Fe and I_2 predisposes to nitrate toxicity.

- Drying
  - Most nitrate is **retained when plants are air-dried** at ambient temperatures (e.g., hays). The nitrate content of hay may even increase during storage due to moisture loss
  - Acid soils
  - Low molybdenum, sulfur, phosphorus, manganese, or magnesium in soils
  - Application of phenoxy (2,4-D like) herbicides
  - Nitrates accumulate in the vegetative tissues of the plant, not in the fruits or grain and concentrations are usually greatest in the stalk than in the leaves.

- Toxicity
  - Acute nitrate poisoning is most likely to occur when forage nitrates exceed 10,000 ppm (1%) (dry weight basis) or when water contains 1500 ppm (0.15%) nitrate. Lethal doses of nitrate and nitrite are included in the following table:

Nitrate	
Source Species	**Lethal Dose in mg/kg of body weight**
Cattle	330 - 616
Sheep	308
Sodium Nitrite	
Pigs	90
Sheep	170

- The amount of preformed nitrite influences toxicity, especially in monogastric species
- *Susceptibility*: dependent upon several factors including
  - Rate of intake
  - Variations in gastrointestinal nitrate reduction (adaptation)
  - Diet (nutrition)
  - Metabolic state of the animal as influenced by age, pregnancy, and disease.

Toxicokinetics

Both nitrate and nitrite are passively absorbed from the gastrointestinal tract and reach their highest concentrations 5 - 6 hours. In addition to conversion of nitrate to nitrite in the rumen, nitrate appears to be converted to nitrite by liver enzymes following absorption, but the rate of the hepatic reduction is slow since no significant methemoglobinemia occurs following the intravenous administration of nitrates.Most nitrate is excreted by the kidney, but some is recycled back into the gastrointestinal tract by salivary and gastrointestinal tract secretion.Nitrite reduction in the gastrointestinal tract is attributed solely to action of microorganisms. In ruminants, this reduction primarily occurs in the rumen, and nitrate, nitrite, and ammonium ions are absorbed directly into the blood. In monogastric species, the stomach contains relatively few microorganisms due to the presence of hydrochloric acid. Monogastric species are, therefore, relatively resistant to toxicosis due to nitrates but are susceptible to poisonings by preformed nitrites.Pregnant ruminants should not be fed over 0.2% nitrates.

Feed Concentration as Nitrate Ion (Dry Matter Basis)	Estimated Toxicological Significance for Cattle
0.0 - 0.44%	Considered safe to feed under all conditions.
0.44 - 0.66%	Safe for nonpregnant animals under all conditions. Limit pregnant animals to 50% of the total dry matter in the ration
0.66 - 0.88%	Limit to 50% of the total dry matter in the ration
0.88 - 1.54%	Limit to 35 - 40% of the total dry matter in the ration. Feeds with over 0.88% nitrate ion should not be used for pregnant animals.
1.54 - 1.76%	Limit to 25% of the total dry matter in the ration. Do not use for pregnant animals.
Over - 1.76%	Do not feed toxic

Toxicodynamics

- Nitrite is the actual toxic compound
- Nitrite oxidizes hemoglobin to methemoglobin
  - 30 - 40% methemoglobin causes mild clinical signs
  - 75 - 90% methemoglobin causes severe clinical signs to death
- Nitrate interferes with hormonal function
- Nitrate interferes with vitamins A,D,B_{12},E,I_2 (thyroid dysfunction)
- The small quantities of methemoglobin formed during (normal) metabolism of physiologic amounts of nitrites or other oxidizing agents are converted to hemoglobin by an enzyme in erythrocytes, methemoglobin reductase. When the formation of methemoglobin exceeds the turnover rate of methemoglobin reductase, abnormally high concentrations of methemoglobin will occur
- 20-40% metHb - hypoxia under stress
- 50% metHb - active animals death
- 75% metHb - resting animals sudden death

Clinical Signs

- Acute (onset within 1/2 - 4 hours after feeding)
  - Abdominal colic

- Direct gastrointestinal irritation - vomiting, salivation, diarrhea.
- Frequent urination initially
- Dyspnoea
- Tremors
- Ataxia
- Rapid, weak heart beat
- Terminal convulsions
- Death in 6 - 24 hours. The number of deaths is increased when animals are stressed due to increased oxygen requirements.

❐ Chronic

Note - These are the results of field observations

- Abortions - "Lowland abortion syndrome"may occur most often at 3 - 5 days after an acute toxicosis
- Ist trimester – implantation of foetus hampered
- Last trimester – death of foetus (the foetus if survives dies soon after birth which in 10-24hrs and those which survive high susceptibility to convulsions and seizures)
- Poor growth and feed efficiency
- Decreased milk production
- Infertility
- Goiter, primarily in sheep (interference with iodine metabolism)
- Increased susceptibility to infections.

Lesions

❐ "Chocolate-brown" blood

❐ Brownish cast to all tissues

❐ Mucous membranes cyanotic

❐ Congestion of ruminal or abomasal mucosa

❐ Placental necrosis suggested by some veterinarians

Diagnosis

Based on

❐ Case history

- Appropriate clinical signs
- Postmortem lesions
- Laboratory analysis of nitrate and/or nitrite of:

Forage/Ingesta	1kg	Ingesta in chloroform or formalin filled air tight container
Water	100ml	
Body fluids	10-20ml	

- Urine (NO_3 stable in urine for around 48 hours)
- Aqueous humor of aborted fetuses may also reveal elevated nitrate concentrations. Except for dry feeds, dry forages, and blood, specimens should be collected as rapidly as possible and shipped to the laboratory in a frozen state
- Blood samples for methemoglobin analysis must be collected within 2 hours of death and rapidly frozen or preferably preserved in phosphate buffer to stabilize the methemoglobin (All samples should be transported with as much air removed as possible
- Serum NO_3 of greater than 20 micrograms (µg) per ml is diagnostic
- Fetal aqueous humor nitrate concentrations above 50 ppm have been considered nitrate toxicosis and 30 - 50 ppm are considered suspect, thus when such levels are encountered diets and water also should be checked for nitrate
- Field Analysis
  - Diphenylamine test for nitrates
  - Alpha-naphthylamine test for nitrites.

Treatment

- Don't stress any more than necessary
- Methylene blue
  - Dogs:4 mg/kg IV in a 1% solution, cattle 15 mg/kg IV in a 1% solution
  - Treatment may need to be repeated
  - Methylene blue 1% w/v solution, @ 8.8 mg/Kg body wt. slow I/V for cattle and sheep. In other species the dosage is 4.4 mg/Kg body wt. slow I/V. Repeat after 30 min. if symptoms persist. Care should be taken while administering methylene blue because it can directly convert haemoglobin into methaemoglobin.

- Function of methylene blue
- Methylene blue is converted into leucomethylene blue in the presence of $NADPH_2$ I and II diaphorase enzyme systems, which in turn converts methaemoglobin into haemoglobin. Multiple doses or a single dose in the absence of nitrite toxicosis, however, may cause Heinz body hemolytic anemia
- Ascorbic acid @ 5-20mg/kg IV
- Antibiotics broad spectrum with 18-20 litres of cold water to decrease the temperature
- Relieve bloat than go for antibiotics
- Adrenergics and adrenolytics are contraindicated
- In case of chronic poisoning supplement with vitamins A,D,B_{12},E,I_2

Prevention

Forages

- Cut forage late in the day on a warm, sunny day
- Analyze forage for nitrate **before** feeding suspected material
  - A diphenylamine-based test for screening can be used
- Wait as long as possible before harvesting, nitrates decrease with maturity of plant
- Wait at least 1 week prior to harvest following a rain immediately after draught
- Ensiling will decrease nitrates by 30 - 50% after 1 - 2 months
- Feed a grain supplement to increase the conversion of nitrates to protein
- Dilute with feed known to be low in nitrate
- Supplement diet with vitamins A, D, and E and iodized salt
- Animals should be well fed before their first access to suspected feed to decrease the initial amount consumed.

Water

- Nitrate additions to ground water can be reduced by limiting nitrogen application, in the form of fertilizer and animal waste that can be taken up by plants
- Minimize or avoid the contamination of water of ponds and lakes with excess nitrate contents and if contaminated avoid the usage of such water for animal husbandry activities

- Nitrate can be reduced in water with ion exchange and reverse osmosis although an economic assessment is often necessary to determine whether this is a practical alternative.

Salt Poisoning

Water Deprivation - Sodium Ion Toxicosis
("water-deprivation-sodium toxicosis-water toxicosis")

Sources

- Salt is an essential nutrient. It is also added to the ration to either increase or decrease palatability. Normally 0.5 - 1% of ration.

High salt intake increases water requirement which increases risk primary problem is usually water deprivation

- Mechanical failure of waterers
- Neglect, overcrowding
- Medicated water unpalatable
- Animals fail to find water (new surroundings).
- Frozen water
- Sodium sulfonamides
- Poultry wet mash made with whey or brine.
- Sodium in water is more hazardous than in feed (water intake exceeds feed intake and no compensatory advantage to drinking more).
- Salt used to control intake of protein block, mineral supplement, etc., esp. if animals unaccustomed.
- Dogs sometimes eat rock salt, usually causes vomiting
- Excessive use of salt as an emetic
- Gastroenteritis, diuresis combine to cause dehydration which increases hazard of excess sodium.
- Aggravated by unlimited access to fresh water following water deprivation or following episode of high sodium intake (water toxicosis)
- More likely in semiarid areas for several reasons:
- Water supplies are lesser, lower humidity and higher temperatures tend to greatly increase water losses from the animals. Water supplied from natural springs and deep wells and water contaminated with run-off may contain high levels of sodium chloride, calcium sulfate, and calcium carbonate.

- Sudden change from fresh water to salt water when animals are thirsty, and water accumulation in salt troughs during drought periods.
- Improperly mixed rations or attempts to limit protein supplement intake by "spiking" it with salt. Also, inadequate trough space increases the likelihood of gorging on concentrate, which may result in excessive sodium intake even with lower amounts of salt in the concentrate.
- Feeding urea can increase the likelihood of Na^+ toxicosis by elevating:
  1. Urinary output
  2. Anhydremia and
  3. Sodium concentrations in the brain
- Saline waters that may be safe for cattle in the winter can be deadly in summer months
- Total salt content of water is more important than any one salt. Total salts in water should not exceed 1.0% for cattle. Older references have suggested up to 1.5% total salts for nonlactating cattle
- Fluorine and magnesium salts have a much greater adverse effect on the alimentary mucosa than does sodium.

Susceptible Species

- Swine > Horses> Poultry> cattle> Dogs >sheep
- Lactating cows are less tolerant of excessive salts in the water or diet than are other cattle.

Toxicity

- Acute oral LD_{50} values
  - Horse, cattle, swine: 2.2 g/kg
  - Dog: 4 g/kg
  - Sheep: 6 g/kg
- Affected by salt concentration and availability of water.

Factors Affecting Toxicity

- *Salt hunger* : animal not provided with sufficient salt become salt hunger and takes excess salt
- *Availability of drinking water*: less availability of water immediately after the ingestion of salt enhances the salt poisoning

- *Species* : poultry most susceptible (taste sense is less and kidney efficiency is less) and swine since exposed to garbage feeding
- *Climatic conditions*: hot and humid conditions also active animals (precipitate salt toxicity).

Toxicodynamics

Assumptions

1) water deprivation

2) Climate hot & humid

- Sodium is rapidly absorbed from gut, distributed throughout body
- Normal animal
  - Plasma Na^+ 135 - 155 meq/1 (mean 143.3 ± 6.5)
  - CSF Na^+ 135 - 150 meq/1 (mean 139.6 ± 5.2)
  - Due to sodium stagnant in nerve cells increased action potential and hyperexcitability is observed in the effected animals
  - Inaddition to CSF Na and water also escapes into other body cavities resulting in increased nasal secretions,hydropericardium,hydrothorax ascites etc.
  - Water deprivation in the presence of normal sodium intake results in serious metabolic disturbances when cattle have lost 10% of their body water. Losses of 20 to 25% of body water are almost always fatal.

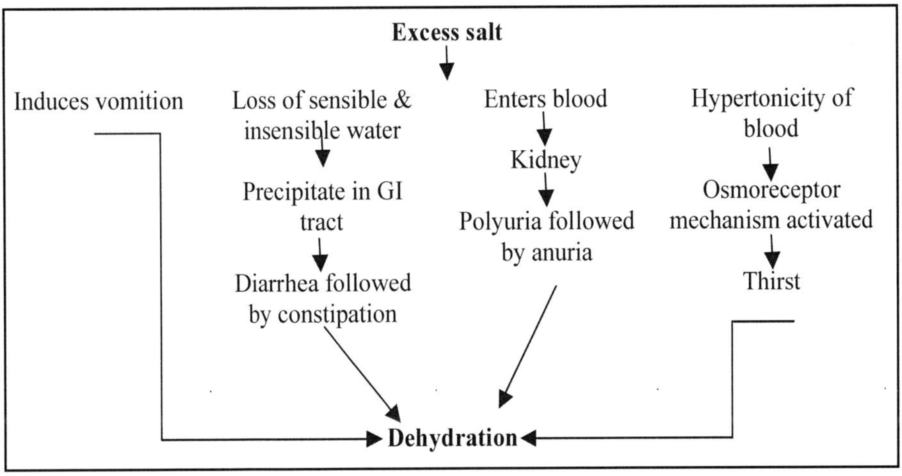

Excess salt in blood

↓

Hypertonicity

↓

Increased vascularity

↓

Initially due to absorption of water
from cells into lumen of blood vessels

↓

Shrinkage of capillary endothelial cells

↓

Sodium and other salts escape into CSF

↓

Na^+ passively diffuses into CSF, but requires active transport
to be removed from the CSF (energy required)

↓

With dehydration, high Na^+ in plasma diffuses into CSF

↓

high Na^+ depresses glycolysis, therefore energy for active transport deprived

↓

Na^+ accumulates in CSF

↓

Sodium trapped in CNS, attracts water due to osmotic gradient.

↓

Irreversible Cerebral edema

In swine esonophilic meningoencephalitis seen

↓

Decreased blood supply to brain

↓

Decreased oxygen supply to brain

↓

Hypoxia

↓

Serious nervous derangement

↓

Behavioural and nervous signs

↓

Ultimately death

Metabolic changes taking place in cattle deprived of water include:

- Loss of weight due to reduction in tissue water and due to actual breakdown of body substance in an effort to furnish water for physiologic needs. First, fat and carbohydrate are used for this purpose and later protein.
- Acid-base disturbances occur usually toward the acid side.
- Obviously hemoconcentration occurs with associated polycythemia, increased plasma protein, and increased chloride and sodium.
- Body temperature, pulse rate, and cardiac output all increase.
- Nonprotein nitrogen increases presumably as a result of increased osmolarity of the blood resulting in decreased glomerular filtrate production and perhaps due to the increased protein catabolism mentioned above.
- Drying out of mucous membranes, subcutaneous tissues and skin takes place.
- Terminally, uremia, exhaustion, and collapse takes place.

Clinical Signs

- Autonomic Signs
  - Vomition
  - Diarrhoea
  - Thirst
  - Colic
  - Increased salivation
  - Polyurea

- Nervous Signs
  - Blindness
  - Deafness
  - Muscle tremors
  - Muscle twichings
  - Convulsions elecitable ,intermittent and generalized
  - Nystagmus
  - Opisthotonus

- Jaw chaping
- Animal rigid when recumbent (at this stage fluid therapy is contraindicated as it may leads to cerebral edema).

- Motor signs
  - Walking backwards
  - Circling movements
  - Walking through fences
  - Jerkey movements of legs
  - Stilted gait
  - Incordination
  - Falling away.

- Behavioural Signs
  - Initially thrist due to stimulation of osmoreceptors later disinclination to take water
  - Initially hyperexcitability later lethargic weak and recumbent does not respond to stimuli
  - Stand with head down ,neck extended and arched back (pressing head against hard objects).

- Dependent signs
  - Secondary to above all clinical signs
  - Generalized seizures
  - Increased temperature due to excessive muscular activity
  - Muffled heart and lung sounds due to fluid accumulations
  - By chance animal recovers there would be permanent blindness or tempermental changes in animal
  - Death within minutes–days (depends on the amount of salt ingested).

Lesions

- Often no gross postmortem findings
- Congested mucosae of the small intestine, omasum, and gall bladder
- Edematous lungs with moderate congestion
- Edema on ruminal surfaces associated with hemorrhages

- Edema around the major bile ducts
- Enlarged liver
- The brain appears firm, white, and swollen
- Polioencephalomalacia
- Decreased clotting of the blood
- Histopathologic findings include
  - Dilation of mucosal and submucosal lymphatics in the duodenum
  - Small foci of necrosis in the liver and renal medulla
  - Leakage of eosinophilic material from glomeruli into Bowman's capsule.
- Swine
  - Cerebral edema, early necrosis, malacia
  - First 48 hours-eosinopenia, eosinophilic cuffs around vessels in cerebral cortex and adjacent meninges (eosinophilic meningoencephalitis)
  - After 3 - 4 days- eosinophils reappear in blood.
- Poultry
  - Edema of tissues
  - Urate nephritis if saline water.

Diagnosis

Based on

- Case history
- Clinical signs
- Postmortem lesions
- Laboratory examination
  - Serum and CSF Na^+ concentrations of over 160 meq/1. In water deprivation/ Na^+ ion toxicosis, CSF Na^+ usually exceeds serum Na^+, unlike the situation in the normal animal
  - Brain (cerebrum) Na^+ usually exceeds 1800 ppm; often 2000 - 3000 ppm
  - Urine chloride increases and specific gravity decreases
  - The PCV does not decrease much.

- *Note: If thorough rehydration has occurred and time has elapsed, the brain Na^+ may be normal. Also water deprivation and excessive serum and brain Na^+ concentrations may result from any other condition which prevents animals from drinking-includes other toxicoses, trauma, encephalitis, etc.*
- Samples to submitted for laboratory examination

Brain	100g
Serum	5ml
CSF	1ml
Feed	1-2kg

- Send half of brain to laboratory frozen (for analysis) and other half to the laboratory fixed in formalin
- Collect a complete set of tissues for toxicology and pathology in case the presumptive diagnosis is incorrect.

Differential Diagnoses

Toxicosis due to lead, organochlorine, organophosphorus or carbamate insecticides, carbon monoxide, cyanide, metaldehyde, nicotine, and certain poisonous plants; as well as encephalitis, trauma, polioencephalomalacia, heat stroke, gut edema.

Treatment

- Eliminate the source i.e.remove source of excess sodium
- Small amounts of water frequently (limit access), try to correct energy balance; i.e., hand feeding, symptomatic supportive care.
- Stomach wash in dogs
- Isotonic/hypotonic salt solution IP for 3 days chances of survival 50%
- In extremely valuable animals or small animals the temporary use of hyperosmotic dextrose or other substance fluids may be worthwhile.
- IV administration of dextrose and electrolytes was effective in saving some cattle after failure with water alone. Thus, hypertonic solutions (low in sodium) are recommended.

Fluoride Toxicosis (Fluorosis)

Fluorine is a reactive nonmetallic element present in varying amounts in soils, water, air, vegetation, and animal tissues. In nature, it is found in a combined (fluoride) form due to its high reactivity. Fluorine is available in the form of organic and inorganic forms.

Inorganic Forms

1. Sodium fluoride - acaricide in swine,wood impregnation,farm pests
2. Calcium fluoride
3. Ammonium fluoride - glass etching ,highly toxic to animals
4. Potassium fluorosilicate -byproduct released in the production of superphosphate releases silicon fluoride gas.

Organic Forms

1. Tri fluoromethane
2. Fluoroacetamide
3. Fluoroacetate
4. DDT

Sources

Acute Fluorosis

- Hydrogen fluoride
- Fluoride in the form of insecticide, sodium fluorosilicate (also called sodium silicofluoride)
- As a swine acaricide (sodium fluoride), also rarely encountered
- In vegetation or feeds containing extremely high levels of fluorine, also rare
- Other fluoride compounds with widely varying toxic properties are also recognized.
- Chronic Fluorosis
  - Forage (especially legumes) and plants grown in soil rich in fluorine. (Herbaceous part accumulates most whereas grains do not accumulate fluorine)
  - Natural sources like fluorspar (CaF_2), cryolite (Na_3AlF_6), rock phosphate ($CaHPO_4$)
  - Natural waters
  - Contaminated pastures due to fluoride fallout from aluminium, super phosphate, enamel, brick industries, thermal power plants and those manufacturing semiconductors and integrated circuits. The fluoride effluent from these industrial sources is carried in the wind and settles on vegetation or into water or feed sources. Herbivores are exposed as a result of ingestion of plants in the contaminated pasture or contaminated feed or water.

- The principal source of fluoride for cattle is drinking water. [39 mg/l]
- Chronic exposure from industrial effluents, fertilizers and mineral supplements is the most common cause of fluoride toxicosis
- The seeds or grains of crops do not accumulate fluorides, but the plant portion (stalk, stem, leaves) will accumulate fluoride. Airborne fluoride may just settle on vegetation as a significant source
- Use of rock phosphate in the diet of animals (rock often contaminated with naturally occurring fluoride) is another possible source
- Ground water and soil normally contain varying amounts of fluoride, and may contribute to a chronic buildup of fluoride in the body
- Volcanic ash may be a source of high fluoride contamination.

Factors Affecting Toxicity

Factors that determine an animal's reaction to fluoride ingestion include:

1. The amount of fluoride ingested: 14ppm –dental changes,100ppm – skeletal and joint effect
2. The duration and variation in amounts of fluoride intake,
3. The solubility of fluoride ingested,
4. The species: cattle 40-50ppm, poultry 200ppm
5. The age of the animal young : Bones & teeth old : Joints
6. The level of nutrition, Health, Emaciation, Malnutrition, parasitic and other disease – increases toxicity
7. Others stressors (simultaneous exposure to other toxic or potentially toxic substances)
8. Individual biological response.

Susceptible Species

Cattle are the most sensitive to skeletal fluorosis followed by >sheep> horses> pigs> rabbits> rats> guinea pigs>poultry.

Toxicokinetics

- NaF is rapidly absorbed from the digestive tract (75 - 90% is absorbed by 90 minutes)
- Fluoride is passively absorbed from the gut into the blood stream, where about half is excreted rapidly in the urine - the rest is stored in calcified

tissues (bones and teeth). Normal adult bones contain from 1000 - 1500 ppm fluoride

- Fluoride is cumulative and potentially toxic as long as constant or increasing amounts are ingested over time, otherwise urinary excretion will tend to maintain body fluoride below toxic levels.

Toxicodynamics

- Acute Fluorosis
  - Depends upon the individual fluoride compound.
  - fluoroacetate combines with oxaloacetate and forms fluorocitrate which inhibits the enzyme aconitase resulting in failure of cell respiration (CNS &CVS are most effected)
  - Fluoride (Fl^-) binds to cations disrupting ionic balance. Fl^- binds to Ca^{++}, Mn^{++}, and Mg^{++}. It also interferes with Na^+/K^+ ATPase.
  - Deaths are primarily due to hyperkalemia and associated conduction changes in the heart, as well to hypocalcemia.
  - Direct irritation to mucous membranes and skin especially from hydrogen fluoride.
  - Inhalation of fluorides causes pulmonary edema and bronchial pneumonia.
  - Interference with calcium metabolism intracellularly and lowering of plasma calcium due to formation of insoluble precipitates of fluoride and calcium.

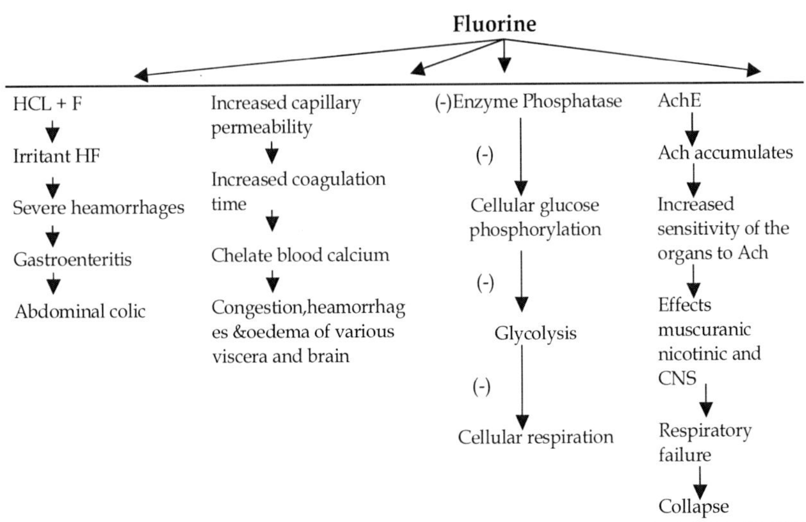

Clinical Signs

- Vomiting, diarrhea, evidence of abdominal pain
- Loss of sensation with tingling of the extremities
- Hypersalivation
- Sweating
- Convulsions
- Pulmonary congestion
- Ventricular tachycardia, with ECG abnormalities such as tall peaked T-waves, small or absent P-waves, wide QRS complexes, and prolonged PR intervals
- Death.

Dogs

- Inaddition to above frenzied running
- Barking and yelping in night
- Intermittent tonic clonic seizures not elicitable
- Opisthotonus
- Coma
- Gapsing
- Death within 2-12hrs.

Treatment

- Orally-administered calcium gluconate (IV), aluminum or calcium compounds (or milk) to bind fluoride before absorption.
- Gyceryl monoacetate 0.1mg/kg-0.5mg/kg IM hrly not to exceed 2-4mg/kg or 8.8ml/kg of 50% ethanol and 55%acetic acid
- Calcium citrate calcium released citrate binds with aconitase
- Symptomatic therapy anticonvulsants
- Quinidine has been used to prevent fluoride-induced hyperkalemia. It blocks K^+ efflux.
- Supportive therapy helps in first 4hrs includes emesis,gastric lavage, catharasis, adsorbants.
- Dialysis to remove fluoride and potassium.
- After onset of hyperkalemia, calcium gluconate may be given via the fluids, and dialysis used to remove fluoride and potassium.

- Chronic fluorosis
  Toxicodynamics
- Teeth

Fluorine
↓
Destroys Ameloblasts & Odentoblats
↓
Delayed mineralization of Pre enamel, Predentine & Pre cementine
↓
Malformation of enamel and dentine
↓
Wear & Tear of Molar & incisors
↓
Uneven erosion of Incisors table
↓
Lesions in mouth
↓
Anorexia

- Oxidation of organic material will stain the teeth brown surrounding the lesion
- Inhibits enzymes neccesary for teeth formation
- Inhibits enzymes necessary for bacterial growth hence used in tooth paste

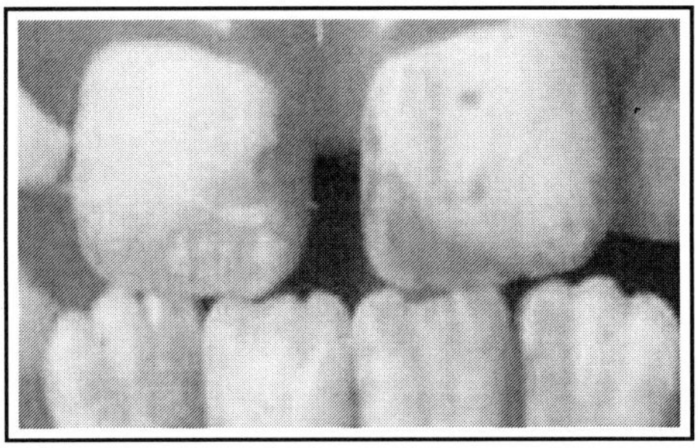

Picture showing the yellow stained tooth with Wear & Tear of Molar & incisors

- Bones

Fluorine
↓
Interferes with osteogenesis
↓
Delayed mineralization
↓
Exostosis
↓
Abnormal bone growth on sides especially medial side palpable
↓
Increased diameter of metacarpals and metatarsals
↓
Wrist & Ankle thickness

- Decreased production of phosphopyruvate
- Impairs glucose & Vit.metabolsim.

Clinical Signs

- Onset takes 2m-years
- Characteristic periodic intermittent shifting lameness
- Enlargement of sternum and lower jaw
- Bony exostosis on medial side form a bridge between two bones and flexor is lost - stiff gait
- Decreased intake to anorexia and teeth deformities
- Rough hair coat and emaciation
- Decreased milk yield.

Lesions

- Teeth uneven
- Bone normal ivory color becomes soft chalky
- Exostosis and protuberances
- Abnormal diameter of Metacarpal ,phalanges & Metatarsals
- Mottling and cavities on teeth unevenly broken teeth
- Gelatinous degeneration & deminished bonemarrow cavity
- Histopathological changes
- Thickened bony trabeculae
- Degenerative changes in kidney,liver,heart muscles and CNS
- Atrophy of spongiosa, irregular calcification of newly formed osseous tissue
- Hypoplasia of enamel and dentine.

Diagnosis

Based on

- Case history (analyze forage, water)
- Clinical signs
- Bone and tooth lesions.
- Considering the animals ages, and recognizing the different times of eruption of incisors, premature wear on different teeth, the bovine

practitioner can readily determine when the exposure occurred (e.g., before or after the animals were purchased Urine fluoride levels (time dependent)

- X - ray examination
- Laboratory examination: Normal concentration in bovine urine is 2-6 ppm. In fluorosis 15-200 ppm fluoride is seen
- Normal Bone F levels 400-1200ppm but in Fluorosis it is 3000ppm
- Samples to be submitted for laboratory examination.

Bone	20g	Ideal sample will be lesion seen in organal bone
Water	100ml	
Forage	100g	
Urine	50ml	

- Bone specimen analysis for fluoride
- Feed and water analysis for fluoride (time dependent).

Differential Diagnosis

- Vitamin D deficiency
- Ca deficiency
- P deficiency
- Parathyroid disease

Treatment

- No specific treatment
- Tolerance Increases by Ca, P, Vit.D & A
- Aluminum sulfate, aluminum chloride, calcium aluminate, calcium carbonate, defluoridated phosphate have been used successfully to reduce the toxic effects of chronically ingested fluoride.
- Salts of Al,Ca & Fe added in concentrates 30g/day
- Fluid therapy
- Symptomatic therapy artharlgia and myalgia use corticosteroids, antibiotics and analgesics
- Livestock with dental lesions and the inability to eat sufficient amounts to sustain high productivity often should be culled from the herd.

Phosphorus

- White or yellow forms of phosphorus are toxic and red phosphorus is non toxic
- The white or yellow types are waxy, whereas the red type is granular, insoluble and not absorbed.

Sources

Accidental ingestion or licking of

- Rodenticides containing phosphorus, bait is usually comprised of phosphorus mixed with grease which prevents the rapid oxidation of the phosphorus and facilitates its absorption
- Phosphorus containing fertilizers either in bags or after applying to fields
- Electrical pastes and in incendiary and smoke bombs
- Ingestion of poisoned rodents
- Dermal exposure may result in burns of serious consequence
- Accidental or malicious.

Toxicokinetics

Phosphorus is first absorbed from the gastrointestinal tract into the blood as phosphorus but is then oxidized to phosphate. Some of the phosphorus is eliminated by the lungs which may give the exhaled air an odour of phosphorus (garlic-like) and the exhaled air may glow in the dark. Similarly vomitus or gastrointestinal tract contents may also be luminous and have the same odour.

Toxicodynamics

- Exact mechanism of action unknown
- Irritation of the gastrointestinal mucosa
- Hepatic degeneration.

Clinical Signs

- Severe abdominal pain
- Profuse vomiting
- Hematemesis
- Apparent recovery of a few hours to 4 days followed by abdominal pain and vomiting recurs, accompanied by jaundice.

- Delirium
- Convulsions in some animals
- Coma and death
- Horses and poultry may exhibit a paralytic-like weakness without other definitive signs
- Oliguria and anuria may occur.

Clinical Pathology

Hypoglycemia, hematuria, and proteinuria.

Lesions

- Inflammation of the gastrointestinal tract, stomach, intestines
- Garlic like odour of the gastrointestinal tract contents
- Inflammatory changes of skin when dermal exposure has occurred
- Fatty degeneration of the liver, muscles and endothelium of blood vessels with secondary extravasation of blood into the subcutaneous tissues, skin and muscle
- Hematoma formation.

Diagnosis

Based on

- Case history of exposure,
- Clinical signs, odour and luminescense of the breath, vomitus, and stomach contents
- Lesions
- Laboratory examination of Phosphorus content in the vomitus or intestinal tract
- In animals surviving the first day, faeces may be preferred over stomach contents (seal in a jar and freeze before transport to the laboratory maintaining a frozen state).

Differential Diagnosis

- Organophosphate compounds
- Heavy metal poisonings like Ar, Pb, Hg causing gastroenteritis and diarrhoea.

Treatment

- Eliminate the source
- No specific antidote is available
- *Dermal exposure*: Brush all traces of dry phosphorus from the skin. The white or yellow phosphorus may then be removed from the skin by washing the skin with a copper sulfate solution. The skin is then repeatedly washed with large volumes of water. Oily substances are contraindicated due to the enhancement of absorption.
- Oral exposure: Careful gastric lavage is preferred to emesis due to the corrosive action of phosphorus.
- Activated charcoal and saline cathartics are highly recommended.
- For hepatic and renal failure, cystine and a high carbohydrate diet which is low in protein are recommended.
- High doses of B-vitamins and ascorbic acid reduce the severity of the liver failure.
- Fluid therapy is indicated to increase the urinary output.
- Hypoprothrombinemia and hemorrhage is treated with vitamin K_1 and, with whole blood or plasma tranfusion(s).

Urea (Ammonia) Poisoning

Urea, biuret and ammonium salts serve as sources of non-protein nitrogen (NPN) for ruminants and are used to furnish up to one-third of the nitrogen protein requirement of ruminant animals. Toxicosis results from the associated build-up of ammonia in the animal. The major NPN source in use today is urea, which is commonly incorporated into feed supplements for mixing or blending, range blocks, range cubes, and molasses-NPN combinations. Extensively used to supplement cattle feeds, although use has declined in recent years.When used as a source of non-protein nitrogen for ruminants, urea is incorporated in rations in amounts not to exceed 1% of the total ration. Biuret, when used as a source of non-protein nitrogen, should not exceed 3% of the total ration.

Sources

Accidental ingestion/ excessive ingestion of

- Improperly mixed raw chemicals or supplements containing high concentrations of urea, biuret, and diammonium phosphate in feeds
- Dry and liquid fertilizers containing ammonia, ammonium salts, or urea
- Ammonium salts used primarily as source of phosphorus,expectorants or in the treatment of urolithiasis

- Currently available non protein nitrogen (NPN) sources and their characteristics are shown in the following table:

Compound	N %	P %	Protein Equivalent %
Urea-pure	46.7	0	292
Urea-feed grade	45.0	0	281
Biuret-pure	40.8	0	255
Biuret-feed grade	37.0	0	320
Monoammonium Phosphate	12.0	27.0	75
Diammonium phosphate	21.0	23.0	131
Ammonium sulfate	21.0	0	131

- One part of urea is equivalent to 2.92 parts of protein and 1% protein is equivalent to 0.34% urea.

Species Susceptible

- All mammalian species are susceptible to urea(ammonia)poisoning.
- Horses, other monogastrics, and ruminants are all of similar susceptibility
- Ingestion of 1.5 grams/kg of ammonium salts are lethal to monogastric animals. 4 grams/kg of urea and 1.4 grams/kg of ammonium salts may cause death in horses. Whereas 0.5 - 1.5 g/kg of urea and ammonium salts cause death in cattle and sheep
- Because of hydrolysis of urea to ammonia by rumen microorganisms, ruminants are much more susceptible to urea than most monogastrics.
- Blood ammonia

  8-13ppm- toxic signs are seen

  20ppm - ataxia

  50ppm - sudden death

Factors Affecting Toxicity

- Failure to gradually adapt ruminants to diets containing NPN predispose the animal to urea toxicosis urea accustomed animals can with stand up to 1g/kg BW where as unaccustomed animals can withstand only up to 0.3-0.5g/ kg BW
- Ruminants susceptible i) feed on plants containing urease ex: raw soya bean ii) alkaline pH (favours hydrolysis of urea)
- Fasting
- Low energy diets
- Elevations of body temperature

- Dehydration
- Stress
- Disease
- Hepatic insufficiency
- Lack of natural protein sources.

Urea

pH of less than 6.2 ↓ amount of urease

Charged ammonium ion (NH^{4+})
highly water soluble and poorly absorbed

At pH 9.0 ↓

NH3/NH^{4+} equals one
and large amounts of ammonia are
available for absorption.

↓

Rumen microorganisms have the ability to form amino acids

↓

Rumen flora microorganisms are overwhelmed by excess ammonia

↓

Ammonia dissolves in rumen fluids

↓

Form ammonium ions and thereby increases the pH.

↓

Concentration of (uncharged) ammonia (NH3)
in rumen fluids and blood increases

↓

Liver

↓ Synthesis of glutamine

↓ Detoxification of Urea (Urea cycle)

↓

When there is saturation of the above two mechanisms

↓

Ammonia (NH_3)

↓ Enters blood → ↓ Crosses blood brain barrier → ↓ Metabolic derangement → ↓ Inhibits citric acid cycle → ↓ Decreases energy production → ↓ Failures of pumps → ↓ Ionic imbalances in the body

↓ Brain → ↓ Postsynaptic inhibition of GABA → ↓ Excitation → ↓ Convulsions (tonic elicitable) → ↓ Death

---

Toxicodynamics

- Ammonia inhibits the Kreb's cycle and there is a compensatory increase in anaerobic glycolysis with resultant lactic-acidemia
- High brain ammonia concentration interferes with cerebral energy metabolism and the sodium-potassium-ATPase pump
- Hyperkalemia has been associated with lethal effects on the heart
- Urea highly irritant to gastric mucosa hence classified as GI poison causes acute abdominal colic.

Clinical Signs

Signs appear when rumen ammonia and blood ammonia concentrations exceed 80 mg/100 ml and 2 mg/100 ml, respectively.

- Behavioural Signs
  - Excitation due to postsynaptic inhibition of inhibitory neurotransmitter GABA
  - Restlessness
  - Dullness
  - Struggling and bellowing in terminal stages
- Nervous Signs
  - Twitching
  - Tremors progress from head to tail (in OP -haphazard)
  - Muscle tremors
- Autonomic Signs
  - Frothy salivation
  - Hyperirritability
  - Grinding of teeth
- Dependent Signs
  - Abdominal pain
  - Increased defecation
  - Polyuria
  - Increased respiratory rate
  - General weakness
  - Bloat and regurgitation of rumen

- Recumbency
- Hyperthermia
- Anuria

- Locomotor Signs
  - Ataxia
  - Prostration
  - Inco-ordinated gait
  - Compulsive hypermotility (not major)
- Gastrointestinal Signs
  - Acute abdominal colic
  - Animals look at abdomen
  - Kicking at abdomen
  - No diarrhoea.

Lesions

- No characteristic lesions
- Odour of ammonia is often noted in rumen contents and tissues
- Pulmonary edema, hydrothorax and hydropericardium may be seen
- Petechial hemorrhages, and generalized congestion are common findings
- Animals bloat rapidly, and carcasses decompose more rapidly than normal.

Diagnosis

Based on

- Case history of acute illness following ingestion of urea or other NPN sources
- Clinical signs
- Postmortem examination
- Laboratory examination : blood ammonia values ranging from 1 - 4 mg/100 ml and rumen ammonia values greater than 80 mg/100 ml. Significant increase in the packed cell volume, blood ammonia, blood glucose, blood urea nitrogen, serum potassium and phosphorus, rumen pH, rumen ammonia and SGPT are noted during urea (ammonia) poisoning.
- Samples to be submitted for laboratory examination.

Whole Blood or serum	5ml	Frozen or add 1-2 drops of saturated mercuric chloride.
Urine	5ml	
Rumen contents	100 g	

Differential Diagnosis

- OP- more gastric discomfort and responds to atropine in urea toxicity salivation stops but other signs remain
- OC - maniacal behavior, clonic -tonic convulsions of flexors (elicitable)
- Heavy metal poisoning.

Treatment

- Eliminate the source
- To reduce the ruminal pH the best treatment for cattle consists of administration of a combination of 19-38 liters of cold water and a 3.8 liters of 5% acetic acid (or vinegar) by means of a stomach tube. Cold water reduces the temperature of the rumen and thus the rate of urease action where as acetic acid reduces the rumen pH and converts the readily absorbed ammonia present in ruminal fluids to the relative less absorbed ammonium ion.
- Intravenous fluids should be administered to insure adequate urine flow.
- When bloat occurs, it should be relieved immediately
- L- argentine and N-carbamyl -L- glutamate stimulates urea cycle
- Rumen lavage via a rumenotomy incision or trochar may be superior to cold water/acetic acid.
- Symptomatic treatment for convulsions.

Contraindications

- Glucose
- Calcium.

Acids and Alkali Poisoning

- Acids and alkalis are also sometimes referred to as caustics or corrosives
- The frequency of serious alkali ingestion is more common than serious acid ingestion.

- Acids include
  - Hydrochloric, sulfuric and (rarely) hydrofluoric acids. Muriatic acid is another name for hydrochloric acid. Naturally there are others, but they are less commonly encountered as toxicants by domestic animals.
- Alkalis include
  - Sodium hypochlorite (Clorox and similar bleach solutions) - One of the more common agents ingested.

Lye, i.e sodium or potassium hydroxide - most common causes of serious toxicoses.

Acid Poisoning in Animals

Sources

Accidental ingestion or exposure to

- Household cleaning products
- Toilet bowl and drain cleaners
- Dishwasher detergents
- Cleaners
- Antirust compounds
- Alkaline batteries

Location, frequency and severity of lesions depends upon:

- Chemical properties of the particular compound.
- Volume and concentration to which the animal is exposed.
- Contact time with the tissues.
- Presence of other ingesta in the gastrointestinal tract at the time of exposure.
- Tonicity of the pyloric sphincter.

Toxicodynamics

Acids produce corrosive burns, resulting in coagulation necrosis, which limits their penetration into deeper tissues. Visible lesions (necrotic scars) are seen on mucous membranes; laryngeal spasm and edema may occur. Alkalis produce liquefaction necrosis, allowing deep tissue penetration that continues until the alkali is neutralized by the tissues.

Clinical Signs

- Irritation of oral mucous membranes
- Salivation
- Oral ulcers or burns
- Oral lesions colored gray, yellow, or black (acids)
- Hematemesis
  - Panting, dyspnoea (especially upper airway although pulmonary edema has been reported)
  - Pain
- Vocalization
- Dysphagia
- Shock
- Perforation of the esophagus (stomach or intestines may perforate but are less likely to do so)
- Pneumothorax
- Peritonitis
- Pleuritis
- Sepsis
- Shock, collapse, and death.

Diagnosis

Based on

- Case history
- Clinical signs
- Postmortem lesions examinations of the oral, pharyngeal and esophageal mucosae are desirable. It is possible to have significant esophageal pathology in the absence of oral damage.
- Alkalis
  - Hyperthermic injury, documented following lye ingestion.
  - Saponification of fats

Toxicity

- Lye tends to penetrate deeply into tissues whereas sodium hypochlorite and acids do not.

- Severity of injury is proportional to the concentration and the volume of the toxic solution.
- Prolonged contact increases the probability of severe injury increasing the risk of perforation.
- A full stomach is less vulnerable to corrosive injury than is an empty one because of dilution of the caustic agent.
- Pylorospasm, which can be induced by the caustic agent, increases the risk of local gastric injury.
- Because dogs and cats lap up materials their exposure to caustics tends to be slower and less of a problem than in children who "drink" such materials in quantity.

Clinical Signs and Lesions

- Alkali
  - Lye commonly injures the oropharynx and esophagus and may injure the stomach as well.
  - Solid lye tends to lodge in the oropharynx or esophagus and tissue injury at the site of contact continues until perforation occurs unless the particles are removed by vomiting or passed into the stomach.
  - Liquid lye often presents a different and even more serious problem than solid lye. Liquid lye seems to cause almost immediate damage and often injures the stomach as well as the esophagus.
  - The most common immediate complication of lye ingestion is an esophageal burn which occasionally goes on to result in perforation. Gastric perforation is unusual but it occurs more often in patients ingesting liquid lye.
  - Respiratory distress occurs secondary to soft tissue swellings of the larynx, epiglottis, vocal cords or as a result of tracheal aspiration.
  - The principle delayed complications are esophageal stricture and pyloric obstruction.
  - Few instances of sodium hypochlorite induced esophageal stricture are on record and, in at least some of these, the history of exposure is of questionable certainty.

Diagnosis

- A history of exposure and appropriate clinical signs are sufficient for a tentative, clinical diagnosis.

- If possible use pH paper to assess the pH of the toxicant in its original container. Commonly, pH papers with a range of 1-12 are available as are high range papers with a range of 12-14. Both should be used if they are available (obtain ahead of time or check with a local hospital emergency department).
- As with other toxicoses, it is important to determine the particular agent ingested, its concentration, the quantity ingested, the duration since ingestion, whether vomiting has occurred since that time and whether a diluent was given thereafter.
- Examinations of the oral, pharyngeal and esophageal mucosae are desirable. It is possible to have significant esophageal pathology in the absence of oral damage, but this would be the exception, rather than the rule.

Treatment

- The use of emesis and lavage are generally regarded as contraindicated in acid or alkali ingestions, because of the possibility of re-exposure of the damaged tissues of the esophagus, because of the risk of rupturing an already weakened stomach, and because of the possibility of aspiration.
- Activated charcoal and saline cathartics are not indicated for ingestions of acids or alkalis because:
  - Activated charcoal is a poor adsorbent for acids or alkalis
  - Tissue injury occurs so fast that, by the time the animal reaches the facility and is administered the treatment, it would do no good and
  - Activated charcoal may limit the ability to characterize any damage endoscopically.
- Corticosteroids are suggested for caustic ingestions in which there has been circumferential mucosal damage in order to limit fibroplasia and thereby minimize stricture formation. In order to be of benefit, the corticosteroid should be given within 48 hours of exposure to the caustic agent. However, care must be taken in selecting patients for corticosteroids use. The xenobiotics are contraindicated in the presence of perforation because of masking of clinical signs and the possibility of reducing the success of surgical correction. Noncircumferential esophageal burns do not require steroid therapy. When used, the steroids are given for a period of several weeks.

- Although disputed by some authors, experimental evidence is in favor of the use of antibiotics when there is a history of perforation and prophylactically when steroids are given.
- Respiratory distress, although serious when it occurs, is very rarely encountered. If severe, endotracheal intubation should be used if the tube can be inserted without causing additional damage to the laryngeal area. If that cannot be avoided, tracheostomy may be required.
- Aspiration into the respiratory tract is also infrequent, but in view of the gastric contents and irritation which may be present, extreme care should be taken to avoid this effect.
- Monitoring blood gases and appropriate measures to alleviate respiratory or circulatory embarrassment leading to anoxia or shock may be of benefit in such patients. These may include artificial respiration, oxygen, and more often, fluids, bicarbonate, and corrective electrolyte solutions.
- An analgesic may be indicated to alleviate pain.
- Survey X-rays may be taken of the thorax and abdomen.
- The use of diluents, especially, milk and water, are often recommended for ingestion of acids or bases although some authors feel that such steps are at best of questionable benefit unless the patient is treated within minutes of exposure.
- Alkalis.
    - Diluents are used with 2 goals in mind:
        1) To remove solid alkali materials from the oropharyngeal and esophageal mucosae; and
        2) To dilute the caustic material and decrease the degree of tissue damage.
    - Acids, such as lemon juice, acetic acid or vinegar are contraindicated in alkali toxicoses, due to the resultant exothermic reaction and associated thermal injury to the mucosae.
    - For solid lye ingestions, the use of milk is preferred over water but if not immediately available water should be administered.
    - For liquid lye ingestions, the use of diluents is more controversial because of a study involving humans, in which such therapy was associated with subsequent vomiting. The author feared that the associated reexposure of the esophageal mucosa would be likely to increase the injury. In view of the relatively infrequent occurrence of esophageal perforation in poisoned dogs and cats, the use of a diluent

may have a more favorable risk/benefit ratio in these species than in humans. Investigation of the prevalence of vomiting and secondary complications in animals ingesting liquid lye with and without the addition of a diluent are needed to make a definitive recommendations.

- Acids
  - Diluents are not known to be of reliable benefit in acid ingestion and, again, there is concern as to the possible increased risk of vomiting. Nevertheless, some of the most commonly relied upon reference systems (e.g., *Poisindex*) for human toxicoses still recommend their use. The use of a diluent is therefore recommended for acid ingestions, especially if the ingestion has occurred minutes prior to presentation.
  - Antacids, especially bicarbonate, are potentially contraindicated due to the release of heat and in the case of bicarbonate, gas bubbles as well.

Chapter 5

PHYTOTOXICOLOGY

Introduction

Plants are the main source of nutrition to farm animals for their maintenance and production. But, under certain conditions, plants intoxicate farm animal life due to the presence of some deleterious substances called phytotoxins. Such plants include a variety of fodder plants (Jowar, wheat straw, Lucerne), grasses (Millet grass), ornamental or fencing plants (Crotons, Nerium sps) and weeds.

(Tribulis) in the farm premises.

Generally, farm animals avoid such plants and weeds due to their unpleasant taste and offensive odor but during fodder scarcity caused by drought, floods or overgrazing, animals consume these plants. In addition, animals introduced into new areas, stall fed animals also sometimes lose their sense of discrimination and ingest such plants containing phytotoxins.

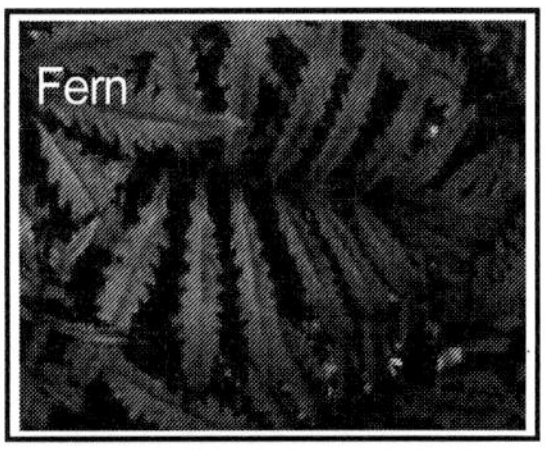

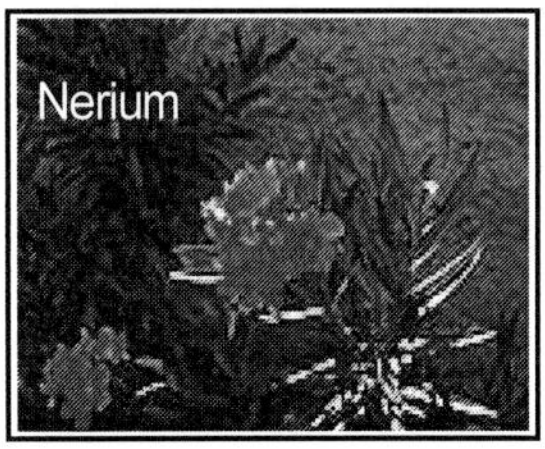

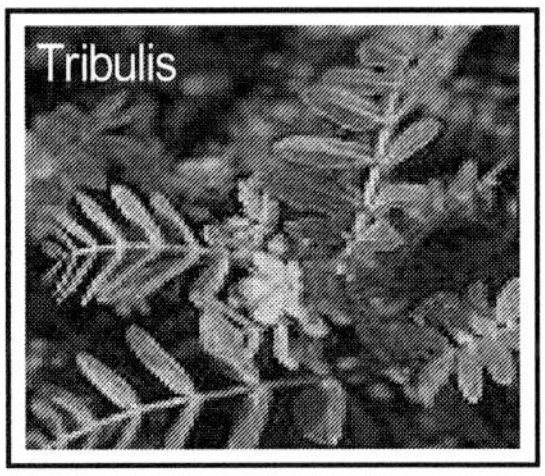

The phytotoxins may be organic or inorganic in nature. Organic phytotoxins are formed as by-products of plant metabolism. They could be alkaloids (strychnine) glycosides (lantadene A) essential oils (croton oil) and resins (podophyllin). Inorganic phytotoxins such as fluorides, nitrates and selenium compounds merely accumulate in the plant due to their translocation from the soil and water rich in these substances. The concentration of phytotoxins depends on the stage of growth, part of the plant, climate and soil composition. Age, sex and health also influence the phytotoxicity in animals.

Clinically, phytotoxicity may be acute or chronic depending on the dose of phytotoxin ingested. In acute cases, gastrointestinal and nervous signs predominate. Animals exhibit off-feed, colic, bloat, diarrhoea mixed with blood and mucous, salivation, convulsions, paralysis and if unattended coma and death may also occur. Chronic phytotoxicity, though not fatal, affects the economy of farmer by rapid fall in production and fertility of animals. In certain cases allergic dermatitis, photosensitisation, haemoglobinuria and agalactia are encountered.

Diagnosis can be made possible by obtaining information on feeding practices, survey of the grazing area and farm premises, symptoms, botanical and toxicological analysis of hay, forage, silage or suspected plant material.

The treatment consists of administration of adsorbents like charcoal, raw white of an egg orally. Antiserum (if the causative phytotoxin is specifically known) and symptomatic treatment such as administration of astringents, antispasmodics, anticonvulsants, fluid therapy etc.

Preventive measures include drying of plants, caution while stall-feeding and manual removal of poisonous plants and weeds from the farm premises.

Cyanide

Cyanide or prussic acid (HCN) toxicosis is a serious and often deadly problem which primarily results when animals are exposed to cyanogenic plants. High levels of exposure usually result in death.

Sources

Accidental ingestion or licking of

- Cyanogenic plants (Cyanogenic means having the ability to produce cyanide from cyanogenic glycosides)

  - Wild black cherry, chokecherry, plum and peach, all of which are *Prunus* spp; especially in seeds.
  - Amygdalin, a cyanogenic glycoside and a constituent of Laetrile, a purported anticancer drug.
  - Sudan, sorghum and Johnson grass, all of which are *Sorghum* spp.
  - Arrowgrass (*Triglochin*).
  - White clover (*Trifolium album*).
- Photographic solutions
- Some silver and metal polishes
- Industrial chemicals
  - HCN is used as fumigant rodenticide.

Species Susceptibility

- All species are affected: cattle, sheep, and horses most often involved.
- Ruminants are more susceptible than monogastrics to the effects of cyanogenic plants because of the rapidity of ruminal hydrolysis of cyanogenic glycosides which liberates HCN.

Production

- Normally cyanogenic glycosides are spatially separated from beta-glycosidase in the intact plant.
- When combined, a multi-step reaction produces HCN.

Factors Favoring Production

- High nitrogen/low phosphorus soils.
- Young plants.
  - Cyanide content decreases rapidly after pollination.
- Leaves and seeds contain more cyanide-releasing potential than stalks.
- Spraying with herbicide.
- Freezing.
- Plant injury or stunting.
- Mastication and digestion (especially in the rumen).

Toxicodynamics

Cyanide ion reacts with Fe^{+3} (ferric) ion of cytochrome oxidase to form a stable complex.

↓

Conversion of Fe^{+3} to Fe^{+2} is thereby prevented so that electron transport and cellular respiration are stopped. The blood is oxygenated, but cannot be utilized by the cells.

↓

The lack of O_2 utilization in chemoreceptors and/or neurons of the brain triggers increased respiratory efforts and the **blood** becomes **hyperoxygenated** ("**bright red**").

↓

End result is nevertheless a functional tissue anoxia

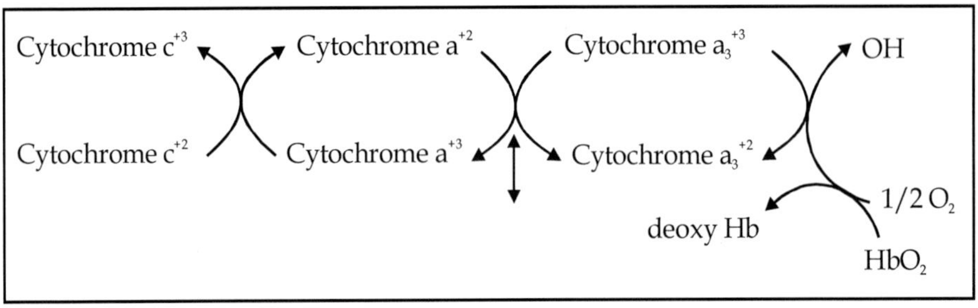

The site of action of cyanide

Clinical Signs

- Clinical course depends on
  - Concentration of cyanogenic glycosides in plant.
  - Time period of consumption (rate and duration of consumption).
  - Amount eaten.
  - Previous hydrolysis to free HCN.
- Large amounts may result in death in a few minutes.
- Smaller amounts may be lethal in 20 - 120 minutes. If animals live longer than 120 minutes, they usually recover.
- Initial Signs
  - Salivation and rapid breathing.

- Progress to
  - Marked dyspnoea, weakness, muscle fasciculations, urination, defecation, rapid heart rate, staggering, mydriasis.
- Terminally
  - Lateral recumbency, convulsions.
  - Death from respiratory paralysis.
  - The heart may beat for several minutes after respiration ceases.
  - With rapid onset of respiratory paralysis, one may occasionally see cyanotic mucous membranes.

Lesions

- Blood is cherry red and often clots slowly unless the necropsy is delayed.
- Tracheal and pulmonary congestion and/or hemorrhage.
- Ruminal distension; contents smell like "bitter almonds".
- Possible gastrointestinal vascular congestion.
- Large exposures may delay carcass decomposition.

Diagnosis

- History of consumption of cyanogenic plants or cyanide salts.
- Analysis of appropriate specimens for cyanide
- Forage, blood, rumen contents, liver, muscle.
- Should be placed in air-tight container immediately and preferably frozen. May quick-freeze using dry ice.
- Rather than freezing, an alternative is immersion in 1 - 3% mercuric chloride.
- Field test of forage or other suspected source materials with "picrate paper."
- In plants, 200 ppm is significant.
- Low concentrations of cyanide in tissues serve as evidence of intoxication.
- Analysis of blood for cyanohemoglobin.
- Differential diagnoses.
  - Nitrate toxicosis.
  - Nitrate poisoning is more common than cyanide toxicosis.

- Nitrate toxicosis causes chocolate-colored blood.
- High levels of nitrate may persist in hay; cyanide is usually low in hay.
- Clinical toxicosis seldom occurs after one feeding.
- Urea toxicosis.
- Urea (ammonia) toxicosis may cause rapid deaths and prominent nervous signs.
- In urea poisoning, there is an ammonia smell to the rumen contents.
- "Cherry red" blood is seen in toxicoses due to:
    - CN
    - CO

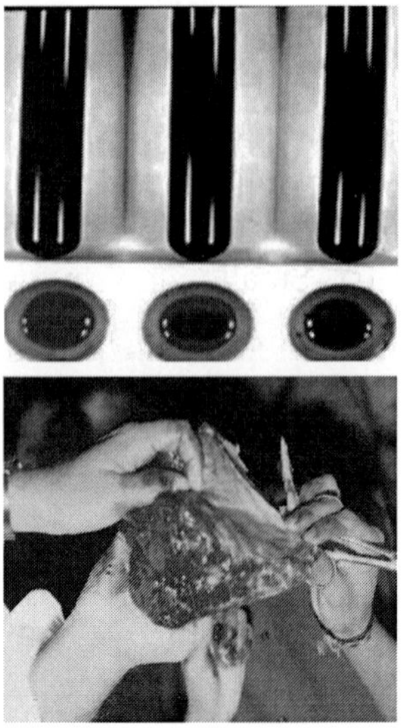

Diagnosis of Poisoning

Treatment

- Activated charcoal may be of significant value, particularly in orally exposed animals.
- Large animals.
    - One protocol for large animals recommends a mixture of 1 ml of 20% sodium nitrite and of 3 ml of 20% sodium thiosulfate at 4 ml/45 kg BW. Commercial solutions for treatment of prussic acid poisoning are available.
    - Sodium nitrite - large animal dose has also been listed as 10 - 20 mg/kg (as a 20% solution).
    - Intended to induce a measured methemoglobinemia such that the Fe^{+3} in methemoglobin will bind CN^- to reduce the amount available and bound at the Fe^{+3} of cytochrome oxidase. This results in the formation of cyanmethemoglobin.
    - Nitrite may also act as a vasodilator.
    - Sodium thiosulfate 30-40 mg/kg (as a 20% solution) is also recommended; and it has recently been suggested that 500 mg/kg is the preferred dose.
    - The enzyme rhodanese causes the sulfur in thiosulfate to react with cyanmethemoglobin to create hydrogen thiocyanate which is excreted in the urine. Thus removing cyanide from the body.

- Thiosulfate may also be given orally to help detoxify cyanide in the rumen contents.
- Although methylene blue IV (not for cats) has been suggested by itself at 4 - 6 grams per 454 kg BW, because of slower detoxification of cyanide, this treatment is not recommended.

❒ Small animals.

- Administer 1.65 ml of a 25% solution of sodium thiosulfate/kg BW and 16 mg of sodium nitrite/kg BW. Repeat dose in 30 minutes if there is no clinical response.

Prevention

❒ Prevent exposure.

❒ Proper forage management.

❒ Don't graze suspect pastures until plants are 2 feet high.

❒ If cyanide concentrations in hay or silage were high at cutting, it is sometimes wise to retest before feeding.If given enough time, cyanide tends to dissipate.

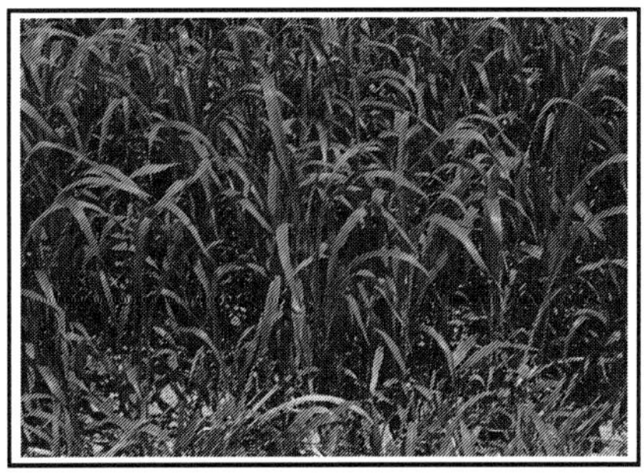

Picture showing the immature *Sorghum vulgare* crop rich in HCN concentrations

Abrus Precatorius

Family - Leguminosae

Abrus precatorius

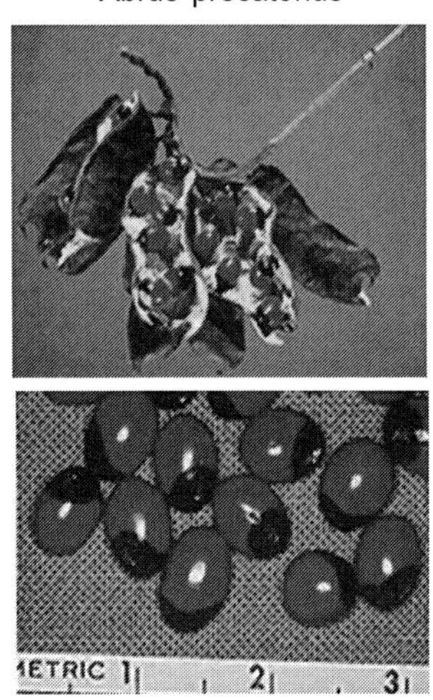

Picture showing the seeds of *Abrus precatorius*

Description

❒ Plant - Perennial vine, climbing on other plants, 10 - 20 feet tall.

❒ Stem - Woody, green when young, slender.

❒ Leaves - Alternate, opposite, pinnately divided, compound. Leaflets are small, oblong, in 8 - 15 pairs and 1/2 inch long.

❒ Flowers - Numerous inflorescences in leaf axils along stem. Racemes, 1 - 3 inch long. Flowers are many, small, red to purple or occasionally white.

❒ Fruit - Legume pod, 1.5 inches long, covered with fine hairs, contains many seeds, hard ovoid, 3/8 inches long. Seeds are bright, glossy, scarlet with jet black mark which covers 1/3 of the seed including the scar of attachment and the seeds are 0.2 - 0.3 inches long. The pod is somewhat septate between the seeds.

Habitat

Tropical locations such as central and western parts of India.

Toxicity

- Seeds are most toxic, seed coat retains the toxin, toxicosis results from broken /chewed seeds.
- Humans and horses are more susceptible followed by goats, cattle, and dogs.

Toxic Principle

1. Abrin -The heat labile phytotoxin (a lectin, also termed a toxalbumin)
2. Abrine (n-methyl tryptophan) - amino acid
3. Heamaglutinin
4. Abralin (baric acid) - glycoside
5. Lipoplytic enzyme.

Toxicodynamics

Abrin

- is a potent cytotoxin
- has a inhibitory effect on protein synthesis by acting on ribosomes
- binds to surface glycoproteins of erythorcytes and cause agglutination (clumping) of RBC's
- is selectively transported through the neurons hence it is called as suicidal transport/poisoning.

Clinical Signs

- General Signs
  - Oral and esophageal irritation, similar to caustic burns, seen by 2 hours.
  - Severe gastrointestinal irritation.
  - Nausea and vomiting, also dehydration.

- Trembling, tachycardia.
- Coma, hemolytic anemia, oliguria and sometimes uremia.
- Incoordination to paralysis.
- Circulatory collapse and death.

- Horses
  - Loss of appetite.
  - Violent purgation.
  - Elevation followed by depression in temperature.
  - In coordination and sometimes paralysis.

- Toxicosis may be seen to occur in 2 general stages
  - Initial stage (2-24 hours after dosing), characterized by oral, esophageal and gastric irritation.
  - Late stage (1-10 days), in which the following may occur:

    i. Ocular hemorrhage (retinal and/or scleral).

    ii. Increased capillary permeability.

Lesions

- Inflammation and ulceration of the GI tract.
- Visceral hemorrhage and thrombi formation.
- Multifocal necrosis in parenchymatous organs.
- Splenomegaly and multifocal necrosis in germinal centers of lymphatic organs.
- Hemolytic anemia and generalized petechial hemorrhage throughout the body.
- Hemagglutination.

Diagnosis

Based on

- Identification of seeds of *Abrus precatorius*,
- Circumstantial evidence of consumption
- Appropriate clinical signs
- Post mortem lesions.

Treatment

- No specific antidotes are available
- Induce emesis unless contraindicated by the condition of the animal.
- Maintain (or establish) respiration.
- Endotracheal intubation preceding gastric lavage.
- Activated charcoal with a saline cathartic, e.g., magnesium sulfate.
- Maintain fluid and electrolyte balance.
- Oral antacids to alleviate local irritation.
- Ascorbic acid increases survival rates.

Note - Drilled seeds as in necklaces are very toxic.

Prevention

Immunization via increasing doses is practiced in India.

Strychnos Nuxvomica

Family : Loganiaceae

Sources

- Strychnine is a bitter tasting indole alkaloid extracted from the seeds of an Indian tree, *Strychnos-nux vomica.*
- Used in "*Nux Vomica*" medications and homeopathic preparations.
- Used in pesticides to control gophers, moles (subsoil use) and rats.
- Accidental poisoning due to
  - Consumption of seeds
  - Consumption of baits containing strychnine kept for foxes, rats, mice etc.
  - Ingestion of birds or rats died due to strychnine poisoning
- Malicious poisoning.

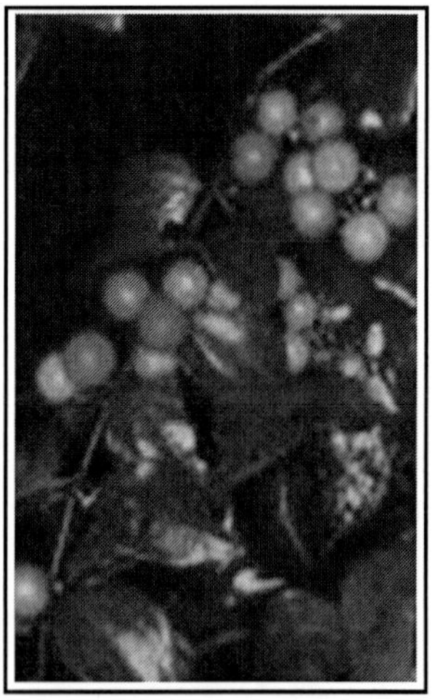

Picture showing the leaves and fruits of *Strychnus nuxvomca*

Toxicity

All species are sensitive; dogs more prone.

- Approximate lethal doses
  - Bovine 0.5 mg/kg
  - Equine 0.5 - 1.0 mg/kg
  - Porcine 0.5 - 1.0 mg/kg.
  - Canine 0.75 mg/kg.
  - Feline 2.0 mg/kg.
  - Rat 3.0 mg/kg.
  - Fowl 5.0 mg/kg.
  - Mallard ducklings 2 mg/kg.
  - Srtychinine undergoes Steep dose-response curve so that any animal displaying clinical signs must be carefully attended and protected for 24 hrs than the prognosis of the animals will be very good.

Toxicokinetics

- Ionized in acid medium (pk1 = 6.0, pk2 = 11.7) and therefore absorbed in small intestine
- Metabolism occurs in liver; metabolites excreted in urine.
- Highest tissue concentrations occur in blood, liver, kidney and stomach contents at death.

Toxicodynamics

Strychnine acts on recurrent inhibitory neurotransmitters(renshaw cells) of the reflex arc in the spinal chord

↓

Acts by competitively and reversibly antagonizing the inhibitory neurotransmitter glycine at postsynaptic neuronal sites

↓

Uncontrolled reflex stimulation, with predominance of more powerful extensors which results in rigidity

Clinical Signs

- Onset: 10 to 120 minutes after ingestion.
- No vomition.

- Anxiety, stiffness.
- Violent tetanic seizures spontaneous or initiated by numerous stimuli, which is a diagnostic feature
- Saw-horse stance/posture of the body
- Opisthotonus and persistent rigid extension of all four limbs
- No paddling, running movements, masticatory activity, or salivation
- Facial musculature contraction causes strained expression
- Rigidity inhibits respiration, apnea results
- Periods of relaxation gradually become fewer and shorter
- Death from anoxia and exhaustion
- Myoglobinuria is evident sometimes.

Lesions

- Rapid rigor, rapid relaxation
- Cyanosis, possible traumatic evidence of seizures
- Dark coloured venous blood
- Engorged lungs and cerebral meninges.

Diagnosis

Based on

- Case history
- Clinical signs
- Postmortem lesions
- Laboratory analysis
    - Baits
    - Frozen stomach contents obtained by lavage
    - Frozen liver
    - Frozen urine. Urine is the primary route of elimination but some animals may die too fast to detect strychnine in the urine.

Differential Diagnosis

- Organo phosphorus insecticides
- Organo chlorine insecticides
- Carbamate poisoning

- Carbon monoxide poisoning
- Metaldehyde poisoning
- Tetanus.

Treatment

- No specific antidote is available
- Detoxification - can shorten course - lessen severity
  - Emetics are generally contraindicated due to the risk of initiation of a seizure and aspiration
- Enterogastric lavage
- Stomach wash with
  - 2% aqueous tannic acid or dilute hydrochloric acid
  - 1:1000 potassium permanganate solution
  - 1:250 dilution of tincture iodine followed by final wash with plain water
- Activated charcoal and a saline or osmotic cathartic
- Fluids, forced diuresis with 5% mannitol in 0.9% normal saline at 7 mg/kg/hour
- Ammonium chloride (100 mg/kg, BID, po) to acidify urine thereby increasing protonation of strychnine to reduce its reabsorption across the renal tubular membrane.

  Note : Ammonium chloride is contraindicated if the animal is acidotic from exertion or from respiratory failure
- Pentobarbital sodium @ 30mg/kg I/V in case of small animals where as 7% chrolahydrate solution in case of large animals
- Glyceryl guaiacolate @ 110mg/kg or Methocarbamol @ 150 mg/kg, IV, initially followed by 90mg/kg may be used as muscle relaxants.

  Note : unnecessary when using pentobarbital
- Artificial respiration if hypoxic
  - Evaluation of glycine and other amino acids is required before they can be recommended
- Cardiovascular effects, if they occur, can be abolished by combinations of alpha- and beta-adrenergic blocking agents and can be reduced significantly by diazepam
- Care must be to maintain animals in undisturbed warm and quiet environment without any manipulation to prevent elicitable muscle contractions.

Contraindicated

- Ketamine - due to motor stimulatory effects
- Morphine - due to respiratory depression, possible stimulation of spinal cord
- Gastric lavage with sodium bicarbonate as it enhances strychnine absorption.

Ricinus Communis

(Castor Bean, Castor-Oil-Plant)
Family - Euphorbiaceae (spurge family)
Description

- *R. communis*
  - Plant - Large, glabrous, annual, shrub-like herb, 3-10 feet tall.
  - Stem - Stout, thick, reddish, green, or purple.
  - Leaves - Alternate, simple, large, palmately veined and lobed, peltate, 4 - 32 inches in diameter. Petiole is stout.
  - Flowers - Imperfect, unisexual, in clusters, no petals; calyx is 3-5 parted; no corolla, stamens are numerous and ovary is 3 celled.
  - Fruit - Capsule - 3 seeded, spiny. Seeds - 1 cm long, smooth and glossy, black or mottled with grey or brown.

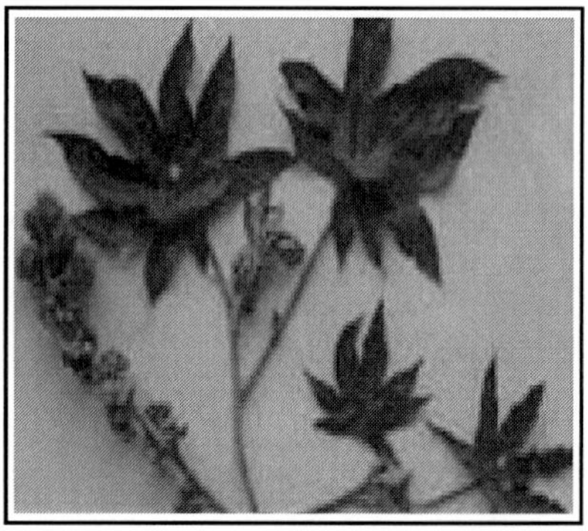

Picture showing the seeds and flowers of Ricinus communis

Habitats

- Commercially grown in India in all states.
- Occurs in roadsides, dumping grounds, barnyards of warmer areas of India but confined to planted sites in cooler areas.
- Used as ornamental outside in summer and less often as a houseplant.
- Toxicosis not only associated with plant, but most often with seed and seed products.

Toxic Principle

- Ricin is the principal toxin, and is a phytotoxin (a lectin, also termed a toxalbumin). Toxalbumins are very toxic proteinaceous compounds of plant origin
- Ricin is 100 times less toxic orally than parenterally
- Orally, ricin is readily absorbed from the stomach and intestine
- Ricin is water soluble and not present in castor oil
- Being a protein, and a fairly large molecule, ricin is heat labile. In castor bean cake, meal, etc. the ricin is generally inactivated by heating. Aging also reduces toxicity
- Ricin may comprise up to 3% of the seed weight
- Another phytotoxin in castor bean, ricinine, is reportedly goitrogenic.

Toxicity

- All parts of the plants are toxic, but especially the seeds.
- Seeds, presscake or meal (if inadequately processed) and foliage are poisonous.
- Castor oil is not poisonous.
- "Presscakes" from castor beans alone or mixed with linseed cakes have caused the most problems in cattle.
- Ricin is also excreted in the milk, which will cause severe purgation in the exposed animals.
- anaphylactic reactions may occur in all species.
- Hens: Are fairly resistant to ricin.
- Poultry general: Beans at 1.4% of BW may cause toxicosis.
- LD_{50} values are

Species	Oral LD_{50}(g/kg BW)	
	Seeds	Oil cakes
Horse	0.10	3.0
Cattle	2.00	3.00
Calf	0.50	-
Sheep	1.25	2.5
Goats	5.50	-
Pigs	1.30	5.0
piglets	2.40	-
Hen	14.00	40.0

Toxicodynamics

- Binds to galacto-lipid and galacto-protein components of plasma membranes which leads to toxin internalization and cell death.
- Toxin internalization relies on binding of mannose components in the ricin molecule (mannose receptor on the cell membrane).
- Protein synthesis inhibition by the A-subunit of ricin by enzymatic de-adenylation of ribosomal RNA, and thus inactivation of 60S ribosomes.
- Ricin exerts primary action via a ribonuclease activity.

Clinical Signs

- Cattle and sheep
  - Usually onset is between 12 hours and 48 hours
  - Nausea, gastrointestinal irritation, abdominal pain, diarrhea which is often bloody, tenesmus, dehydration
  - Anorexia, cessation of rumination
  - Excessive thirst
  - Weakness, muscle twitching
  - Dullness of vision, convulsions, dyspnoea, opisthotonus, coma and death
  - Sometimes clonic convulsions and decreased tendon reflexes are observed
  - After convulsions, death may result from paralysis of the respiratory center
  - Clotting time may be prolonged, possible hypoprothrombinemia
  - Cyanosis.
- Horses
  - Trembling, sweating, dyspnoea, incoordination
  - Vigorous heart contractions
  - Shivering, cold extremities
  - Depression, increased body temperature
  - Weak pulse
  - Constipation or diarrhea, convulsions.

- Poultry
  - Depression
  - Roughened feathers, droopy wings
  - Greyish wattles and combs
  - Egg production ceases
  - Emaciation
  - Death.

Lesions

- Generalized congestion
- Catarrhal to hemorrhagic gastroenteritis
- There may be petechial serosal hemorrhages on the viscera in body cavities and in the subepicardium
- Liver and kidney- swelling
- Fatty and hydropic degenerative changes in liver
- Birds- yellow discoloration (fatty liver) and hemorrhage
- Mesenteric lymph nodes are usually oedematous
- Pulmonary oedema.

Diagnosis

Based on

- Case history
- Circumstantial evidence by identification of *Ricinus* or products and evidence of consumption
- Clinical signs
- Postmortem lesions
- Laboratory analysis

Treatment

- Early - Use an emetic in appropriate species followed by activated charcoal and a saline cathartic unless contraindicated; e.g., due to marked diarrhea
- A gastrointestinal tract protectant such as kaolin-pectin and fluid therapy are used as indicated. Appropriate fluid and electrolyte therapy can greatly increase chances of survival.

- Ricin is not dialyzable.
- Judicious use of anticonvulsants if indicated.
- Monitor renal and hepatic function and electrolyte - Fluid balance.
- Maintain (or establish) respiration, fluid, and electrolyte balance.
- Oral antacids to alleviate local irritation. Ascorbic acid increases survival rates.
- Forced alkaline diuresis has been suggested to prevent nephrosis.

Prevention

- Do not plant castor bean plants where animals may have any access
- Clip heads before they mature when used as an ornamental
- Allow castor-oil-cake to stand or heat treat before feeding.

Nicotiana Spp.
(Tobacco)
Family - Solanaceae

N. tabacum - tobacco, burley tobacco

N. attenuata - coyote tobacco, wild tobacco

N. trigonella - desert tobacco

N. glauca - tree tobacco.

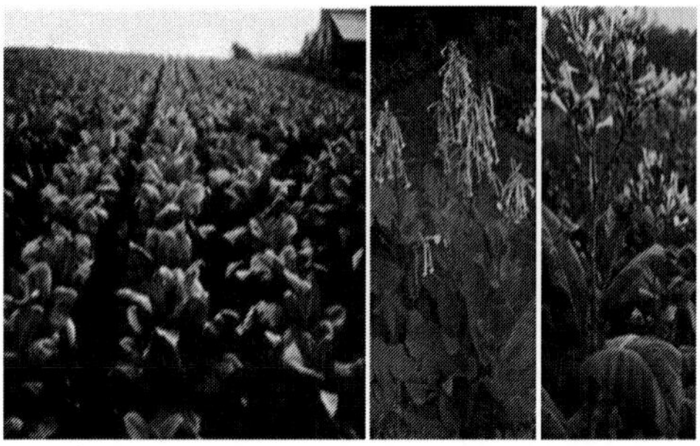

Picture showing the leaves and flowers of *Nicotiana tobaccum*

Description

- Acrid herbs, annual or perennial, shrub or small tree, 1-4 feet tall
- Sticky haired stem, with alternate leaves
- Lower leaves are oblong to egg-shaped but upper leaves are more lanceolate with sharp or blunt tips. Leaves are simple and opposite, usually have smooth edges, broad, hairy, and sticky
- Flowers are terminal or branched, 5-lobed, tubular and about 2 in. long, greenish-white, yellowish or lavender
- Fruit is a 2 celled capsule with many seeds.

Toxic Principle

1. Alkaloids nicotine

2. Teratogenic agents anabasine, anatabine, and anabaseine.
3. Carcinogenic polycyclic aromatic hydrocarbons such as benzo(a)pyrene are produced during combustion.

Toxicokinetics

Nicotine in pesticides is rapidly absorbed from gastrointestinal tract and skin. Nicotine and other alkaloids, when present in tobacco, may be absorbed more slowly.

Toxicity

- Tobacco plants are unpalatable and animals generally avoid consumption
- The entire plant is poisonous, foliage contains a high content of nicotine; tops are most toxic
- Because tobacco stalks are high in nitrogen, they are often returned to the soil to increase fertility and may poison foraging animals
- Small animals ingest tobacco, which causes centrally mediated vomiting, therefore, tobacco poisoning is infrequently fatal
- Fatalities are common in cattle. The minimum lethal dose of *N. trigonophylla* is approximately 2% of body weight on a green-weight basis
- LD_{50} in sheep 2.3 - 3.4 mg/kg of anabasine.The minimum toxic dose is 1.5% of the body weight and the lethal dose is 3.25% of BW.

Susceptible Species

- Cattle, swine, sheep, horses, and birds following ingestion of tobacco plants
- Small animals (dogs, cats) following ingestion of tobacco containing products.

Toxicodynamics

- Initially stimulate ganglia of sympathetic and parasympathetic nervous systems by direct action on ganglion cholinergic receptors
- Followed by ganglionic blockade due to persistent depolarization
- Initially CNS stimulation (tremors, convulsion) followed by depression
- Death due to respriatory failure from neuromuscular blockade.

Clinical Signs

Gastrointestinal Signs

- Vomition, salivation, abdominal cramps, bloat, frequent urination, colic, diarrhoea.

Musculoskeletal Signs

- Muscular weakness, staggering, tendency to fall on forelimbs, lameness, trembling, shivering, spasms, muscle tremors, blindness, dullness, stupor.

General Signs

- Irregular, weak pulse, or violent palpitation of the heart.
- Prostration, opisthotonus, diaphragmatic spasms.
- Elevated body temperature, but extremities cold.
- Dyspnoea, respiratory paralysis and death.

In swine, the primary problem is teratogenesis. Pregnant sows eating tobacco stalks may give birth to pigs with arthrogryposis. Arthrogryposis is aflexion, anterior or posterior of limbs with medial deviation of limbs. Sows may not show signs of toxicosis before giving birth to malformed pigs. Sometimes over 50% the pigs on a farm are born abnormal. Unable to nurse normally, piglets may die from hypoglycemia.

- No effect on fertility of sows
- No increase in abortions.

Lesions

- There may be ingesta in the trachea or lungs from aspiration.
- In ruminants, the abomasum may be congested, and there may be engorgement of subcutaneous blood vessels. Obviously, these lesions are non-specific.
- Arthrogryposis: Affects primarily the appendicular skeleton, but the spinal column and mandible have been affected. There may be clubbing of one or more feet and acute kyphosis (humpback) and brachygnathia. Affected bones become thickened, curved, twisted, or shortened, and there may be malallignment of joints.

Diagnosis

Based on

- Case history

- Circumstantial evidence by identification of nicotine or products and evidence of consumption
- Clinical signs
- Postmortem lesions
- Laboratory analysis.

Treatment

- No specific antidote
- Emetics if no contraindications exist
- Lavage followed by administration of activated charcoal and saline cathartic
- Artificial respiration and oxygen therapy if required.

Lathyrus spp.

(Sweet pea-poor mans dal)

Source

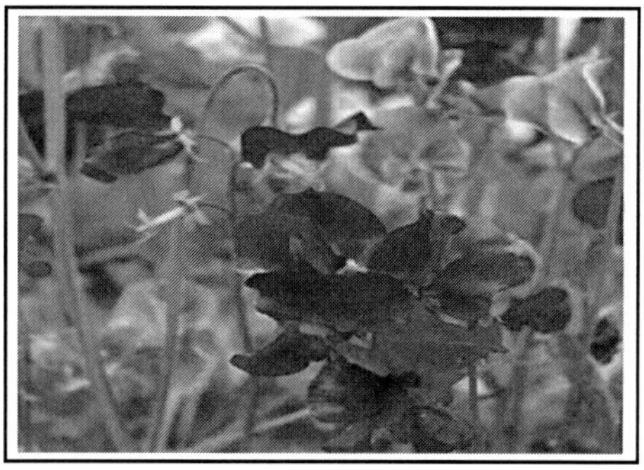

Picture showing the flowers and stems of *Lathrus odoratus*

- These outbreaks, which are now generally of historical interest, arose primarily from conditions of poverty and drought in which people were forced to subsist on a diet composed largely of *Lathyrus* sp. seeds. Large quantities of these seeds in the diet can produce a paralytic syndrome in man and livestock.
- Toxic species of *Lathyrus* are: L.*sativus*, L.*cicera*, L.*odoratus*, L.*pusillius*

Susceptible Species

- Different species of livestock vary considerably in susceptibility. The horse is particularly sensitive to the toxic principle and is most often poisoned.
- Osteo lathyrism - Cattle and other ruminants
- Neurolathyrism - Horses and monkeys.

Toxic Principle

- Osteolathyrism : caused by L.*odoratus*,L.*pusillius* toxic principle is beta-(gamma-L-glutamyl)-aminopropionitrile (BAPN). It is localized primarily in the pea or seed of the plant. Once ingested this compound may be converted *in vivo* to beta-aminoproprionitrile, which appears to be the substance responsible for the toxic effects
- Neurolathyrism : caused by L.*sativus*, L.*cicera* toxic priniciple is β-N-oxalyl-L-a-g-diaminoproprionic acid (ODAP)
- Neurotoxin is heat labile and can be destroyed by cooking.

Toxico Dynamics

Osteolathyrism
↓
BAPN
↓
Inhibits lysyl oxidase
↓
No formation of cross linkages in bones
↓
Bony structure effected
↓
Fractures
↓
Severe skeletal abnormalities
↓
Aortal aneurism (blood vessels effected)

Nuero lathyrism
↓
ODAP
↓
inhibits uptake of glutamate into synaptic vesicles
↓
demyelination of nerves (skeletal muscles are demyelinated)
↓
paralysis of nerves
↓
rapid fall of transmission of impulse
↓
wasting of muscle (muscle atrophy especially of hindlimb, rectum, bladder)
↓
In advance stage effects vagus nerve innervating larynx and pharyngeal muscles
↓
dyspnoea (intercoastal and diaphragm effected)
↓
death

- During pregnancy, the developing feotus is especially sensitive to the poison.

Clinical Signs

Osteolathyrism Predominately Affects Livestock

- Lameness in cattle may appear between the 3rd and 5th day of consumption when seeds are present at the time of poisoning. Lameness may rarely be severe.

Neuro Lathyrism Predominately Effects Horses

- Weight shifted to front legs
- Hind legs held forward and a hopping gait
- Seem normal when in a recumbent position
- When get up, pain is associated with locomotion and may appear as if "tied up" due to stiffness in hindquarters
- Sometimes the head is held low
- Paralysis of recurrent laryngeal nerve leading to dyspnoea and roaring and respiratory problems.

Lesions

- No specific pm lesions in osteo lathyrism
- Neuronal degeneration in the spinal cord and nerves to the hind legs is observed in neurolathyrism.

Diagnosis

Based on

- Case history
- Circumstantial evidence by identification of Lathyrus seeds or products and evidence of consumption
- Clinical signs
- Postmortem lesions
- Laboratory analysis.

Treatment

- No specific antidote is available

- If large quantities of the seed have been ingested, induce emesis and perform gastric lavage
- Administer activated charcoal and a saline cathartic
- Symptomatic
- Supportive.

Cotton (*Gossypium* spp.)
(Cottonseed, and Gossypol)

Family : Malvaceae

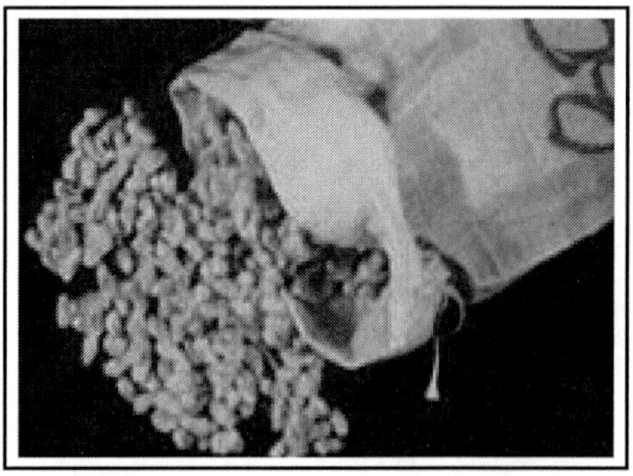

Picture showing the cotton seeds

Cottonseed, cottonseed meal, and cottonseed cake are high protein materials used in animal feeds. Cottonseed contains about 20% protein and 20% oil where as the meal made from it contains about 40% protein and 7% oil. Cotton seeds contain a highly toxic polyphenolic binaphthalene pigment called gossypol in the glands of the seeds which appear as tiny black spots which are retained in the seed after decortication (hull removal). The pigment glands contain approximately 50% gossypol, which accounts for 2 - 5% of the weight of the seed and is comprised of 3 isomeric forms. Gossypol is also associated with 2 other pigments, gossypurpurin and gossyverdurin; the latter being more toxic than gossypol. The gossypol content of cottonseed varies considerably with the strain of cottonseed, the location in which it is grown, the particular climatic conditions that year, and on the extraction procedure. The cellulose walls of the pigment glands are quite tough and although gossypol is soluble in a number of solvents and reactive with a variety of compounds, it is not extractable nor does it react in most milling or rolling processes unless the glands are first ruptured by the addition of water which ruptures the seams of the seeds. With the traditional cottonseed-oil extraction, the seed is heated to relatively high temperatures for comparatively long periods of time before mechanical pressing to expel the oil. During this cooking, the majority of the pigment glands are ruptured and their contents released into the meal. Free (toxic) gossypol is inactivated (bound) to form a nontoxic molecule in time by reactions which occur in the meal spontaneously or during the milling process. The amount of free gossypol present in the meal is dependent upon the degree to which the glands have ruptured and the degree of subsequent inactivation of the gossypol. Delinted cottonseed, sometimes referred to as "delinted cotton" or "whole cotton", may be made by treating cottonseed with sulfuric acid. This treatment may impart a yellow color to the dark seeds. Delinted cottonseed is sometimes added to cattle diets.

Toxicity

The acute toxicity of gossypol is low with the LD_{50} being on the order of 5 gm/kg. However, the ingestion of small amounts over long periods of time leads to illness and death.

Susceptible Species

- Monogastrics are usually readily poisoned
- The horse is relatively resistant
- Dogs and swine quite sensitive
- Ruminants are not usually very susceptible except young calves before the rumen is fully functional. The resistance of adult ruminants has been attributed to the binding of gossypol to soluble proteins in the rumen to form a nontoxic molecule which resists subsequent digestion
- Broiler Diets - Tolerance to gossypol may be affected by age and strain of birds, level of dietary protein, iron salts, and alkaline materials. Levels up to approximately 400 ppm (0.04%) may be fed successfully if ferrous sulfate is added at 1:1 iron to free gossypol weight ratio
- Layers - Egg production is not affected by dietary-free gossypol at up to 200 ppm (0.02%). Dietary concentrations of free gossypol up to 40 to 50 ppm may be fed without consequential egg yolk discoloration. When higher levels of free gossypol are fed (up to 150 ppm), protection against yolk discoloration can be provided by supplementing with iron in a 4:1 weight ratio to gossypol.

Toxicokinetics

- Gossypol is highly lipid soluble. Primarily eliminated via faeces; minor amount leaves as a conjugate in the urine.

Toxicodynamics

- Inhibits protein synthesis
- Anemia may result from the chelation of iron to gossypol
- Binds to proteins and amino acids rendering them unavailable during the digestive process

- Interferes with oxidative processes and prevent the release of oxygen by hemoglobin
- Undecorticated cottonseed meal or cottonseed cake contains up to 25% indigestible fiber which may cause trouble from intestinal impaction
- Cottonseed meal is so low in vitamin A that a deficiency may occur in animals unless adequately supplemented. Cattle with blindness, ataxia, swollen joints and anorexia may sometimes respond to vitamin A
- Inhibits testicular lactic dehydrogenase (LDH) enzymes via a competitive inhibition of a cofactor required for LDH activation.

LDH

$$\text{Lactate} + NAD^+ \rightarrow \text{Pyruvate} + NADH + H^+$$

LDH function

- Inhibits glutathione S-transferase and decreases detoxification of other xenobiotics.

Clinical Signs

Cattle

- Signs tend to begin after the animals have been on cottonseed meal for 4 weeks to as much as a year
- Inappetence, weight loss, and poor feed conversion
- weakness, dyspnoea, emaciation, generalized oedema and death.

Swine

- Dyspnoea, gasping or thumping, froth or bloody froth at the mouth
- Emaciation and weakness
- Cyanosis immediately prior to death.

Dogs

- Very sensitive to antifertility effects.

Poultry

- Weight loss, anorexia, decreased hatchability, discolored egg yolks and whites and abnormal texture of the egg whites.

Lesions

- Generalized congestion and oedema

- Large quantities of straw-colored fluid in peritoneal, pericardial, and thoracic cavities
- Swollen and congested ventral body wall, lungs, kidneys, mesenteric lymph nodes and other organs
- The lungs are oedematous with foam in the trachea leading to pneumonia
- Liver severely congested with degenerative changes
- White coloured patches on the skeletal muscle
- Heart is oedematous, flabby, dilated, and on histologic section, areas of necrosis are present.

Diagnosis

Based on

- Case history
- Circumstantial evidence by identification of cotton or products and evidence of consumption
- Clinical signs
- Postmortem lesions
- Laboratory analysis
- Quantification of free gossypol in the feed and characteristic lesions.

Differential Diagnosis

- Mulberry heart disease (selenium deficiency)
- Coal tar poisoning (phenolics)
- Selenium toxicity
- Monensin and lasalocid poisoning

Treatment

- No specific antidote
- Eliminate the source
- Alleviate pulmonary oedema and congestive heart failure.
- Withdrawal of cottonseed from the diet
- Supplementation of vitamin A to exposed animals
- Supplementation with vitamin A, iron, lysine and protein are recommended
- High protein intake is protective against the effects of gossypol.

Prevention

The toxicity of gossypol may be neutralized by the addition of iron, in the form of ferrous sulfate to the diet at a rate of 1 part iron to 1 part gossypol. Generally, for swine and poultry, the concentration of gossypol in the diet must be less than 0.01% to be safe.

Crotalaria spp.
(Rattlebox)

Family - Leguminosae (Pulse or Bean Family)

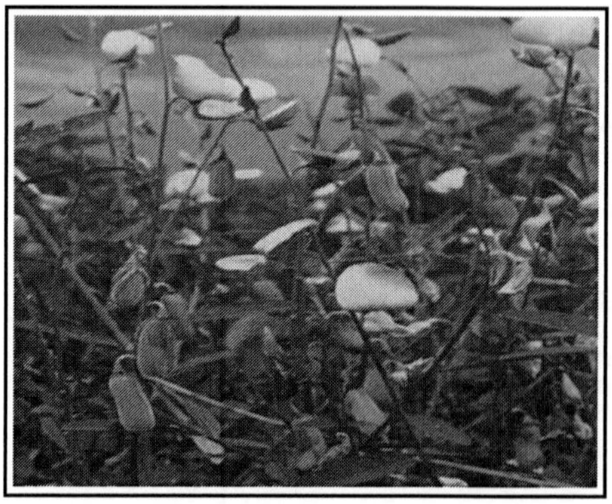

Picture showing the flowers and stems of *Crotalaria juncea*

Other species

Crotalaria sagittalis - Arrow Crotalaria, rattle box, wild pea

C. spectabilis - Showy Crotalaria

C. retusa

C. mucronata var.giant-striate

C. incana

C. rotundifolia

C. burkeana

C. juncea

C. dura

C. equorum

C. globifera

Susceptible Species

- *C. sagitallis* - Horses are more susceptible than cattle.
- *C. spectabilis* - Poultry, cattle, horses and swine are more sensitive than sheep goats and mules.
- *C. retusa* – Poultry are known to be susceptible to several species of *Crotalaria*

Toxic Principle

- The pyrrolizidine alkaloid, monocrotaline Monocrotaline is a diester of monocrotalic acid and the nitrogen-containing rectroecine.

Toxicity

- Alkaloid is most concentrated in the seed, but it is also present in the leaves and stem
- Also toxic when dry (as in hay)
- *Crotalaria* turns green early and remains green when other forage turns brown; consequently, most cases of poisoning occurs as a result of ingestion early in spring or late in fall.

Toxicodynamics

- Monocrotaline is a pyrrolizidine alkaloid, acts on the DNA, especially of hepatocytes
- Causes constriction of the lumen in the medium and small veins of the hepatic portal system
- pneumotoxic causes mast cells in the lungs to release 5-hydroxytryptamine which is responsible for pulmonary vascular lesions.

Clinical Signs

Horses

- Toxicity is also known as Bottoms disease
- Slow emaciation, weakness, stupor
- Incoordination, aimless walking and pushing against objects (head pressing) for hours
- Delirium, excitement, apparent blindness
- Icterus, weakness and stupor
- Death

Cattle

- Three types: acute, intermediate, chronic
- In acute - Signs appear in 1 day and death in 4 days where as in intermediate signs appear in 2 months and death in 2 - 3 months animal exhibits weakness, emaciation, incoordination, constipation or diarrhea
- Chronic - Signs develop in a few days or months and consist of loss of appetite, poor condition, tenesmus, nervousness, excitability, blood in faeces, prostration, bloody nasal discharge and death.

Swine

- Signs appear in several weeks
- Loss of hair, unthriftiness.

Poultry

- Characteristic comb discoloration in 29 hours
- Severe greenish-yellow diarrhea
- Depressed with ruffled feathers.

Lesions

- Generalized Congestion and hemorrhage in various visceral organs
- Degenerative changes in liver and spleen
- Stomach is abnormal with full of undigested food
- Acute - Profuse hemorrhage on the serous membranes of the abdominal and thoracic cavities
- Intermediate - Hepatic cirrhosis, ascites, petechiae on the intestinal serosa
- Chronic - Widespread hemorrhage, petechiae or ecchymoses in nearly all tissues; ascites, oedema in the mesenteries, occasional icterus; degeneration of parenchymatous organs, liver indurated and bluish-gray.

Swine

- Ascites
- Firm indurated liver
- Hemorrhages of heart

Poultry

- Thickened air sacs and pericardial sacs
- Atrophic spleen
- Petechial hemorrhages of serous membranes of abdominal and thoracic cavities
- Petechial and ecchymotic hemorrhage of the visceral fat, heart and musculature
- Swollen kidneys
- Dark, small, marbled liver

- Liver may be ruptured
- Enlarged gallbladder
- Distended abdomen due to ascites.

Diagnosis

Based on

- Case history
- Circumstantial evidence by identification of crotolaria spp. and evidence of consumption
- Clinical signs
- Postmortem lesions
- Laboratory analysis.

Treatment

- No specific antidote
- Treatment has little value after signs appear
- Symptomatic therapy
- Supportive therapy.

Lantana spp.

Family - Verbenaceae (Verbena Family)

Description

- *Lantana* spp.
  - Plant - Erect or spreading shrub
  - Stem - Ridged, angular, prickly
  - Leaves - Opposite, ovate, crenated or serrated margin, veined from base, spreading hairs, 1.5 - 5 inches long
  - Flowers - Small, tubular, spreading lobes, long axillary peduncles, yellow or pink changing to orange or bright red
  - Fruit - Fleshy, drupe-like, 2-celled or 2 one-seeded.

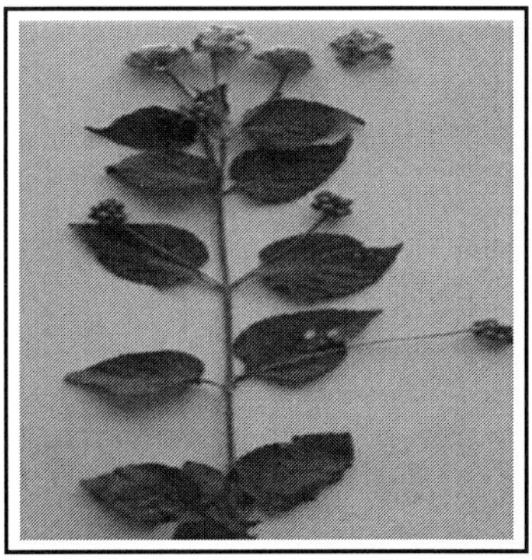

Picture : *Lantana* - The oval, toothed, and veiny leaves; the square prickly stems; the terminal flower clusters; and the black berries are characteristic of this attractive ornamental shrub.

- L. camara
  - Plant - Low, perennial shrub, 3 - 6 ft tall.
  - Stem - Square, sparse weak spines, occasionally vine-like, hairy.
  - Leaves - Opposite or in whorls of 3, ovate, petioled, crenatedentate, 2 - 4 inches long, 1.2 - 2.4 inches wide, toothed, aromatic, rough above, hairy beneath; leaf stalks, 0.4 - 0.8 inches long.
  - Flowers - Small, tubular, yellow or pink changing to bright red, 0.4 - 0.5 inches long, 0.24 - 0.31 inches across; in flat-topped clusters, axillary umbels, 1.6 - 2.4 inches across.
  - Fruit - Greenish-blue or black, fleshy, berry-like, 0.24 - 0.31 inches diameter, glossy; seeds, oval, 0.16 -0.2 inches long, 0.12 - 0.14 inches thick, grooved on 2 sides, brown, rough, irregular.

Habitat

- General – all major states of India
- Fence rows, ditch banks, fields, waste areas, pastures, sandy soils, potted; cultivated as outdoor annual, dry woods.

Toxic Principle

- Pentacyclic triterpene acids, including lantadene A and B, reduced lantadene A, dihydrolantadene A, and icterogenin
- Hepatogenous photosensitizer
- Gastrointestinal irritants.

Susceptible Species

- Sheep, cattle

Toxicity

- *Lantana camara*
  - Foliage and ripe berries contain toxic substance
  - Green berries have a higher concentration of the toxin
  - Three-fourths to 1 kg of dry leaves may cause toxicosis of a 400 kg bovine (1% of animals weight) (green weight basis)
  - Fifty to 90% of animals newly exposed are affected
  - High mortality of affected animals (90%)
  - All species of *Lantana* should be considered poisonous
  - Poisoning commonly occurs among grazing animals.

Toxicodynamics

Ingestion of the plant by the animals
↓
Digestion of the plant in the rumen
↓
Absorption of the toxin from the rumen and small intestine
↓
Transportation of the toxin in the liver
↓
Secretion of the metabolites into the bile
↓
Metabolites injure the bile canalicular membranes
↓
Cholestasis

↓ Retention of bilirubin → ↓ Jaundice

↓ Retention of phylloerythrin → ↓ Photosensitization

↓ Ruminal stasis → ↓ Retention of toxin in the rumen → ↓ Absorption of toxin from the rumen → ↓ Further injury to liver

Clinical Signs

- Acute Toxicosis
  - Photosensitization, the onset of which takes place in 1 to 2 days after consumption of a toxic dose (1% or more of animal's body weight)
  - Jaundice
  - Decreased appetite due to decreased digestive tract motility and constipation
  - Sluggishness
  - Weakness and transient
  - Bloody diarrhea
  - Death occurs in 2 to 4 days.
- Subacute and Chronic Toxicosis
  - Subacute poisoning is more common.
  - Photosensitized surface areas are susceptible to invasions by fly maggots and bacteria.
  - In severely affected cattle, Death may occur after 1 to 3 weeks of illness and weight loss.

Lesions

- General
  - Highly pigmented liver
  - Icterus, general oedema
  - Gallbladder paralysis and distention
  - Necrosis of renal tubules, hemorrhages in some organs
  - Myocardial damage and intestinal paralysis
  - Lesions may appear at the muzzle, mouth, and nostrils Ulceration may be present in the cheeks, tongue, and gums, while swelling, hardening, peeling of mucous membranes, and deeper tissues occur in the nostrils.

Diagnosis

Based on

- Case history
- Circumstantial evidence by identification of Lantana spp. and evidence of consumption
- Clinical signs
- Postmortem lesions
- Laboratory analysis

Treatment

- No specific antidote
- Prevent the effected animals from exposure to direct sunlight
- Hepato protective agents
- Surgical intervention through rumenotomy to remove the toxic weed from the rumen
- Supplementation of ruminal contents with fresh rumen cud of healthy animals
- Saline purgatives to remove from gastro intestinal contents
- Activated charcoal (5g/kg) to adsorb the toxin and prevent further absorption
- Symptomatic therapy like antihistamines and antibiotics
- Physostigmine may initiate dramatic reversal of some of the signs within minutes.

- Contraindications for the use of physostigmine include: asthma, gangrene, cardiovascular disease, mechanical obstruction of the gastrointestinal or urogenital tracts.
- Supportive therapy
- Fluid therapy.

Introduction to Solanaceae

Solanine is a glycoalkaloid (sugar attached to an alkaloid). Because of the structure of the alkaloid portion solanine also referred as steroidal alkaloid. The aglycone (sometimes called an alkamine aglycone) is called solanidine. The word aglycone simply means the compound remaining after the sugar moiety has been removed.

Sources

Solanaceae family.

Toxicity

- Glycoside (solanine) more toxic than aglycone (solanidine)
- Rapid faecal and urinary excretion.

Toxicokinetics

Solanine is poorly absorbed from GI tract.

Toxicodynamics

- Principle effects of solanine alkaloid poisoning are gastrointestinal tract irritation and CNS impairment.
- Inhibits cholinesterase activity.
- Exerts weak cardiotonic activity.
- Depression, recumbency occurs in horses, cattle, swine.
- Ulcerative stomatitis, conjunctivitis, diarrhea, and eczema of legs in cattle and pigs.

Clinical Signs

- The signs of poisoning due to solanine and atropine are parallel and both produce pupillary dilation, ataxia, muscular weakness, restless or thrashing movements, and body temperature elevation
- They differ in that solanine often produces gastroenteritis, depression, salivation, sweating in capable species and dyspnoea.

Lesions

- Gastroenteritis
- Congestion of cerebral membranes and kidneys.

Some members of the Solanaceae have primarily solanine-type alkaloids (solanine, solanidine, etc.); others have atropine or atropine-like compounds; and still others may have both solanine-type as well as atropine-like constituents which complicate therapeutic considerations. Jerusalem cherry (*Solanum pseudocapsicum*), black nightshade (S. nigrum and other species), jessamine (*Cestrum* spp.) ground cherry (*Physalis* spp.), and tomato leaves and unripe fruit (*Lycopersicon*) often contain both solanaceous and atropine-like alkaloids and clinical signs from either may predominate. Potato (S. *tuberosum*) may also contain both types of alkaloid; however, the atropine-like constituents tend to predominate. In addition to the alkaloids mentioned above, Jerusalem cherry (S. *pseudocapsicum*) also contains solanocapsine, which produces marked bradycardia. These considerations are alluded to in the following sections.

Atropa Belladonna

(Deadly nightshade, nightshade, sleeping nightshade)

Family: Solanaceae member

Description

A. belladonna is a coarse herb with a thick root, and with highly branched stems which grow from 0.6 - 1.6 m tall. The leaves are large (approximately 15 cm [6 inches] long), ovate, and alternately inserted but develop so rapidly that they may appear to be inserted in pairs at the same point with one member of each pair larger than the other. Flowers are solitary, almost 2.5 cm long, 5 parted, with a 5-pointed calyx, a tubular corolla, and dull purple. Single berries (1 - 1.3 cm in diameter) are purple to black when ripe. Reddish sap.

Toxicity

- Atropine, which is present throughout the plant, increases maximum at maturity
- Ingestion of berries is fatal.

Clinical Signs

- Poisoning is rare

- Trembling, excitement, followed by prostration
- Tachycardia, weak pulse
- Extreme mydriasis with difficulty in short range vision (accommodation)
- Dyspnoea
- Gastric and/or intestinal atony
- Coma and death.

Diagnosis

Based on

- Case history
- Circumstantial evidence by identification of Atropa bellodona spp. and evidence of consumption
- Clinical signs
- Placing a drop of urine into a cat's eye causes mydraisis
- Postmortem lesions.

Treatment

As for atropine ingestion

Hyoscyamus Niger

(Henbane)

Synonyms

- Black henbane, henbane, stinking nightshade, poison tobacco, fetid nightshade, and insane root.

Description

An annual or biennial, coarse, hairy, erect herb, 1 - 4 feet tall with coarsely toothed, oblong leaves 3 - 8 inches in length. Flowers are single on short pedicels or in the leaf angles becoming crowded near the tips. Flowers are 5 lobed with greenish-yellow or yellowish-white with a purple throat and veins. Fruits are enclosed in a 5 lobed capsule. Spindle-shaped roots.

Habitat

- Primarily found in the northeastern states
- Common in some areas of the southern states especially near mountains
- Usually in dry soils, in roadsides, other "waste areas".

Toxicity

- Atropine and scopalamine
- The seed is poisonous.

Susceptible Species

- Livestock
- Poultry from eating seed.

Clinical Signs

- Similar to other anticholinergic poisoning
- Poisoning is rare, perhaps because the plant is distasteful.

Treatment

As for atropine ingestion.

Datura Stramonium

(Jimson Weed)

Synonyms

- Jamestown weed, thornapple, devil's trumpet, mad apple, and stink weed.

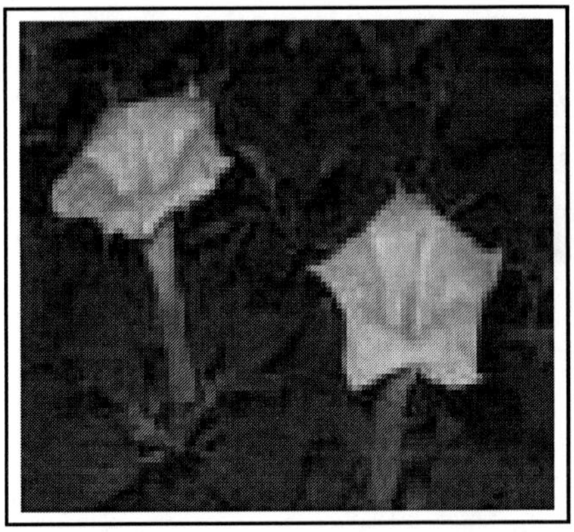

Picture :*Datura stramonium* - L. 1, upper portion of plant; 2, flower; 3, seed pod; 4, seed. Annual, reproducing by seed. Roots thick, shallow, extensively branched. Stems smooth, thick, erect, branching widely in upper part, 2 to 4 feet (0.6 to 1.2 m) tall. Leaves alternate, large, course, smooth, ovate, with irregularly toothed edges and a distinctive rank odor. Flowers large, funnel-shaped, white to pinkish, 2 to 5 inches (5 to 12.5 cm) long, borne singly on short stalks in the axils of the branches. Seed pod about 1 inch (2.5 cm) in diameter, egg-shaped, covered with short, sharp spines. Seed dark brown to black, kidney-shaped, flattened, surface irregular and pitted. Found in cultivated crops on rich land and especially in old feedlots. This plant contains poisonous materials.

Description

Plant is a stout, coarse, annual herb which is 0.6 - 1.6 m tall with spreading branches and simple alternate leaves (15 - 20 cm [6 - 8"] long) which are coarsely and irregularly toothed with a rank odor.Flowers are large, white or purple and tubular; 5 - 10 cm (2 - 4") long.Fruit is a spiny capsule 2.5 - 5 cm (1 - 2") in diameter which can be split into four parts. Sheds small brown to black seeds; seeds contaminate corn, etc.

Habitat

- Fertile soils where other plants are scarce - e.g. barnyards, fertile cultivated fields

Toxic Principle

- Tropane alkaloids
  - Hyoscyamine = an isomer of atropine.
  - Scopalamine = L-hyoscine = epoxidized hyoscyamine.

Toxicity

- Poisoning occurs primarily when hungry animals are turned into an area where better forage is absent.
- Poisoning may also result when a large amount is present in hay.
- Palatability may increase when sprayed with 2,4-D or similar herbicides.
- Possible poisoning as a result of seeds in grains and feeds (seeds contain 0.05% alkaloid by weight).
- Entire plant is toxic, seeds most often implicated.
- Pigs appear to be very sensitive to seeds, 2.2 - 2.7 mg/kg/day reported to cause toxic signs.
- Toxic signs seen in cattle given seeds at 0.06 - 0.09% bw/day.

Clinical Signs

- Hypothermia in animals
- Depression, anorexia, weight loss, tachypnea, tachycardia, mydriasis, polyuria, polydipsia, diarrhea.

Cattle

- Excitability, tremors, rumen atony, nervousness, bloat, tenesmus, and anorexia.

Goats

- Tachypnoea, tremors, drowsiness, recumbency, and altered locomotion

Sheep

- Ataxia, inability to stand, tachypnoea, reduced drinking and mild tremors
- Death from respiratory paralysis.

Diagnosis

Based on

- Case history
- Circumstantial evidence by identification of Atropa bellodona spp. and evidence of consumption
- Clinical signs
- Placing a drop of urine into a cat's eye causes mydraisis
- Postmortem lesions.

Treatment

As for atropine ingestion.

Solanum spp.
(Nightshade Group)

Family – Solanaceae

Other Species

S. nigrum, S. americanum, S. ptycanthum - black nightshade, deadly nightshade, nightshade

S. tuberosum - Irish or white potato

S. carolinense - horse nettle, Carolina horse nettle, bull nettle, tread salve, sand briar *elaegnifolium* – silver leaf nightshade

S. rostratum - buffalo bur, Kansas or Texas thistle

S. dulcamara - European bittersweet

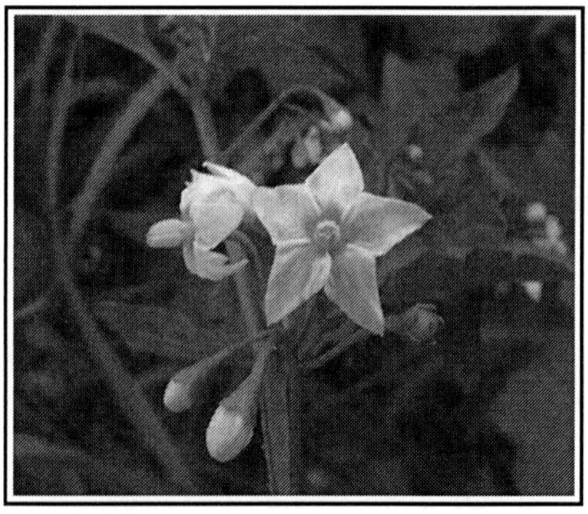

Picture showing the leaves and flowers of *Solanum nigrum* plant

S. gracile - graceful nightshade
S. pseudocapsicum - Jerusalem cherry, natal cherry
S. triflorum - cutleaf nightshade
S. villosum - hairy nightshade
S. melangena - egg plant
S. intrusum
S. aculeatissium (S. capsicoides) - devil's apple, sode-apple, love apple
Lycopersicon - tomato.

Description

- *S. nigrum*
  - Climbing perennial herb reaching up to 3 m tall, but usually 0.3 - 1 m tall, annual, erect. Leaves are alternate, simple or deeply lobed, wavy-toothed or oval- to lance-shaped, stalked and long, 3.8 - 10 cm. Flowers are white with large yellow anthers, which extend from the leaf axils in small drooping clusters with 2 - 20 blossoms. Flowers are small (0.6 - 1 cm across) with 5 white or pale violet petals. Fruits are round, 0.6 cm thick, purple-black when fully ripened, green when unripe, and contain many seeds.
- *S. carolinense*
  - Perennial herb, 0.3 - 0.6 m tall, with yellow spines on the stems and simple, oblong, irregular or lobed leaves. Flowers are pale violet or white. Fruits are yellow berries about 1.2 cm in diameter.
- *S. eleagnifolium*
  - Perennial, 0.3 - 1 m tall, with a white hairy stem, and simple, thick, lanceolate to linear leaves with short, stiff spines. The leaves are silvery white in color. Flowers are violet or blue, and fruits are yellow or orange berries. Plant has long creeping rootstalks.
- *S. pseudocapsicum*
  - A shrub or potted plant growing up to 1.3 m tall, with dark green, shiny, waxy leaves, oblong in shape and 10 cm long. Flowers are white, in clusters, or alone, and 1.2 cm wide. Fruits are globular, 1.2 cm in diameter, scarlet or yellow, and resemble miniature tomatoes.
- *S. malacoxylon*
  - A shrub, up to 1 - 1.5 m tall, smooth with sharp pointed, lanceolate somewhat fleshy leaves on comparatively long stems.

- *S. dimidiatum*
  - Perennial, 1 m tall, with short, rounded, leaves of 15 cm in length. Fruit are pale yellow berries of ~3 cm in diameter.

Susceptible Species

- Sheep, goats, calves, adult cattle, chickens, ducks, horses, rabbits, dogs, swine (especially).

Toxic Principles

- Contain steroidal glycoalkaloid solanine, upon hydrolysis, yields a sugar and the alkaloid solanidine. The free (unconjugated) steroidal alkaloid (the aglycone) is the primary form acting on the nervous system.
- Other aglycones include dihydrosolanidine, tomatidine and strophanthidin.
- Some plants may also contain saponins.
- Some of these plants also have cardiac effects, e.g., Jerusalem cherry (*S. pseudocapsicum*) contains an additional alkaloid, solanocapsine, which produces bradycardia. The plant may also irritate the skin.
- In some plants, atropine-like constituents predominate, e.g., potato (*S. tuberosum*), and some strains and stages of black nightshade (*S. nigrum*).
- *Solanum malacoxylon* contains toxic amounts of 1,25-dihydroxy-cholecalcified glucoside.

Toxicity

- Poisoning occurs under conditions of overgrazing
- Leaves and green fruits are toxic. The juice in the wilted leaves is especially toxic, and may be deadly if ingested
- Silverleaf nightshade (*S. eleagnifolium*) is exceptional in that the ripe fruit is more toxic than the green. *S. eleagnifolium* is toxic at only 0.1% of the body weight
- Toxicity is not lost upon drying and Solanine content increases up to maturity
- Solanine is reportedly destroyed by cooking except potatoes
- Potato (*S. tuberosum*) peelings contain the major portion of the toxic principle in the tuber, and leaves, sprouts, vines

- Spoiled potatoes and peelings have also caused severe poisoning. Cooking does not appear to destroy all the alkaloids in greened potatoes. Toxicity may vary with the soil, climate and other variables. Animals may browse potato plants or eat sprouted potatoes, leading to toxicity.

Toxicodynamics

- Solanine is a direct irritant of the esophageal and gastric mucosae
- Acts as inhibitors of acetylcholinesterase
- neurotoxic and often cause ataxia and depression
- Atropine-like alkaloids from some *Solanum* species competitively inhibit acetylcholine at muscarinic receptors.

Clinical Signs

- Salivation, anorexia, severe gastrointestinal disturbances, with hemorrhagic diarrhea
- Intestinal stasis and constipation
- Hemolysis and anemia.
- Apathy, drowsiness, depression, confusion, progressive muscular weakness, numbness, dilated pupils, trembling, labored breathing, nasal discharge, rapid heartbeat, weak pulse, bradycardia
- CNS depression and incoordination accompanied by paralysis of the rear legs
- Terminal signs include unconsciousness, shock, paralysis, coma, circulatory and respiratory depression, and death.

Lesions

- No Specific lesions
- Oedema around the kidneys with clots
- Tubular necrosis of kidneys when examined histologically.
- Hyperemia, hemorrhage and ulceration of the alimentary tract
- Congested liver with gallbladder distended
- Oedema of the ventral body wall
- Congestion and emphysema in the lungs
- Hemorrhages and congestion in the heart and spleen

- *S. dimidiatum* is unique among Solanacea in causing necrosis of Purkinje cells of the cerebellum.

Diagnosis

Based on

- Case history
- Circumstantial evidence by identification of Solanum spp .and evidence of consumption
- Clinical signs
- Postmortem lesions.

Treatment

- No specific antidote
- Induce vomition unless contraindicated
- Establish respiration
- Activated charcoal, saline cathartic
- Fluid therapy to maintain body fluid and electrolyte balance
- Symptomatic and supportive treatment
- Dermatitis may be relieved by washing with soap and water and application of corticosteroids
- If signs suggesting cholinesterase inhibition consider cautious (!) treatment with atropine
- Cattle surviving 24 hours will generally recover.

Prevention

- The pasture should be mowed before the seeds ripen to control propagation of the weeds
- Keep animals out of areas with heavily concentrated weeds, especially if forage is not abundant
- Hungry animals should not be allowed to graze areas where an abundance of nightshade is growing
- Use Herbicides to control nightshades
- When in hay and animals are preferentially eating the other plants, consistent overfeeding of the hay and daily removal of the "wasted" (uneaten) poisonous plants may sometimes be an economic necessity.

Amaranthus spp.
(Pigweed)

Family -
Amaranthaceae
Amaranth Family

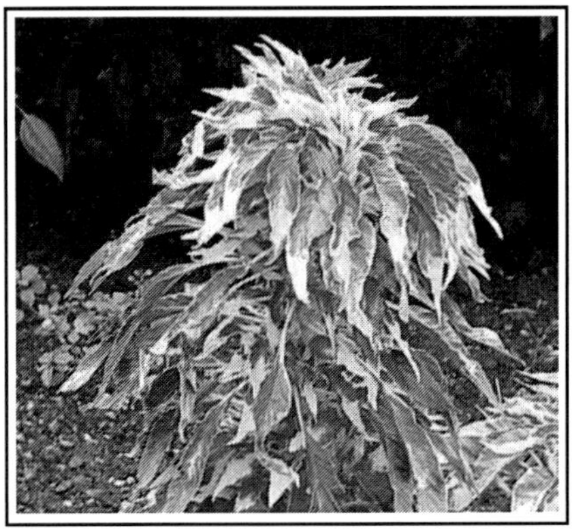

Amaranthus retroflexus L. 1, lower stem and roots; 2, upper stem with leaves and flower clusters; 3, flower; 4, seed. Annual, reproducing by seeds. Taproot shallow, reddish. Stems erect, up to 6 feet (1.8 m) high, rough, branching freely if not crowded. Leaves dull green, usually at least 6 inches (15 cm) long when mature, ovate to lanceolate. Flowers green, small, in thick, stiff, paniclelike terminal spikes with many short, crowded lateral branches. Bracts much longer than sepals and utricles. Sepals longer than utricle, curved, rounded, often with small notch at end. Seeds shiny black, lens-shaped, ovate, notched at the narrow end, about 1mm in diameter. Found in cultivated fields, yards, fence rows, and other waste places. Other species, such as smooth pigweed and Powell amaranth, are similar to redroot pigweed in morphology and weedy habits, and may often be found in the same area. Redroot pigweed is also commonly known as rough pigweed.

Other Species

Amaranthus retroflexus - Rough Pigweed, Redroot Pigweed
A. palameri - Redroot Pigweed
A. gangeticus.

Description

- Annual reproducing by seeds
- Stems erect, branching above
- Leaves alternate, simple with long petioles, ovate or rhombic, with a wavy margin
- Flowers in dense thick spikes, crowded in a close, stiff terminal panicle. Flowers are polygamous, small and green with 3 stiff, spine-like persistent bracts, 4 - 6 mm long; calyx with 5 sepals, 5 stamens, and 1 pistil which is 1-celled
- Fruit is a utricle, opening with a lid. Seed is lens shaped, ovate, 0.9 - 1.3 mm long, glossy and black.

Habitat

Roadsides, fields, barnyards, and other areas rich in organic matter and natural pastures.

Toxic Principle

- Oxalate (up to 30%, dry weight): Leaves have 3 times as much oxalate as the stems
- Nitrate (concentrations at different life stage range from 0.04 to 2.9%)
  - Green plant at rapid stage of growth (0.066% KNO_3)
  - Plants that stop growing due to inadequate moisture (0.828% KNO_3)
  - Plants that wilted due to lack of moisture (2.874% KNO_3)
- Hay contaminated by pigweed can be dangerous.

Susceptible Species

- Swine are most often poisoned
- Growing calves, cattle.
- Sheep may also be affected.

Clinical Signs

Swine (Perirenal Oedema Syndrome)

- Swine raised in confinement with access to contaminated pasture develops perirenal oedema
- Posterior incoordination, weakness, trembling, and knuckling at the pasterns
- Sternal recumbency, flaccid paresis, especially in the rear limbs and unable to rise even when stimulated
- Distended abdomen
- Coma with death within 48 hours after the onset of clinical signs.

Cattle

- Nephrosis
- Dyspnoea and depression.

Lesions

- Retroperitoneal oedema in the perirenal connective tissue is the pathognomonic lesion
- Oedema of the ventral abdominal wall and perirectal area

- Blood tinged oedema fluid
- Kidneys are normal or small in size and pale with subcapsular petechiae
- Toxic tubular nephrosis with degeneration of proximal tubules
- Necrosis and dilation of the convoluted tubules and a large number of proteinaceous tubular casts with oxalate crystals.

Diagnosis

Based on

- Case history
- Circumstantial evidence by identification of *Amaranthus* spp and evidence of consumption
- Clinical signs
- Postmortem lesions
- Presence of oxalate crystals in kidneys will **not** be consistent

Treatment

- No specific antidote
- Eliminate the source of plant from the vicinity of the animal
- Symptomatic therapy
- Supportive therapy
- Avoid stress and dehydration to the effected animals.

Prevention

- Mow, then spray with 2,4-D or similar herbicide
- Spraying plants with 2, 4-D may intensify nitrate accumulation
- Therefore, remove all animals from pasture for 1 week following spraying to avoid exposure to plants until they have dried out.

Nerium spp.

Family - Apocynaceae (dogbane family)

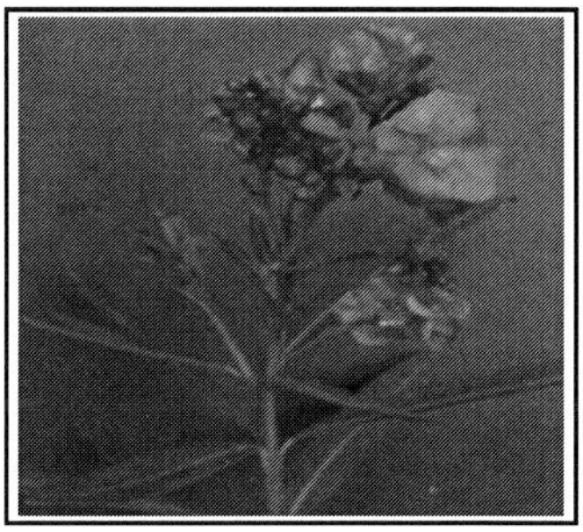

Picture :Oleander (*Nerium indicum*) - The narrow leathery leaves, the colorful flowers, and the hairy seed and slender seed pod (lower right) are characteristic of this deadly plant

Other Species

Nerium oleander - Common pink oleander

N. odorum - Rose laurel, adelfa

N. indicum - Rosenlorbeer.

Description

- Plant - Evergreen shrub about 5 - 25 feet tall, looks like a small tree if all but one stem is cut; gummy, sticky sap.
- Stem - Bark smooth, green until several years old.
- Leaves - Simple, evergreen, leathery, narrow, entire, smooth edges, oblong lanceolate, sharply pointed, 4 - 12 inches long, whorled or sometimes opposite.
- Two primary parallel veins run perpendicular to the midrib.
- Flowers - Spring or early summer, showy, white, pink, yellowish, rose, deep red, large cluster.
- Fruit - Pods, several inches long, narrow, contain many seeds; seeds have a tuft of brown hairs.

Habitat

- Native to Asia,an ornamental shrub in Southern and Southwestern India
- Used as a houseplant in the majority of the states in India.

Susceptible Species

All species of animals

Toxic Principle

- Highly toxic cardiac glycoside similar to digitoxin
- The cardiac glycosides: nerioside, oleandroside, oleandrin, digitoxigenin, neriin and folinerin, oleandromycin (antibiotic), and rosagenin (strychnine-like).
- *N. indicum* contains odoroside (a steroidal glycoside).

Toxicity

- Stems, flowers, leaves all are toxic
- Toxicity is not lost on drying

- Garden cuttings thrown into feeder troughs are a major cause of poisoning
- The glycosides are distributed throughout the plant, but growing tops are most toxic; dried leaves and bark are also poisonous.
- Males may be more sensitive to toxic effects.
- Contact may produce dermatitis in sensitive individuals.
- Oleandrin is water soluble, so leaves falling in a pond can poison the water, but the water is usually made unpalatable, so animals may avoid it.
- Plant is bitter and usually avoided.
- Ld_{50} values

Dog	150 - 225 mg/kg
Cat	220 and 450 mg/kg
Goats	200 mg/kg
Sheep	of just 2 or 3 leaves
Cattle	1 - 20 grams (green) or 15 - 25 grams (dry) leaves.

Toxicodynamics

- Inhibition of Na/K ATP-ase enzyme system causing increased intracellular sodium and decreased potassium concentrations.
- Bradycardia and/or tachycardia.
- Severe hyperkalemia with marginal hypocalcemia and hypoglycemia

Clinical Signs

General

- Local irritation of the mucous membranes of the mouth and stomach.
- Abdominal pain, nausea, vomiting, sweating in some species.
- Anorexia.
- Digitalis-like effects on the heart (pulse rapid and weak or slow and strong, depending on the stage of the disease).
- Constriction of the blood vessels, cold extremities.
- Pupillary dilation, blurred vision, fever.
- Dizziness, drowsiness, ataxia.
- Colic, bloody diarrhea (may be severe).

- Cardiac arrhythmias, unconsciousness, hypotension, hypothermia, bradycardia.
- Respiratory paralysis, dyspnoea, shallow breathing.
- Tremors followed by progressive paralysis, coma and death (fibrillation in terminal stages).
- Goat
  - Bleating and suppressed ruminations
  - Excessive salivation, nausea, vomition, mydriasis, incoordination, depression, prostration, convulsions, dyspnoea, cyanosis; contact dermatitis.

Lesions

- Severe catarrhal or hemorrhagic gastroenteritis
- Generalized congestion
- Agonal hemorrhages are commonly encountered on the heart and serous and mucous membranes.
- Clear or blood-stained fluid present in the serous cavities.
- Microscopically indications of hepatitis and nephrosis
- Cortical tubules exhibit coagulative necrosis and heamoglobin stained albumin casts.

Diagnosis

Based on

- Case history
- Circumstantial evidence by identification of Nerium spp and evidence of consumption
- Clinical signs
- Postmortem lesions

Treatment

- No specific antidotes
- Emetics (apomorphine)if no contraindication exists
- Osmotic or saline cathartics ($MgSo_4$ and Na_2So_4)
- Gastric demulcents
- Treat as for other cardioglycoside toxicosis

- Administer atropine in conjunction with propranolol
- Give phenytoin or lidocaine to improve atrio-ventricular conduction
- Provide artificial respiration
- Dipotassium edetate has been used in the treatment of Oleander toxicosis and acts by antagonizing the cardiotoxicity via increasing membrane permeability through reduction of the calcium ion concentration and, consequently enhanced re-entry of potassium ions into the cardiac myofibers.

Contraindication

Infusion of calcium containing fluids.

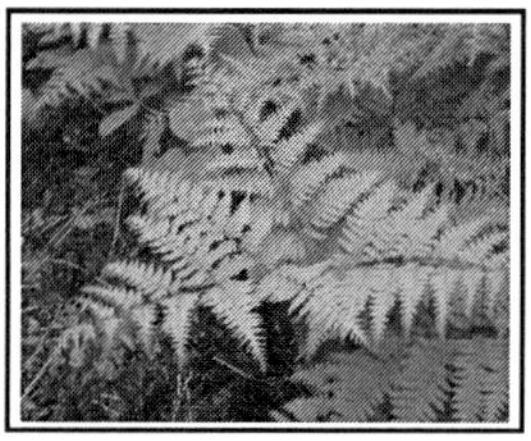

Pteridium Aquilinum

(Bracken Fern)

Synonyms - Brake fern, hog brake

Description

- Perennial herb, which spreads by means of a deep, stout, especially toxic horizontal rhizome. The rhizome is often below plow depth and results in growth of large patches of the plant.
- Triangular coarse, leaves (fronds) tend to be erect. Fronds are palatable.
- Up to 6 feet tall.
- Spores in late summer; sporangia are protected by the rolled under edges of the blades.

Habitat

- Worldwide, especially forested areas, common where recently cleared, in abandoned fields, open woods, chiefly on dry sandy soils or gravelly areas.
- Often in dense stands.

Species Affected

- Seasonal tendency - Late summer to early rainy.
- Horses and cattle are primarily affected, and the syndromes differ:
  - Horses - Mainly neurologic.
  - Cattle - Mainly bone marrow damage.
- Sheep and swine rarely eat bracken, but exposed swine produce a thiaminase mediated syndrome.

Toxic Principles

Four toxic principles are recognized:

- Thiaminase
- Aplastic anaemia factor or bone marrow toxin also known as ptaquiloside
- Factor causing heamaturia
- Carcinogen

Toxicity

- Poisoning may occur at any time of year, but is more often in late summer when other forage is depleted, or in winter when contaminated hay is fed. Levels of thiaminase in the plant will be peak in the late summer.
- Toxic principles are present in both fresh and dried plant materials.
- Young plants and rhizomes are more toxic.

Toxicodynamics

- Toxicity in horses (and rats) is due to a thiaminase (destroys thiamine in the digestive tract before it can be absorbed), resulting in central nervous system dysfunction and damage.
- Thiamine deficiency results in impaired pyruvate utilization. Blood pyruvate levels rise. Animal suffers from abnormal energy metabolism due to inadequate ATP production.
- Toxicity in cattle is due to an unidentified toxic principle and not thiaminase. At least part of the problem is due to a carcinogen.

Clinical Signs

Ruminants

Cattle

- Considered a "radiomimetic" disease in cattle and sheep.
- Thiamine production in the rumen results in resistance to the thiaminase syndrome seen in horses.
- Disease develops as a result of bone marrow suppression.
- Early fever (106 - 108° F).
- Loss of condition, anorexia.
- Anemia
- Bracken fern-induced hematuria in cattle is known as bovine enzootic haematuria.

- Leukopenia, thrombocytopenia with blood-tinged nasal discharges, bloody or "tarry"coloured faeces, blood clots in faeces, hematuria. Prolonged clotting times, defective clot retraction.
- Dyspnoea.
- Bladder and upper gastrointestinal carcinoma in cattle exposed to bracken fern for 1 - 6 years.

Sheep

- Bright blindness in sheep due to progressive retinalatrophy and is characterized by permanent blindness and the pupils of the effected eyes respond very poorly to light.

Non -ruminants

Horse

- Emaciation.
- Loss of weight occurs
- Lethargy.
- Incoordination, especially when forced to walk.
- Wide stance, arched back, crouched stance.
- Severe tremors, unable to arise, injuries from attempts to get to feet;
- Bradycardia with arrhythmias seen in early stages
- Hyperthermia, Convulsions, recumbency, opisthostonus with weak and fast pulse in terminal stages.

Swine

- Depressed growth rate, dyspnoea, weakness, recumbency, and death.
- Clinical signs are the result of thiamine deficiency.
- Elevated pyruvate levels.

Lesions

Ruminants

Cattle

- Generalized hemorrhages, anemia, aplastic bone marrow
- Ulceration of the abomasum
- Lesions in urinary tract and bladder ranging from hyperplastic and hemorrhagic inflammation to neoplasias.

Sheep

- Loss of rods and cones and outer nuclear layers in eyes
- Hemorrhagic syndrome similar to cattle.

Non- ruminants

Horses

- Generalized heamorrhages and congestion in gastrointestinal tract
- Pericardial and epicardial hemorrhages

Swine

- Enlarged, mottled heart, congestive heart failure.
- Lungs oedematous, ascites, and enlarged gall bladder.
- Degenerative changes of cardiac muscle fibers

Diagnosis

Based on

- Case history
- Circumstantial evidence by identification of brackenfern sp. and evidence of consumption
- Clinical signs
- Postmortem lesions
- Thiamine analysis of whole blood (avoid hemolysis) of monogastrics may help support the diagnosis.

Differential diagnosis

- Septicemia,
- Anaplasmosis,
- moldy sweet clover ingestion,
- Leptospirosis.

Treatment

Ruminants

Cattle

- No specific antidotes
  - DL-batyl alcohol: Treatment with DL-batyl alchohol
  - Preparation of DL-batyl alcohol for intravenous administration: add 5 grams of Tween-80 or Tween 20 emulsifier to 100 ml saline and

dissolve in a water bath. After heating, add 2 grams of DL-batyl alcohol and shake vigorously periodically until homogeneous. After cooling in cool water, the mixture should be only mildly opalescent. If not, reheat with shaking and cool again. This approximately 2% batyl alcohol solution may be given intravenously.

- Preparation for subcutaneous administration: the concentrated alcohol may be diluted in olive oil at a rate of 1 gram DL-batyl alcohol to 10 ml of the oil.
- The dose administered is 1 gram of DL-batyl alcohol intravenously or subcutaneously daily for five days.

- Blood transfusions - as per requirement
- Protamine sulfate (1%), a heparin antagonist administered as a 10 ml injection, in conjunction with blood transfusions may be of benefit.
- Broad spectrum antibiotics.

Non–ruminants

Horses

- Saline cathartic.
- Activated charcoal.
- Thiamine HCl - At a dose of 0.25 - 0.5 mg/kg, IV or IM, daily for several days, up to 2 weeks.subcutaneous administration of 100-200mg daily for 6 days is also successful.

Swine

Treatment is similar to that described for horses.

Bracken Fern. Note the large pinnately divided leaf-like frond, the spore-bearing frond (lower left), fiddleneck (lower center), unfolding fiddleneck (lower right), and the underground rootstock (lower right) of this primitive plant.

Senecio spp.

(Ragwort-Groundsel)

Family - Compositae

Other Species

S. jacobaea - Ragwort, stinking Willie, tansy ragwort

S. ridelli - Riddell's groundsel

S. longilobus - Threadleaf groundsel, wooly
S. spartioides - Broom groundsel
S. integerrimus - Lamb's tongue groundsel
S. burchellii
S. douglasii
S. erraticus
S. glabellus
S. ilicifolius
S. lobatus
S. plattensis
S. vulgaris - Common groundsel
S. confusus
S. pauperculus - Prairie groundsel.

Description

Senecio spp. Mostly perennial herbs, approximately 3 feet tall. Leaves are palmately dissected, narrow segmentations are present; leaves are whorled, but bracts are not overlapping and form a cup under the head. Flowers are yellow, in heads clustered at the top of the plant and are numerous. The seeds are in both the disc and in the ray florets.

Habitat

- The *Senecios* tend to grow in rangelands.
  - *S. jacobaea*
  - *S. riddellii*
  - *S. longilobus*
  - *S. spartioides*
  - *S. integerrimus*
- *S. jacobaea* grows in roadsides, pastures and waste places. The plants increase in number when pastures are overgrazed.

Toxic Principles

- *S. jacobaea* - Jacobine, jacodine, senecionine.
- *S. ridelli* - Ridelliine.
- *S. longilobus* - Longilobine.

- *S. spartioides* - Seneciphylline.
- *S. integerrimus* - Integerrimine.
- *S. vulgaris* - Senecionine, seneciphylline, retrorsine.

Susceptible Species

- Cattle and horses are most often poisoned; sheep and pigs require a longer time to show signs. Although sheep were, at one time, used in reducing the *Senecio* contamination of pastures, they may be poisoned on some strains at doses only slightly higher than those affecting cattle.
- Young, growing animals are more susceptible to the hepatotoxic effects of those compounds than are adults.
- Chronic pyrrolizidine alkaloid poisoning occurs worldwide causing extensive livestock losses.
- Of over 100 known pyrrolizidine alkaloids, only a few have proven to be toxic.

Toxicity

- Dry leaves retain their toxicity.
- 'In the field, acute poisoning is rare, but chronic poisoning is common. In this instance, 12 - 56% of the animal's weight must be eaten before symptoms appear.
- Poisoning tends to occur as a result of ingestion of contaminated hay
- Poisoning may also occur during the growing season when good forage is scarce and the animals are forced to eat these plants
- *S. longilobus* is evergreen and may be eaten in winter. Young leaves are believed to be of greater toxicity than more mature leaves and stems.
- Ensiling hay containing pyrrolizidine alkaloids does not ensure detoxification and multiple deaths have occurred in cattle consuming contaminated silage. However, the addition of molasses to the green chopped plants during the ensiling process may lessen the risk.

Toxicokinetics (Applies to all Pyrrolizidine Alkaloid Plants)

Pyrrolizidine alkaloids are rapidly absorbed from the intestine and thereby expose the liver first via the portal circulation. They are also rapidly excreted in body fluids such as milk and urine. Since pyrrolizidine alkaloids are considered to be carcinogens, there is a potential public health problem. In addition, the alkaloids pass across the placenta and can thereby affect the foetus.

Toxicodynamics (Applies to all Pyrrolizidine Alkaloid Plants)

Pyrrolizidine alkaloids

↓

Dehydrogenation of pyrrolizidine alkaloids by hepatic microsomal enzymes

↓

Pyrrole derivatives

↓

Alkylates macromolecules in the hepatocyte

↓

DNA, which impairs cell division

↓

Prevents the hepatocyte from undergoing binary fission to regenerate hepatocytes.

↓

Hepatocytes continues to grow although unable to divide

↓

Hepatocytomegaly and karyomegaly

↓

Necrosis of the Hepatocytes occurs

↓

Necrosis triggers a regenerative response accompanied by bile duct proliferation

↓

Cell reaches a critical mass and dies

↓

Generalized hepatic insufficiency syndrome.

Clinical Signs

- Acute poisoning
  - Dullness, weakness, abdominal pain and death in a few days to weeks.
  - Horses may exhibit extreme nervous excitement.
- Chronic poisoning
  - Clinical signs often may not appear for 2 - 8 months after the first ingestion of pyrrolizidine alkaloids containing plants.
  - Animals lose condition over months and develop icterus.
  - In the later stages, cattle may exhibit nervous derangement and mania.

Horses

- Exhibit nervous signs, especially yawning, drowsiness and staggering. The condition in horses is called "sleepy staggers" and "walking disease".
- Stand apart and lose appetite.

- An unpleasant, sweetish odor may emanate from the skin.
- Chew fences and walk aimlessly.
- Pressing of head due to hepatoencephalopathy.
- Death within about a week of onset.

Cattle

- Exhibit secondary photosensitivity: subcutaneous oedema, dry, scaly muzzle, rough hair coat, and tenesmus associated with diarrhea or constipation with prolapse.

Swine

- Pyrexia and severe respiratory signs.

Lesions

- Enlargement and congestion of the liver, necrosis and hemorrhage in lobules.
- Liver may be enlarged and cirrhotic.
- Patchy gastroenteritis.
- Ascites
- Hepatitis
- Intestinal oedema
- Enlarged hepatic lymph nodes
- Toxic tubular nephrosis
- Cerebral oedema

Histologic Lesions

- Hepatocytomegaly and karyomegaly.
- Hepatic necrosis.
- Bile duct proliferation.
- Fibrosis and cirrhosis of liver

Diagnosis

Based on

- Case history
- Circumstantial evidence by identification of Senecio sp. and evidence of consumption

- Clinical signs
- Postmortem lesions
- Detection of pyrrolizidine alkaloids in plant materials and liver of exposed animals.

Treatment

- No specific antidote
- Eliminate the source or prevent the animals from access in areas infested with Senecio sp.
- Laxatives
- High protein, low carbohydrate diet
- Symptomatic therapy
- Supportive therapy.

Goitrogenic Substances

Introduction

Goitrogens are substances that suppress the function of the thyroid gland by interfering with iodine uptake which can, as a result, cause an enlargement of the thyroid.

- *Goiter* - Defined as any nonmalignant enlargement of the thyroid gland as a whole, accompanied by either hypo- or hyperthyroidism due to increase in the amount of thyroid tissue (hyperplasia), or due to increase in the amount of colloid causing a distension of acini.
- *Hyperplastic goiter* - Hyperplasia is the first morphologic response to iodine deficiency. With reduced thyroxine production the pituitary releases increased amounts of thyrotropic hormone, which is the stimulus for hyperplasia.
- *Colloid goiter* (simple goiter) is characterized by enlargement and distension of the acini (which are filled with colloid). The colloid contains very little iodine and thyroxine, symptoms are those of hypothyroidism. Milder goitrogenic substances (e.g., soybeans) are likely to cause this type of goiter.
- *Goitrogenic substances* - Any substance which can lead to an increase in the size of the thyroid gland. Ex: thiouracil (therapeutically used to treat hyperthyroidism), glucosinolates, cyanides, sulfocyanates, thiocyanates, and some sulfonamides.

Source

Goitrogenic drugs

Chemicals that have been shown to have goitrogenic effects include:

- Sulfadimethoxine, propylthiouracil, potassium perchlorate, and iopanoic acid.
- Thiocyanate overload especially if also in conjunction with selenium deficiency.[2] Reliance on cassava as a carbohydrate provides a source of thiocyanate in some areas.

Goitrogenic foods

These foods include

- Soybeans (and soybean products such as tofu)
- Pine nuts
- Peanuts
- Millet
- Strawberries
- Peaches
- Spinach
- Bamboo shoots
- Radishes
- Horseradish
- Vegetables in the genus *Brassica*
  - Bok choy
  - Broccoli
  - Broccolini (Asparations)
  - Brussels sprouts
  - Cabbage
  - Cauliflower
  - Chinese cabbage
  - Choy sum
  - Collard greens
  - *Kai-lan* (Chinese broccoli)
  - Kale

- Kohlrabi
- Mizuna
- Mustard greens
- Rapeseed (*yu choy*)
- Rapini
- Rutabagas
- Tatsoi
- Turnips.

Toxicodynamics

Thyroid nodule genesis may be considered as an amplification of thyroid heterogeneity due to genetic and/or epigenetic mechanisms. Thyroid nodules can be five types with distinct histological features: hyperplastic, neoplastic, colloid, cystic and thyroiditic nodules.

Hyperplastic: Thyrocyte proliferation is under the control of TSH but several other paracrine and autocrine factors are secreted by follicular cells, the stromal apparatus and the lymphocytes, which are implicated in initiation and perpetuation of thyroid hyperplasia. Growth occurs mainly through TSHR, cAMP and PKA. Constitutive cAMP overproduction has been shown to be due to point mutation of the TSHR or Gs protein, producing overgrowth and hyperfunction.

Neoplastic: Several activated oncogenes have been identified in thyroid malignancies. Oncogenes relevant to the thyroid carcinogenesis are: mutated TSHR and gsp (constitutive activation of cAMP); TRK (receptor for NGF); RET/PTC (phosphorylation of tyrosine kinase receptor)–an isoform of this oncogene is induced by radiation: ras (it encodes Gs proteins transducing mitogenic signals); and c-MET (receptor for hepatocyte growth factor). The evolution of a differentiated thyroid cancer towards an undifferentiated cancer is due to a mutation of a family of proteins (i.e., p53), which acts as a brake, preventing the genomic instability of cancer. It is suggested that a tumor initiates by RET or ras and possibly progresses–as a result of additional mutations and by p53 mutation–to anaplastic carcinoma.

Colloid: Flattening of the epithelium and dilatation of follicles containing viscous material–made up by a concentrated solution of thyroglobulin (hTg)–is the characteristic of the colloid nodule. A defect of intraluminal reabsorption of hTg has been suggested but not proven. Experimentally, a load of iodine is able to change thyroid hyperplasia to a colloid feature; however, a load of iodine is rarely found in the clinical history of patients. A new clue to the pathogenesis comes from the finding that a relevant part of the colloid (10–20%) is made up of insoluble globules, where hTg is compacted in a polymeric form. It is suggested that stocking hTg into globules is defective in colloid nodules, leading to enormous enlargement of the follicle.

Cystic: It is estimated that between 15 and 40% of thyroid nodules are partly or entirely cystic. The 'true cyst' is rare; most of the so-called cystic nodules are 'pseudocysts', which follow necrosis and colliquation. Necrosis issues as an imbalance between growth and the precisely regulated process of angiogenesis. More recently, the VEGF/VPF has been found to be at the origin of recent and recurrent cysts. Immunotoxic and apoptotic mechanisms have also been suggested. Chemical analysis of cystic fluid showed a 'denatured' and 'serum-like' pattern suggesting different mechanisms in the pathogenesis of the pseudocystic thyroid nodules.

Thyroiditic: Nodular lymphocytic thyroiditis (NLT) includes two different entities: 1) lymphocyte thyroiditis growing as a nodule in a hyperplastic or normal gland, and 2) lymphocyte thyroiditis associated in the same nodule with other nodular diseases of the thyroid: papillary thyroid carcinoma and lymphoma have been found to be associated to chronic lymphocytic thyroiditis.

The transformation of the normal fully differentiated thyroid follicular cell to the rapidly growing undifferentiated anaplastic thyroid carcinoma cell involves a number of stages which have been defined morphologically and are now being related to various growth pathways and to molecular biological defects. The two main factors involved in this transformation are growth stimulation and mutagenesis. Growth stimulation alone, through elevated TSH, can lead to the development of thyroid tumours, usually benign, and retaining TSH dependency in some cases. Mutagens alone, if growth is suppressed, do not produce tumours, the combination of mutagens and increased growth is a potent carcinogenic regime. Non-genotoxic carcinogenesis in the thyroid involves growth, without mutagenesis the agent often causes this through affecting one component of thyroid hormone synthesis or metabolism, leading to a fall in thyroid hormone levels and a rise in TSH. Growth stimulation increases the rate of cell division, and therefore increases the chance of a mutation. Continued growth increases the change of subsequent events, in particular loss of heterozygosity in a tumour suppressor gene. p53 is involved in the progression of either papillary or follicular adenoma to an undifferentiated carcinoma. In experimental thyroid carcinogenesis, ras is again involved, with a link between the mutagenic agent used and the type of ras gene showing mutation. Analysis of the involvement of different growth factors and oncogenes in thyroid carcinogenesis suggests that genes related to the two receptors concerned with normal TSH stimulated growth, TSH receptor and the IGF1 receptor may be involved in the progression of thyroid tumours of follicular pathology. Several tyrosine kinase receptors with unknown ligands or of uncertain physiological function are linked to papillary carcinoma.

Certain plants are known to be goitrogenic when consumed ex: Soyabeans and members of the Brassicas (cabbage, rape, kale, and turnips). Goitrogenic substances from these plants have been transmitted through the milk (glucosinolates). Cooking, heating, or processing (e.g., soybeans) destroys the goitrogenic substances in these plants.

Glucosinolates are -D-thioglucoside glycosides found in members of the genus Brassica. The primary significance of glucosinolates in animal nutrition is that oils from these plants are occasionally used as protein supplements. The glucosinolates are hydrolyzed by the enzymes glucosinolase or thioglucosidase. The enzymes required for this activation are present in the plant and are produced by ruminal microorganisms.

A major effect of the hydrolysis products of glucosinolates is inhibition of the thyroid gland.

Antithyroid Agents have 4 General Effects

1) They may interfere with iodine uptake by the thyroid gland (e.g., thiocyanate),
2) Can interfere with tyrosine iodination
3) Suppress thyroxine secretion
4) Function as a metabolic antagonist to thyroxine in the tissues.

Clinical Signs

- Diminished power of concentration.
- Emotional upsets
- Depression
- Irritability
- Swelling of the thyroid gland.
- Breathing problems, if the goitre is large enough to press on the windpipe (trachea).
- Swallowing problems, if the goitre is large enough to press on the oesophagus.

Diagnosis

Thyroid Function Tests

The thyroid function test measures the amount of certain hormones in the blood. An excessive amount of the two hormones produced by the thyroid gland - thyroxine and triiodothyronine - would indicate an underlying condition that is making thyroid gland over-active, such as Grave's disease.

If thyroid gland is under-active, another gland, known as the pituitary gland, will produce a hormone known as thyroid stimulating hormone (TSH). TSH is released by the body in order to stimulate thyroid gland. So a high level of TSH in blood would indicate that thyroid gland is under-active.

Radioactive Iodine Scan

During a radioactive iodine scan, a small amount of radioactive iodine is injected into vein. The iodine then builds up in thyroid gland and can be studied using a special camera.

The scan can provide more information about the structure and function of thyroid gland. The amount of radiation that is used is perfectly safe for most animals, although it may not be suitable if animal is pregnant.

Ultrasound Scan

An ultrasound scan can be used to build up a picture of the inside of thyroid gland, assess its size, and check if there are any enlarged nodules that have not been found during the physical examination.

Treatment of Goitre

- Goitres are often removed because of cosmetic reasons or, more commonly, because they compress other vital structures of the neck including the trachea and the oesophagus making breathing and swallowing difficult
- Benign thyroid nodules - are shrunk with medications, destroyed with radioactive iodine treatment or surgically removed, depending on the type.
- is treated by surgical removal of the gland, followed by radioactive iodine treatment
- If have a small goitre that is not due to a cancerous nodule, and thyroid is making the correct amount of thyroxine and T3, then may not need any treatment.
- If have cancer of the thyroid, will probably need surgery.

If these fail to work, part or all of the thyroid gland is surgically removed alternatively, some or all of the thyroid's hormone-producing cells can be destroyed with radioactive iodine treatment.

Oxalate Poisoning

Oxalic Acid

COOH
COOH is corrosive because acid

Soluble Oxalates

1) Potassium acid oxalate
   COOK
   COOH
2) Sodium oxalate
   COONa
   COONa
3) Ammonium oxalate

Insoluble oxalates include calcium and magnesium salts.

Sources

1. Ethylene glycol (antifreeze) is metabolized to oxalates - kittens and puppies at risk
2. Plants - usually 10% or higher oxalic acid on a dry weight basis - most are palatable
   a. Oxalate ion, pH of 6
1. *Halogeton* - can be 34% soluble oxalates on DM basis
2. *Sarcobatus* (greasewood) - 10 to 20% oxalates
3. *Amaranthus* - usually nitrates
   b. Acid oxalates, pH 2
4. *Rumex* (dock)
   c. Both or unspecified
5. *Rheum* (rhubarb) - petiole contains malonic acid
6. *Beta* (sugar beets) at green and leafy stage, also may have toxic level of nitrates
7. *Aspergillus* - oxalate producing fungi may elevate oxalate content to toxic level in some moldy feeds.

d. Calcium oxalate crystals - insoluble, but once theorized that sharp, cause intense burning if bite plants. Now suspect proteolytic enzyme.

8. *Arisaema* (Jack-in-the-pulpit)
9. *Dieffenbachia* (dumbcane - house plant)
10. *Symplocarpus* (skunk cabbage)
11. *Philodendron* - house plant
12. *Caladium* - house plant.

A Large Amount of Oxalates Must be Eaten to Cause Poisoning Because Most Either

1. Made insoluble as calcium oxalate, if sufficient calcium in diet or
2. Digested to bicarbonate; rumen can handle this metabolism better than simple stomach, also increases in ability to metabolize oxalates with continued ingestion - adapts. Oxalate metabolized to formate and then to CO2.

Results of Oxalate Poisoning Vary According to the Ion

1. GI irritation if eat large amount:Diets with more than 6% oxalates cause diarrhea in sheep - secondary fungal invasion of rumenitis and hepatitis lesions may follow.
2. Removal of calcium from blood - precipitated as calcium oxalate, leads to a hypocalcemic muscle weakness syndrome with hemorrhages (Na oxalate is an anticoagulant because it binds calcium). Hypocalcemia contributes to great decrease in GI motility. Oxalates also have effect of immobilizing calcium in the gut if already on calcium deficient diet.
3. Acute nephrosis and uremia if calcium oxalate crystals precipitate in and block many tubules of the kidney - cumulative damage is possible; more tubules blocked with further exposure.
4. Oxalate calculi in kidney, bladder, urethra if smaller amounts over longer time.
5. Osteodystrophia fibrosa - metabolic bone disease.

Clinical Signs

- Diarrhoea. Colic in Halogeton poisoning.
- Dullness, sheep lags behind others, head drooped at 45 degrees. Signs occur 2-6 hours after ingesting toxic amount - get weakness, muscle tremors, staggering, go down; rapid weak pulse, rapid labored

respiration; rumen atony, dilated pupils; hemorrhages; may see excess salivation, froth at mouth. Coma and death about 10 hours after ingestion. Must differentiate in sheep from Hypocalcemia at parturition or with starvation or forced exercise, also lactation tetany.

- Toxic indigestion - history of overload of grain - splashy, atonic rumen; cold, comatose, hypocalcemic.
- Pregnant and lactating animals are most susceptible to oxalates because greater demand for calcium
- Depression, anuria, may strain to urinate if calculi in urethra. Foul smell from mouth when uremic. Urine may be red-brown.

Diagnosis

- Serum calcium - total may be normal; just unavailable because tied up as calcium oxalate. Ionic, available calcium may drop to 20% of normal at time of death
- Better to assay suspected plant for oxalate level.
- Albuminuria, hematuria from kidney damage. Elevated BUN, creatinine.
- G. Postmortem - no characteristic signs.
  - Cystitis, urethritis, ureteritis
  - Calculi in urethral process of ram, sigmoid flexure of bull and ram.
- Swollen kidney, dark red cortex and medulla of kidney separated by line of gray where oxalates accumulated.
- Histologically, crystals in renal tubules - small, rhomboid, nearly transparent crystals or rosette of crystals occluding lumen of tubule. Crystals in rumen wall also.
- Splashy hemorrhages due to anticoagulant action.

Treatment

- Calcium borogluconate: 50-100 ml in sheep, 500 ml in cows, IV or SC. Usually not enough to save animals because imbalance of other ions has occurred. Na^+ and K^+ liberated when Ca^{++} precipitated, may get alkalosis. Also oxalates have interfered with enzymes activated by calcium and magnesium, thus interfering with energy metabolism. Halogeton sheep don't respond to calcium, but still try.
- Fluids to flush kidneys - dextrose solution IV, force feed water.

Prevention

- Ruminants safer than monogastrics physiologically (detoxify, making carbonates and bicarbonates in the rumen) but management endangers. Sheep are kept on that kind of range, readily eat the oxalate plants.
- *Halogeton* most toxic with rapid growth in autumn after dry summer.
- Sheep vulnerable, when eat indiscriminately:
  - trailing thought dense growth of oxalate plants
  - unloaded into dense growth of oxalate plants
  - watering thirsty animals where plant abounds
    - Salt hunger may predispose, so supply ample salt in diet.
    - Ample water for kidney function
    - Safer if full rumen, so don't trail hungry sheep
    - Can become adapted: switch slowly to high oxalate diet if nothing else to feed;
    - Prophylactic dicalcium phosphate during times of exposure;
  - 1/4 - 1/2 pound alfalfa pellets with 5% dicalP/day (protects 2-4 hours)
  - salt free choice that is 25% dicalP
  - alfalfa hay

Photosensitisation

- Photosensitivity reactions or Photosensitization is a clinical condition in which skin (areas exposed to light and lacking significant protective hair, wool, or pigmentation) is hyperreactive to sunlight due to the presence of photodynamic agents. Molecules of photosensitizing agents present in the skin are energized by light. When the molecules return to the less energized state, the released energy is transferred to receptor molecules that quickly initiate chemical reactions in various skin components. Tissue injury is thought to result from the production of reactive oxygen intermediates or from alterations in cell membrane permeability. Photosensitization can be difficult to differentiate clinically from actual sunburn, though it is totally unrelated to sunburn.

  These reactions are due to the accumulation of photosensitive compounds beneath the skin. These compounds can be the metabolites of drugs or photodynamic substances seen in plants which gain entry to the body after ingestion and get accumulated in the system either unchanged or after metabolism inside the body.

- In some other cases, the photodynamic substances can be produced in the body itself due to some inborn errors of pigment metabolism, especially those involving the heme synthesis. Photosensitivity reactions are usually seen in herbivorous or omnivorous animals, though such reactions are not uncommon among carnivores

  Cattle suffer from this condition when they feed on water damaged alfa alfa hay, drink water from ponds with algae, feed on pasture crops such as lucerne and millet grass. Accidental ingestion of weeds such as lantana and tribulis species and drugs such as carbontetrachloride, tetracyclines, sulfonamides and corticosteriods cause this condition. It is also seen after leptospirosis. Fungal toxins like aflatoxins and rubratoxins which damage the liver, are involved in its etiology.

  The photosensitivity reactions are characterized by the formation of severe inflammation of the skin with depigmentation and ulceration. In some cases, there will be excretion of pigments, which may be fluorescent in nature, through urine or deposition of such pigments in hard tissues such as bones and teeth causing discolouration. The affected animals should be protected from direct sunlight, until the photodynamic compounds have been completely eliminated from the body or appropriate treatments have been given.

Classification of Photosensitivity reactions

Based on the origin, the photosensitivity reactions have been classified into four types - Type I, Type II, Type III and Type IV.

Type I (Primary) Photosensitivity

- It occurs when the photodynamic compounds are directly accumulated under the skin of the body following ingestion. Primary photosensitization occurs when the photodynamic agent is absorbed either through the skin or from the GI tract unchanged, reaching the skin in its native form.
- Such compounds need not undergo metabolism to get activated.
- Examples of primary photosensitizers are hypericin (from *Hypericum perforatum* [St. John's wort]) and fagopyrin (from *Fagopyrum esculentum* [buckwheat]). Plants in the families Umbelliferae and Rutaceae contain photoactive furocoumarins (psoralens), which cause photosensitization in livestock and poultry. *Ammi majus* (bishop's weed) and *Cymopterus watsonii* (spring parsley) have produced photosensitization in cattle and sheep, respectively. Ingestion of *A majus* and *A visnaga* seeds has

produced severe photosensitization in poultry. Species of *Trifolium* , *Medicago* (clovers and alfalfa), *Erodium* , *Polygonum* , and *Brassica* have been incriminated as primary photosensitizers. Many other plants have been suspected, but the toxins responsible

- Some drugs like phenothiazine or its derivatives can also lead to photosensitivity reactions, commonly in sheep. The phenothiazine is converted into phenothiazine sulfoxide, which is the photodynamic compound.

Type II Photosensitivity

- It occurs due to inborn errors in the metabolism of some biological pigments. Due to absence of some key enzymes of metabolism, the products of intermediary metabolism get accumulated.
- Type II photosensitivity due to aberrant pigment metabolism is known to occur in both cattle and cats.
- In this syndrome, the photosensitizing porphyrin agents are endogenous pigments that arise from inherited or acquired defective functions of enzymes involved in heme synthesis. bovine erythropoietic protoporphyria are the most commonly reported diseases in this category.
- They are either eliminated through the urine and body fluids or are deposited in some body tissues like bone and teeth.
- A common condition seen in animals is congenital porphyria due to the accumulation of Uroporphyrin. This compound get deposited in the teeth and bones giving them a pink discolouration. Some times, this compound may get excreted through urine, showing a pinkish fluorescence under ultra violet light.

Type III (Hepatogenous) Photosensitivity

- It is also known as secondary or hepatic photosensitivity, the most common type of photosensitivity reaction seen in animals
- The photosensitizing agent, phylloerythrin (a porphyrin), accumulates in the plasma due to impaired hepatobiliary excretion. Phylloerythrin is derived from the breakdown of chlorophyll by microorganisms present in the GI tract. Phylloerythrin, but not chlorophyll, is normally absorbed into the circulation and is effectively excreted by the liver into the bile. Failure to excrete phylloerythrin due to hepatic dysfunction or bile duct lesions increases the amount in the circulation. Thus, when it reaches

the skin, it can absorb and release light energy, initiating a phototoxic reaction. This condition is exacerbated in the presence of hepatic parasites

- Phylloerythrin has been incriminated as the phototoxic agent in the following conditions: common bile duct occlusion; facial eczema; lupinosis; congenital photosensitivity of Southdown and Corriedale sheep and poisoning by numerous plants including *Tribulis terrestris* (puncture vine), *Lippia rehmanni* , *Lantana camara* , several *Panicum* spp (kleingrass, broomcorn millet, witch grass), *Cynodon dactylon, Myoporum laetum* (ngaio), and *Narthecium ossifragum* (bog asphodel).
- Photosensitization also has been reported in animals that have liver damage associated with various poisonings: pyrrolizidine alkaloid (eg, *Senecio* spp, *Cynoglossum* spp, *Heliotropium* spp, *Echium* spp ; cyanobacteria (*Microcystis* spp, *Oscillatoria* spp), *Nolina* spp (bunch grass), *Agave lechuguilla* (lechuguilla), *Holocalyx glaziovii, Kochia scoparia, Tetradymia* spp (horse brush or rabbit brush), *Brachiaria brizantha, Brassica napus, Trifolium pratense* and *T hybridum* (red and alsike clover), *Medicago sativa, Ranunculus* spp, phosphorus, and carbon tetrachloride. Phylloerythrin is likely the phototoxic agent in many of these poisonings.

Type IV (Idiopathic) Photosensitivity

- It is another type of photosensitivity reaction which occurs following the ingestion of some plants like alfalfa. The reason is obscure or idiopathic.
- Photosensitivity where the pathogenesis is unknown is classified as type IV. Examples include winter wheat (cattle), *Medicago* spp (alfalfa), *Brassica* spp (mustards), and *Kochia scoparia* (fireweed).

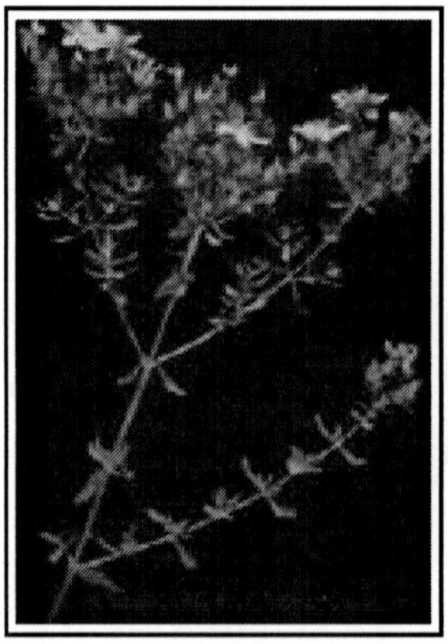

Hypericum perforatum

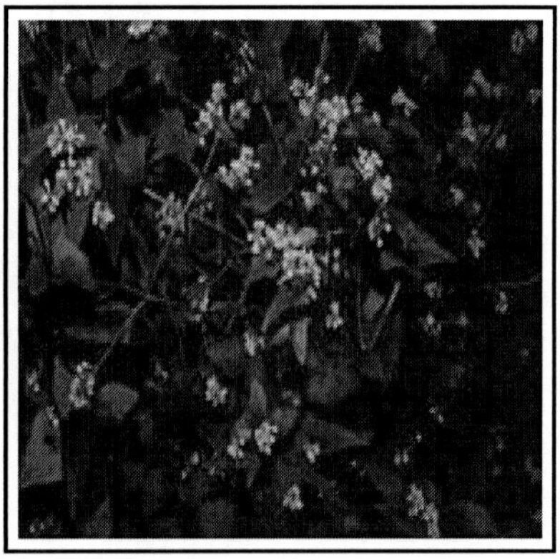

Fagopyrum esculentum

Clinical Findings and Lesions

The clinical signs associated with photosensitivity are similar regardless of the cause. Photosensitive animals are photophobic immediately when exposed to sunlight and squirm in apparent discomfort.

- They scratch or rub lightly pigmented, exposed areas of skin (eg, ears, eyelids, muzzle). Severe phylloerythrinemia and bright sunlight can induce typical skin lesions, even in black-coated animals.
- Erythema develops rapidly and is soon followed by edema. If exposure to light stops at this stage, the lesions soon resolve.
- When exposure is prolonged, serum exudation, scab formation, and skin necrosis are marked.
- In cattle, and especially in deer, exposure of the tongue while licking may result in glossitis, characterized by ulceration and deep necrosis.
- Activation of photodynamic substance liberates histamine, which causes redness, swelling, leakage of serum from damaged capillaries, death of tissue and sloughing of skin. Intense itching makes the animal restless and rub against objects causing tissue injury and secondary bacterial infection.
- Conjunctivitis is prominent.
- In addition to the above, Depending on the initial cause of the accumulation of the photosensitizing agent, other clinical signs may be seen. For example, if the photosensitivity is hepatogenous, icterus may be present. In bovine congenital erythropoietic porphyria, discoloration of dentin, bone (and other tissues), and urine often accompanies the skin lesions. Photodermatitis is the sole manifestation observed in bovine erythropoietic protoporphyria.
- Liver damage results in off feed, diarrhoea, jaundice and decreased production of milk, meat and wool.

Diagnosis

- Clinical signs are easily recognized in cases of marked photosensitivity but are similar to the primary actinic effects of sunburn in early or mild cases.
- Reference to the specific diseases in which photosensitization is an objective sign may assist in diagnosis of the underlying disease.
- Evaluation of serum liver enzymes and liver biopsies may be necessary to confirm the presence of hepatic disease.
- Examination of blood, faeces, and urine for porphyrins can also be performed.

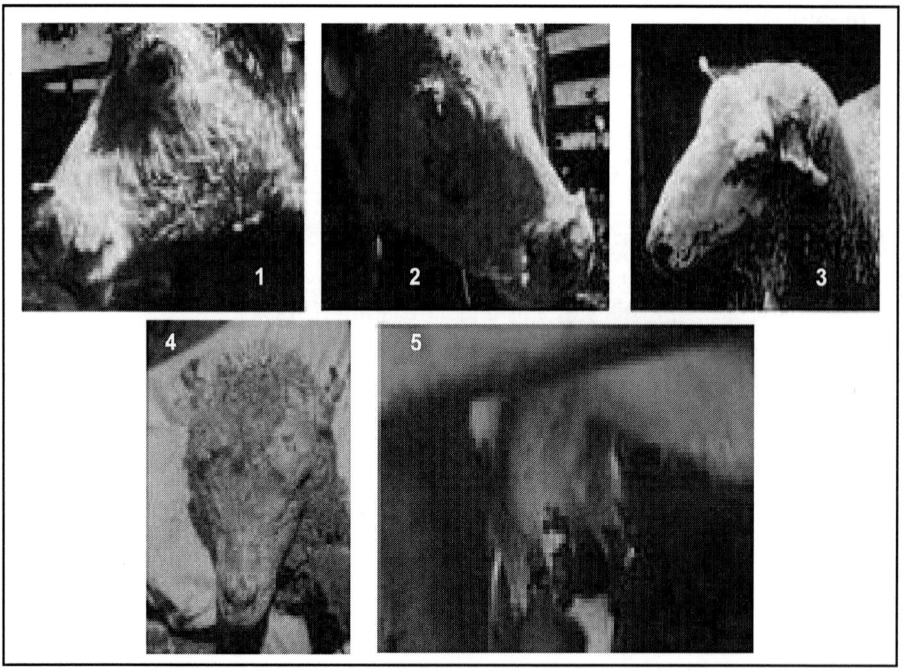

1 & 2 Cattle with conjunctivitis and muzzle being effected
3 & 5 Sheep affected in non-hairy areas, **4.** Udder affected with congestion

Treatment

The prognosis and eventual productivity of an animal is related to the site and severity of the primary lesion and/or hepatic disease, and to the degree of resolution

Treatment involves mostly palliative measures. While photosensitivity continues, animals should be shaded fully or, preferably, housed and allowed to graze only during darkness. The severe stress of photosensitization and extensive skin necrosis can be highly debilitating and increase mortality. Corticosteroids, given parenterally in the early stages, may be helpful. Secondary skin infections and suppurations should be treated with basic wound management techniques, and fly strike prevented. The skin lesions heal remarkably well, even after extensive necrosis.

- Stop feeding the suspected feed / drug. The affected animals should be transferred to shade, indoors.
- To overcome shock, corticosteroid therapy and fluid infusions may be tried

- Antihistamines are also useful.
- Liver tonics
- Skin ointments
- Antibiotics.

Anti-Nutritional Factors, The Potential Risks of Toxicity and Methods to Alleviate Them

Introduction

The anti-nutritional factors (ANFs) may be defined as those substances generated in natural feed stuffs by the normal metabolism of species and by different mechanisms (e.g., inactivation of some nutrients, diminution of the digestive process or metabolic utilization of feed) which exert effects contrary to optimum nutrition. Being an ANF is not an intrinsic characteristic of a compound but depends upon the digestive process of the ingesting animal. Trypsin inhibitors, which are ANFs for monogastric animals, do not exert adverse effects in ruminants because they are degraded in the rumen The utility of the leaves, pods and edible twigs of shrubs and trees as animal feed is limited by the presence of ANFs. In fact, plants contain thousand of compounds which, depending upon the situations, can have beneficial or deleterious effects on organisms consuming them. These compounds, with the exception of nutrients, are referred to as 'allelochemicals' ANFs may be regarded as a class of these compounds, which are generally not lethal. They diminish animal productivity but may also cause toxicity during periods of scarcity or confinement when the feed rich in these substances is consumed by animals in large quantities.

The ANFs which have been implicated in limiting the utilization of shrub and tree forages include non-protein amino acids, glycosides, phytohemagglutinins, polyphenolics, alkaloids, triterpenes and oxalic acid.

Mimosine

Mimosine, a non-protein amino acid structurally similar to tyrosine, occurs in a few species of *Mimosa* and all species of closely allied genus *Leucaena*. Concern has arisen because of the importance of *L. leucocephala*, in which the level of mimosine in the leaf is about 2–6% and varies with seasons and maturity.In non-ruminant animals; mimosine causes poor growth, alopecia, eye cataracts and reproductive problems. Levels of *Leucaena* meal above 5–10% of the diet for swine, poultry and rabbits generally result in poor animal performance. The mechanism of action of mimosine in producing its effect is

Anti-nutritional factors in the leaves of tree and shrubs documented as being used in livestock feeding (Table 1).

	Anti-nutritional substances	Species
1.	Non-protein Amino acids	
	Mimosine	*Leucaena leucocephala*
	Indospecine	*Indigofera spicta*
2.	Glycosides	
	(A) Cyanogens	*Acacia giraffae* *A. cunninghamii* *A. sieberiana* *Bambusa bambos* *Barteria fistulosa* *Manihot esculenta*
	(B) Saponins	*Albizia stipulata* *Bassia latifolia* *Sesbania sesban*
3.	Phytohemagglutinins	
		Bauhinia purpurea
	Ricin	*Ricinus communis*
	Robin	*Robinia pseudoacacia*
4.	Polyphenolic compounds	
	(A) Tannins	All vascular plants
	(B) Lignins	All vascular plants
5.	Alkaloids	
	N-methyl-B-phen	
	ethylamine	*Acacia berlandieri*
	Sesbanine	*Sesbania vesicaria* *S. drummondii* *S. punicea*
6.	Triterpenes	
	Azadirachtin	*Azadirachta indica*
	Limonin	*Azadirachta indica*
7.	Oxalate	*Acacia aneura*

not clear but it may act as an amino acid antagonist or may complex with pyridoxal phosphate, leading to disruption of catalytical action of B6-containing enzymes such as trans-aminases, or may complex with metals such as zinc The main symptoms of toxicity in ruminants are poor growth, loss of hair and wool, swollen and raw coronets above the hooves, lameness, mouth and oesophageal lesions, depressed serum thyroxine level and goitre. Some of these symptoms may be due to mimosine and others to 3, 4 dihydroxypyridine, a metabolite of mimosine in the rumen. Toxic signs like skin lesions also resemble Zn deficiency. Reduction in calving percentage due to *Leucaena* feeding has also been noted. A solution to the mimosine problem could be the development of low mimosine cultivars. However, low mimosine types are found to be unproductive and of low vigor. The other approach is to feed *Leucaena* mixed with other feeds. The use of *Leucaena* fodder may be restricted to 30% of the green forage in the case of cattle and buffalo, and 50% for goats. The effect of *Leucaena* and mimosine can be reduced by heat treatment by supplementation with amino acids or with metal ions such as Fe^{2+}, Al^{3+} and Zn^{+2}.

Cotton Seed Cake (Gossypol)

Not to be fed more than 1 kg/animal/day in ration. The amount of gossypol varies with the method of production. Contra-indicated in young animals as it retards growth and in pregnant animals as it causes teratogenicity.Symptoms are seen after 1-3 months.Signs include loss of appetite, restlessness, gastroenteritis, diarrhoea, dyspnoea and spasms. Animal is weak and reluctant to get up.In poultry - not recommended as gossypol stains yolk - red and egg yield is decreased.Pigs - acute toxicity- anorexia, respiratory symptoms followed by death. Chronic toxicity - vomiting and bloody diarrhea. Rx: Stop feeding cotton seed cake, replace with an easily digestible diet with increased vitamin-A content. Glucose - I/V. Adding Ca.carbonate, which binds gossypol, can reduce toxicity.

Gossypium herbaceum Cotton	Gossypol in cotton seed cake (sheep are susceptible. Hypovitaminosis A.increases susceptibility.	Prolonged feeding for 1-3 months	Cardiac myopathy and hepatic necrosis. Anorexia, dyspnoea and weakness are characteristic. Haematuria.	Prevention is by cooking or by addition of 1% CaOH. or 0.1% ferrous sulfate

Rapeseed Cake (Sinigrin, a cyanogenetic glycoside).

Never exceed 0.5 kg/day in adult cattle. Contra-indicated in pigs, horses and young stock. Sinigrin under optimum temperature, humidity and enzyme-myrosin releases allyl mustard oil (toxic in nature)

Linseed cake (Linamarin, a cyanogenic glycoside).

High quality feed used in young breeding animals and dairy cattle @ 0.2-2kg /head/day.

Cyanogens

Cyanogens are glycosides of a sugar, or sugars, and cyanide containing aglycone. Table 1 provides a few examples of fodder trees and shrubs containing cyanogens.

Cyanogens can be hydrolysed by enzymes to release HCN which is volatile gas. However, the glycosides occur in vacuoles in plant cell and enzymes are found in the cytosol. Damage to the plant results in the enzymes and glycoside coming together and producing HCN. The hydrolytic reaction can take place in the rumen by microbial activity. Hence ruminants are more susceptible to CN toxicity than non-ruminants. The HCN is absorbed and is rapidly detoxified in the liver by the enzyme rhodanese which converts CN to thiocyanate (SCN). Excess cyanide ion inhibits the cytochrome oxidase. This stops ATP formation, tissues suffer energy deprivation and death follows rapidly.

The lethal dose of HCN for cattle and sheep is 2.0–4.0mg per kg body weight. The lethal dose for cyanogens would be 10–20 times greater because the HCN comprises 5–10% of their molecular weight .For poisoning, forage containing this amount of cyanogens would have to be consumed within a few minutes and simultaneous HCN production would have to be rapid. Recorded accounts of livestock poisoning by cyanogenic plants show that such situations do arise.

Cyanide can cause goitrogenic effects due to thiocyanate produced during detoxification. Poor animal performance due to *A. sieberiana* pod feeding has been attributed to cyanogens Cyanogens have also been suspected to have teratogenic effects.Post-harvest wilting of cyanogenic leaves may reduce the risk of cyanide toxicity. Animals suffering from cyanide must be immediately treated by injecting a suitable dose of sodium nitrate and sodium thiosulphate.

Saponins

Saponins are glycosides containing a polycyclic aglycone moiety of either C_{27} steroid or C_{30} triterpenoid (collectively termed as sapogenins) attached to a carbohydrate. They are widely distributed in the plant kingdom. Table 1 includes some of the fodder trees in which they may have nutritional significance.

Saponins are characterised by a bitter taste and foaming properties. Erythrocytes lyses in saponin solution and so these compounds are toxic when injected intravenously. The anti-nutritional effects of saponins have been mainly studied using alfalfa saponins. In non-ruminants (chicks and pigs), retardation of growth rate, due primarily to reduction in feed intake, is probably the major concern. Such effects have also been noted when *Sesbania sesban* leaf meal (saponin 0.71%) was incorporated in a chick diet.

In ruminants, saponins were implicated in causing bloat. Furthermore, because saponins may also undergo bacterial degradation in the rumen, they may not retard the growth of ruminants. Nevertheless, recent studies indicate that they inhibit microbial fermentation and synthesis in the rumen. The adverse effects of saponins can be overcome by repeated washing with water which makes the feed more palatable by reducing the bitterness associated with saponins

Phytohemagglutinins

Phytohemagglutinins, otherwise referred to as lectins, are proteins which agglutinate red blood cells. They have been shown to occur in some important fodder trees (Table 1). The highest concentrations of lectins are found in seeds but, in the leaves, their concentration is low due to translocation. The biological effects of lectins probably result from their affinity for sugars. They may bind to the carbohydrate moieties of cells of the intestinal wall and cause a non-specific interference with nutrient absorption. In fodder trees, the lectins of interest are robin and ricin.

Robin, a lectin from *Robinia pseudoacacia*, has been reported to cause symptoms of anorexia, lassitude, weakness and posterior paralysis in cattle.Ricin occurs in castor beans (*Ricinus communis*) which have been reported to cause poisoning in all class of livestock. Due to ricin, deoiled castor seed cake (CP 35%) is seldom used as a livestock feed. However, the mature leaves of *R. communis* have been found suitable for feeding to sheep; hence precautions against bean contamination are necessary. Castor bean meal can be detoxified by autoclaving at 20 psi for 60 minutes for incorporation in sheep diets.

Tannins

Tannins are water soluble phenolic compounds with a molecular weight greater than 500 and with the ability to precipitate proteins from aqueous solution. They occur almost in all vascular plants. Hydrolysable tannins and condensed tannins (proanthocyanidins) are two different groups of these compounds. Generally tree and shrub leaves contain both types of tannins. The two types differ in their nutritional and toxic effects. The condensed tannins have a more profound digestibility-reducing effect than hydrolysable tannins, whereas the latter may cause varied toxic manifestations due to hydrolysis in rumen. Animals like mule deer, rats and mice have been shown to secrete proline-rich proteins in saliva which constitute the first line of defence against ingested tannins. Nevertheless, deleterious effects and episodes of toxicity suggest the inadequacy of defence against high quantities of dietary tannins.

The anti-nutritional effects of the tannins present in tree leaves are summarised in Table 2. The mechanism of dietary effects of tannins may be understood by their ability to form complex with proteins. Tannins may form a less digestible complex with dietary proteins and may bind and inhibit the endogenous protein, such as digestive enzymes. Tannin-protein complexes involve both hydrogen-bonding and hydrophobic interactions; the precipitation of the protein-tannin complex depends upon pH, ionic strength and molecular size of tannins. Both the protein precipitation and incorporation of tannin phenolics into the precipitate increase with the increase in molecular size of tannins. However, when the molecular weight is very large (>5000), the tannins become insoluble and loose their protein precipitating capacity. Hence the measurement of the phenolic profile in terms of total phenols, condensed tannins, their protein precipitating capacity and degree of polymerization becomes imperative to asses the role of tannins in ruminant nutrition. In tree leaves tannins are present in NDF and ADF in significant amounts which are tightly bound to the cell wall and cell protein and seem to be involved in decreasing digestibility. Hence, there is a need to account for these tannins in estimating the nutritive value of tree leaves. number of methods have been tried to overcome the deleterious effects of tannins. Alkali treatments include ferrous sulphate and polyethylene glycol-4000 (PEG-4000); the last was found to be effective for deactivation of tannins in tree leaves. However, using PEG-4000 in routine feeding may not be economic. Three months feeding of *P. cineraria* leaves and *Cenchrus* spp. (50:50) with 1% urea has been found to maintain adult sheep. In such a feeding system, urea not only provides extra nitrogen to the animals but also deactivates the leaf tannins. Therefore, the use of urea to overcome the deleterious effects of tannin may be of practical value.

Other Anti-Nutritional Factors

Apart from the ANFs discussed in preceding sections, shrub and tree forage may contain alkaloids, terpenoids, oxalate, indospecine, lignins (Table 1) and certain other ANFs. Alkaloids such as N-methyl-a phenethylamine cause locomotor ataxia of the hindquarters in sheep. Sesbaine causes haemorrhagic diarrhoea. The terpenoids azadirachtin and limonin impart a bitter taste and the leaves of *Azadirachta indica* are therefore not relished by cattle. Oxalate in the leaves of *Acacia aneura* may limit the Ca availability and a negative correlation between digestibility and lignin content has been observed.

Table 2

Fodder Tree/Shrub	Predom-inant Tannin*	Animal	Nutritional Effect
Acacia aneura	CT	Sheep	Reduction in N digestibility decreased wool yield and growth, decreased S absorption
A. cyanophylla	CT	Sheep	Reduced feed intake, negative N digestibility, loss in weight
A. nilotica (pods)	CT	Sheep	Low growth rate, reduced N and NDF digestibility
A.sieberiana (Pods)	HT	Sheep	Low growth rate, reduced N and NDF digestibility
Albizia chinensis	CT	Goat	Reduced *in sacco* N digestibility
Leucaena leucocephala	CT	Poultry	Poor N retention, low apparent metabolisable energy value
Manihot esculenta	CT	*In vitro*	Inhibits digestibility
Prosopis cineraria	CT	Sheep	Reduction in feed intake protein, digestibility, decreased wool yield & growth, decreased iron absorption
Robinia pseudoacacia	CT	Rat	Reduced protein digestibility
		Rabbit	Reduced feed intake & growth, cecotrophy increased protein digestibility
Ziziphus nummularia	CT	Sheep	Reduction in feed intake protein and DM digestibility

Studying the ANFs: A Challenge

As previously noted, most of the ANFs belong to a group of related compounds with similar mode of actions. There are about 8,000 polyphenols,

270 non-protein amino acids, 32 cyanogens, 10,000 alkaloids and several saponins which have been reported to occur in various plant species. Studying such a vast number of compounds is bound to provide major challenges.

1. *Detection*: This can be approached either by evaluating animal performance or by chemical analysis. Certain ANFs can be detected through chemical analysis but it is not easy to look for all possible allelochemicals in a single plant. Furthermore, lesser known fodder trees and shrubs may contain unknown ANFs and their presence would only be revealed through feeding trials, not by chemical analysis directed at known compounds.
2. *Quantification*: There is wide variation in the reported concentration of ANFs in the same plant species. This may be either real, because of the changes occurring due to environmental conditions, or may arise because of lack of standardization of methods between laboratories, as well as their destruction in assays.
3. *Assessment of biological effects*: It is often observed that sensitivity to ANFs varies between species of animals, different ages and physiological stages. Furthermore, the leaves of a particular tree or shrub may contain different group of ANFs and it becomes difficult to separate their biological effects.

Methods to Alleviate: An Overview

1. The uncertainty of quantification and the imperfectly understood biological effects of ANFs impede the development of methods to alleviate their effects. The simplest approach of dilution, i.e., feeding allelochemical containing leaves in mixtures with other feeds, may certainly reduce the risk of toxicity but simultaneous nutritional benefits may not accrue. Moreover the required degree of dilution is difficult to recommend because of uncertain quantification.
2. Tannin-rich leaves, in combination with concentrate rations, could be fed to animals without any adverse effect. This happens because animals consume protein in excess of their requirement from the concentrate and therefore, the antinutritional effects of tannins were masked.
3. The utility of management practices involving lopping/harvesting of tree leaves at times when the concentration of ANFs are lowest, is limited because pattern of changes in concentration of various allelochemicals

may not be same. For a particular ANF, the effect of season also varies between plant species. It has also been noted that, as leaves mature, both the ANF and nutrient contents decrease.

4. Another approach of supplementation, e.g., polyethylene glycol-4000 with tannin-rich leaves, may be suitable during acute shortage to avoid livestock losses. These cannot be used routinely because of prohibitive costs. However, metal ions and urea supplementation could be recommended to farmers after thoroughly assessing their alleviating effects against highest possible reported concentrations of allelo-chemicals.

5. Many ANFs are heat labile. Hence simple heating or autoclaving has been found useful in removing the effects of allelochemicals. This practice can be used by the feed industry but not by farmers. Unfortunately, heating would substantially increase the cost due to the energy involved both in the treatment and transport. The efficacy of wilting in reducing the risk of cyanide toxicity needs to be tested before it is recommended to farmers. Simple washing with water removes the soluble allelochemicals but nutrients also leach out.Since ANFs have a major role in plant defence, selecting for low ANFs lines may have undesirable effects on the plant.

6. Alleviation By Rumen Microbial Activity : Ruminant animals have a symbiotic relationship with rumen microorganisms. The rumen environment (slightly acidic pH:E° = -0.35V; 10^{10} microbes/ml) provides many reductive and hydrolytic reactions which, in the majority of cases, decrease the biological activity of the allelochemicals before their absorption from the tract. Rumen bacteria and fungi capable of degrading lignin have been isolated. Anaerobic degradation of flavonoid and hydrolysable tannins by mixed rumen microbes has also been demonstrated. Such rumen microbes are present in small numbers and their growth rate is slow. Anaerobic microbial degradation of condensed tannins has also been demonstrated. Dietary oxalate can be degraded by rumen microbes into CO_2 and formic acid. Ruminants adapted to diets with high oxalate content can tolerate oxalate levels that are lethal to non-adapted animals. Evidence also exists that rumen microbes can be genetically manipulated. These findings imply that towards identification of the various anaerobic and rumen microbes capable of dissimilating ANFs, so that genetic manipulation of rumen bacteria can be effected for the useful fermentation of ANFs.

List of Phytotoxins with their Toxic Priniciples Clinical Signs and Treatment

Botanical Name	Toxic Principle	Clinical Signs	Treatment
Abrus precatorius	Abrin	Intensive irritation, inflammation, oedema, ecchymoses, necrosis at the site of roduction. Anorexia, salivation, incoordination, muscular spasms and convulsions.Animal dies in2-3 days.	Activated charcoal, demulcents, saline purgatives, fluid therapy
Adhatoda vasica	Vasiciinne	PersistentBronchodilation, hypotension, uterotonic, abortifacient, cardiac depression	Symptomatic
Allium cepa Onion	n-propyl disulfide	Haemoglobinuria. Anaemia. In extreme cases onion odour in urine and tissues.	Symptomatic
Areca catechu betel-nut palm	Arecoline	Emesis, exaggerated catharsis, colic, diarrhea, restlessness, convulsions	Atropine sulphate 0.044mg/kg BW
Argemone mexicana	Sanguinarine	Glaucoma, ascites	Diuretics, supportive therapy
Atropa belladonna Datura stramonium Solanum nigrum	Atropine Atropine, hyoscine and hyoscyamine Solanine, solanidine, tropeine	Mydriasis,cycloplegia,anorexia, muscular spasms, dryness of mouth,tachycardia respiratory depression and nervous symptoms.	Emetics – to empty stomach contents. Mild cholinergics, sedatives / hypotics to medullary stimulatnts-Nikethamide, Leptazole)
Beta vulgaris Amaranthus viridis, Chenopodium albua, Solanum spp., Trianthema spp. Oxalis spp, Calandrinia, Atriplex spp.	Oxalates	Vomiting, depression, ataxia, weakness, dehydration, thirst, renal failure due to haematuria/anuria, coma	Antiemeticis, antihistaminics, gastric lavage with 5% soda bicarb. solution, lime water, dicalcium PO_4 in feed
Brassica nigra	Sinigrin	Acute gastroenteritis,colic,dyspnoea	symptomatic
Calotropis gigantica	Gigantin (a glycoside)	Gastro intestinal upset, loose stool, vomiting, cardiac arrhythmia	Rest, control arrhythmia with anti arrhythmics like Phenytion, Lignocaine, Propranol, Potassium chloride 0.6-1mg orally followed by 0.3-0.5g (Dogs) in every 2hrs.
Calotropis procera	Glycoside (digitalis like action on heart)		
Capsicum annum	capsaicin	GI irritant, vomiting and diarrhoea. Not likely to be lethal.	Symptomatic; irritation relief—cool water irrigation, topical or oral mineral or vegetable oil. Rarely topical anesthetics.
Cassia tora	anthraquinone	Colic,Diarrhoea,Ascites	Symptomatic
Crotolaria juncea	Monocrotaline or related pyrrolizidine alkaloids in seeds.	Bloody faeces, salivation, nasal discharge, jaundice, dyspnoea, and colic.	Symptomatic
Croton tiglium	Crotonalic acid Tiglicacid	Nausea,tympanitis, colic and diarrhoea.	Symptomatic, demulcents,. astringents and anti peristaltic agents like Loperamide

contd...

Table contd...

Digitalis purpurea	Digitalis	Gastro intestinal upset, loose stool, vomiting, cardiac arrhythmia	Rest, control arrhythmia with anti arrhythmics like Phenytion, Lignocane, Propanol, Potassium chloride 0.6-1mg orally followed by 0.3-0.5g (Dogs) in every 2hrs.
Equisetum arvense	Thiaminase	Excitement, nervous signs, nystagmus, opisthotonus, weakness, diarrhea, crouching stance	Thiamine parenterally
Eupatorium odoratum	Sterols, Flavones	Nephrotoxic and hepatotoxic signs,	Saline purgatives, fluids, , liver tonics
Gossypium herbaceum	Gossypol	Cardiac myopathy and hepatic necrosis.Anorexia, dyspnoea and weakness are characteristic. Haematuria.	Symptomatic Prevention is by cooking or by addition of 1% CaOH. or 0.1% ferrous sulfate
Hypericum perforatum Fagopyrum esculentum Lantana camara Tribulus terrestris Medicago sativa lucerne	hypericin fagopyrin Lantadene saponins	photosensitisation. signs redness, swelling, serous fluid oozing from skin surfaces, oedema and sloughing of skin. Intense itching causing tissue injury and secondary bacterial infection. Eartip, nose muzzle,udder, teats are affected Conjunctivitis , liver damage signs	topical demulcent, antibiotics, corticosteroids, antihistamines, antibiotics, DNS, saline purgatives and liver tonics
HysocyamusNiger	Hyoscyamine	Delerium, Vocalisation, Terminal Convulsions	Symptomatic & Anticonvulsants
Ipomoea carnea	Ipomeanols. (toxic saponin). Photosensitive principle	Pulmonary emphysema and oedema.Lysis of RBC, anaemia and lumbar paralysis in S&G. Hepatic derangement	B-complex vit. Nervine tonics lipotropics & haematinics.
Jatropha curcas	curcin	Drastic purgation, nausea, vomition, sedation	Symptomatic
Lathyrus odorata	Betaine(β-minopropio nitrite lathyrine)	Leg weakness leading to paralysis (Neuro-osteo-angio lathyrism), rapid, irregular pulse, resp. distress	Symptomatic treatment, calcium supplementation
Leucaena leucocephala Mimosa pudica	Mimosine	Mimosine is antimitotic, goitrogen, depilatory agent. Alopecia in all species Anorexia, salivation, vomition, inco-ordinated gait, loss of body wt. Mucosal ulceration, ear and eye lesions, scaly skin.	Supplement with L-phenylalanine and L – tyrosine. Treat leucaena meal with 0.05 N sod. acetate.
Lobelia spp.	Lobelin	Depression,Diarrhoea,oral ulcers,Heamorrhages,tremors,paralysis	Symptomatic
Meliolotus spp.	Dicumarol	Extensive sub-cultaneous haemorrhages, impaired clotting	Symptomatic treatment, calcium supplementation
Nerium oleander	Oleandroside, nerioside, nerin in leaves, pods and fruit	Violent vomition, diarrhoea, ruminal atony and bloat, colic, cardiac arrhythmias and convulsions.	Symptomatic. Atropine 0.5 mg /kg. i/v. along with propranolol 5 mg/kg. i/v.

contd...

Table contd...

Nicotiana tobaccum	Nicotine	Clonic-tonic convulsions, depression, OP poisoning like symptoms	Oxygen therapy, caffeine and symptomatic
Papaver somniferum	Morphine	CNS stimulations, seizures, gastro intestinal disturbances	Narcotic antagonists like Naloxone 0.04 mg/kg BW (Dogs) IV/IM, sedatives
Parmetia perlata	Usnic acid	Incordination, depression, paralysis	Symptomatic treatment
Parthenium hysterophorus	Histaminergic/ allergic.	Photosensitisation. rash, swelling on face, dewlap, neck and various parts of body. Intense itching causing open wounds.	Anti-histaminics. Antibiotics. Corticosteroids.
Ricinus communis <u>Castor plant</u>	Ricin	Bloody diarrhea in cattle. (Horses - tumultous heart beat).	Specific antiserum Sedatives Shock therapy. Prevention –boiling the cake, ricin coagulates.
Robinia pseudoacasia	tannins	Colic, neurosis	Symptomatic treatment
Sesbania grandiflora	Saponine	Colic, depression, salivation	Symptomatic treatment
Solanum tuberosum	L-chalconine, solanidine, solanicin, solanine	Severe colic, salivation, depression, trembling, paralysis, coma	Gastric lavage, demulcents, symptomatic treatment
Strychnos Nuxvomica	Strychnine and brucine	Spinal convulsions.Signs – Muscular spasms, convulsions, opisthotonus, dilated pupil, asphyxia, paralysis of respiratory muscles.	Sedatives,hypnotics nticonvulsants. Gastric lavage with dil. $KMnO_4$/ Tannic acid.
Thevetia peruviana	Thevetin and other cardiac glycosides	Toxic to heart violent vomition, diarrhoea, ruminal atony and bloat, colic, cardiac arrhythmias and convulsions.	Symptomatic. Atropine 0.5 mg /kg. i/v. along with propranolol 5 mg/kg. i/v.
Withania somnifera	withaferine	CNS depression signs	symptomatic

Chapter 6

PESTICIDAL TOXICOLOGY

Introduction

In the thirst of modernization and industrialization man has contributed pollution to the life and ecology of plants, animals and microbes. Increased demand for food and fiber has lead to the chemicalization of agriculture we have reached to such a stage that modern agriculture is dependent on high yielding varieties, which can only be grown under the influence of fertilizers and pesticides. Pesticides are the man made chemicals which are being used to produce enough cheap food. In India, 90,000 MT of technical grade pesticides are used annually to control pests and plant diseases. The pesticides are classified as insecticides, fungicides, weedicides, herbicides, nematodicides and rodenticides; of which insecticides constitutes 77% of the total pesticides used in different agricultural and animal husbandry practices and in public health operations.

History of pesticides

- 1000 : B.C. Sulfur
- 900s : Arsenic
- 1700s : Rotenone, Pyrethrins
- 1800s : Copper sulfate, nicotine, Mercury
- 1940s : DDT, Ops, Warfarin
- 1950s : OC, Carbamates, Chlorophenoxy
- 1960s : Triazines, Paraquat, Alachlor, Dithiocarbamates
- 1970s : Pyrethroids, Glycophosphate
- 1980 : Neonicotinoids
- 1990s : Phenylpyrazoles
- 1990s : Genetically Modified Seeds

Majority of these pesticides are beneficial when used for specific purposes, handled properly and applied as per the recommendations of the manufacturer. However, over the years, there has been a mounting fear and concern that indiscriminate and improportionate use of pesticides may lead to their residues in food chain which may exert their harmful effects in human beings and animals. In an ideal pesticide application, the chemical should fall exactly on the target and be degraded completely to harmless compounds but this never occurs and only some part of the pesticide hits the target pests while remaining drifts into the environment.

If we look retrospectively, we find that the use of pesticides started during second world war when these hazardous and toxic poisons were considered as chemical weapons. Paul Muller, a swiss scientist, invented DDT in the year 1939 which was considered as a wonder chemical that kills the insects, pests and was found wonderful in malaria control programmes. But soon after the discovery of DDT, its harmful effects also came into the knowledge of the scientists. In 1944, A famous biologist found harmful effects of DDT in birds, which produced thin shelled eggs, easily broken in nests resulting into failure of reproduction and decline of bird population.

Since then pesticides are increasingly used by farmers as wonder chemicals that kills the insects, weeds, fungus and helps in getting rid of the insect transmitted diseases. In India, the insecticide consumption increased from 2000 MT in 1955 to 90,000M tons in 1998-99 which is only 400-450 gm per hectare in comparison to Japan 12000 gm/hectare. DDT and BHC have been banned in other countries. India has categorised it as restricted pesticide to be used only in ublic health operations. Inspite of this, India amounts to 777 of DDT and 95% of BHC out of their total production in the world. In spite of ban, DDT and BHC are still produced in India and we have 77% DDT and 95% BHC in India out of their total production in world.

Consumption of Pesticides

1. India - 400 g/hectare
2. Mexico - 750 g/hectare
3. USA - 3000 g/hectare
4. Germany - 3000 g/ hectare
5. Japan - 12000 g/hectare

The amount of pesticide used in India is very low in comparison to other developed nations. Even then we have much higher polluted food in our country, it may be because of following reasons which needs to be looked into for the control of pesticide induced problems :

1. Indiscriminate use of pesticides
2. Inproportionate use of pesticides
3. Lack of education
4. Lack of extension activities
5. Inadequate literature supplied by the manufacturers
6. To increase production
7. To get more profit
8. Lack of safer pesticides
9. Use of banned pesticides
10. Negative role of Developed Nations
11. Man is ultimate consumer.

Status of Pesticide Residues in India

The presence of pesticide residues have been detected in various items and in food chain. The levels of the pesticides are found much higher than expected level because of heavy contamination of environment. A list of commodities is given in which very significant levels of pesticides are recorded see (Table 1). Besides, human milk, fat or tissue samples screened for the presence of pesticide residues were also found to have very significant levels of harmful pesticides. The BHC has been found from 0.120 to 1.22 ppm in human fat samples. Heptachlor, an organochlorine pesticide was found to be 0.425 ppm and DDT from 0.195 to 1.695 ppm. Even human breast milk is not free from DDT, which was found to be upto 2.39 ppm levels. Similarly human blood was found to have a much higher concentration of 12.00 ppm as against of 0.050-ppm safe levels (no effect levels).

Table 1: Pesticide residues in food chain

S.No.	Items	Pesticide residues detected
1.	Soil and water	Permethrin, cypermethrin, fenvalerate, deltamethrin, DDT, Aldrin, Dieldrin , BHC, Heptachlor, Lindane, Endosulfan
2.	Air	DDT. BHC
3.	Fodder (Lucerne)	Monocrotophos, Phosphomidon, Endosulfan
4.	Cattle feed	Cypermethrin, DDT, BHC
5.	Pasture & Hay	DDT. Aldrin, Dieldrin, BHC, Heptachlor., Lindane .
6.	Rice, wheat flour, oils	DDT, BHC
7.	Dairy Products, baby milk powder, butter, ghee, cow/ buffalo milk	DDT, BHC, HCB, PCB, Heptachlor
8.	Meat, Eggs	DDT, heptachlor, PCB, Carbaryl
9.	Liver, Kidneys, Hair, skin	Cypermethrin
10.	Vegetables	Endosulfan
11.	Adipose tissue of man	BHC, DDT, PCB, HCB, Heptachlor, Aldrin
12.	Human breast milk	BHC, DDT, Aldrin, Heptachlor, HCH
13.	Blood of man	BHC, DDT, Aldrin, Heptachlor, HCH

The primary concern of the chronic low dose toxicity in man and animals is related to the carcinogenic, teratogenic, mutagenic, immunotoxic, immunopathological and/or neuropathic effects of pesticides. The perusal of literature in this regard reveals the studies directed towards only one or two pesticides while in nature, when a large number of pesticides are present and their combined effect has not been measured; which of course will give very dangerous view. Various Pathological effects of low doses of pesticides in animals and man are as under.

1. Immunopathological effects:
    a) Acquired Immunodeficiency
    b) Autoimmunity
    c) Hypersensitivity
2. Carcinogenic effects
3. Mutagenicity
4. Teratogenicity
5. Neuropathy
6. Nephropathy
7. Hepatotoxicity
8. Reproductive Disorders.

Strategies to Combat with Pesticide Residues

1. The farmers should be advised about the harmful effects of pesticides so that they should minimize the use of pesticides in crops. They should judiciously use the pesticide in terms of their quantity and frequency.
2. It should be assured that the pesticides produced in country should be distributed proportionately so that the indiscriminate and improportionate use can be avoided.
3. All emphasis must be laid on the development of Bio-pesticides like viral, bacterial or fungal pesticides or pesticides of botanical origin like Neem or Tulsi, which can be used on crops to kill the insect pests without polluting the environment.
4. The harmful pesticides like some organochlorines, organophosphates and carbamates must be banned strictly in India, their production, import or use should be completely banned.
5. To reduce the effect of pesticide residues, some herbal preparations should be developed which can overcome the immunopathological, neuropathic or nephropathy effects, there are many herbs mentioned in our Indian ancient literature, which can be scientifically validated to prevent and control the harmful effects of pesticides. This will certainly give a new direction to the world not to depend on synthetic things.

Classification of Pesticides

1. Insecticides

a) Organochlorine Compounds

i) Dichlorodiphenyl ethanes : DDT, Dicofol
ii) Chlorinated Cyclodienes : Aldrin Endosulfan, Dieldrin
iii) Hexchlorcyclohexanes : Lindane
iv) Arl hydrocarbons : BHC, kepone, mirex

b) Organophosphorus Compounds

i) Phosphates & pyrophosphates : Paraoxan, TEPP, Dichlorovos, schraden
ii) Phosphonates : Trichlorfon
iii) Phorothiolates: Profenophos, echothiophate
iv) Phosphoramidates : Phospholan mephospholan
v) Phosphorohalides : Sarin, DFP (diisopropylphosphorofluoridate)
vi) Phosphorocyanides : Tabun
vii) Phosphorothionates : Parathion, fenthion, Diazinon
viii) Based on action : Direct acting dichlrovos, DFP, TEPP

2. Indirect acting : Malathion, Parathion, Triazophos

c) Carbamate Insecticides

i) Naphthyl carbamates : Carbaryl (sevin)
ii) Phenyl Carbamates : Propoxur
iii) Heterocyclic methylcarbamates : Pyrolan
iv) Heterocyclic dimethyl carbamates : Carbofuran, furadan
v) Oximes : Aldicarb, thiodicarb

d) Pyrethriods

i. Natural : Pyrethrum extracts
ii. Synthetic : Cypermethrin, flumethrin, permethrin, deltamethrin.

e) Formamidine Insecticides : Amitraz

f) Natural Insecticides : Rotenone, Nicotine

3. Herbicides

I) Inorganic

i. Arsenicals : Sodium arsenite
ii. Chlorates : Sodium chlorate

II) Organic

i. Dinitrocompounds : Dintrophenol
ii. Phenoxyacetic acids : 2,4-D,-2,4,5-T
iii. Bipyridinium compounds : Paraquat, diquat
iv. Triazenes : Atrazine, propazine
v. Choroalipathic acids : Dalapan
vi. Substituted ureas : Diuron, isoprotouron
vii. Substituted dinitroanilines : Pendimethalin
viii. Carbamates : Barban, propham
ix. Uracils : Bromacil, isocil
x. Chlorobenzoic acids : Chloramben, dicamba
xi. Diphenyl esters : Nitrofen, lactofen.

4. Rodenticides

i) Inorganic Rodenticides

a. Arsenic compounds : Arsenic trioxide, sodium hydrogen arsenite
   i. Fluorine compounds : Sodium fluorosilicate
   ii. Bariumcarbonate
   iii. Elementary phophorus
   iv. Thalium sulphate
   v. Zinc phosphide

ii) Organic Rodenticides

1. Anticoagulants : Warfarin
2. ANTU
3. Sodium fluoroacetate
4. Bromethalin
5. Cholicaliceferol
6. Strychinine
7. Redsquil
8. Norbormide
9. Crimidine.

5. Fungicides

1. Inorganic Compounds

- Sulphur & Chemicals like copper sulphate Cadmium Chloride, Bordeaux mixture ($CuSo_4$ + $CaCl_2$)

2. Organic Compounds

i) Organomercurial compounds : Phenyl mercuric chloride
ii) Dithiocarbamates : Zineb, maneb
iii) Chlorophenols : Trichlorophenol, pentachlorophenol
iv) Phathalimides : Captan, folpet
v) Benzimidazoles : Benomyl, thiophantamethyl
vi) Organic tin compounds : Methyl bromide organotin, triphenyltin
vii) Miscellaneous : Cyclohexmide, pyrozophos, terrazole

6. Fumigants

i) Inorganic : Aluminium phosphide, HCN, SO_2, carbondisulphide
ii) Organic: Methylbromide, ethyleneoxide, ethylenedibromide, chloropicrin

Insecticides

Organochlorine Insecticides

Organochlorine insecticides (OCs) are chlorinated hydrocarbon insecticides. These compounds appear to share the same mechanism with regard to neurotoxicity.

Sources

- DDT type (diphenyl aliphatic) - includes DDT, methoxychlor, perthane, and dicofol
  - Methoxychlor is used a lot, including products for use around gardens, animals.
- Miscellaneous (mirex, kepone, paradichlorobenzene).
- Paradichlorobenzene.

DDT Type Organochlorine Insecticides

Toxicodynamics

Peripheral Nerves and Brain

- Slows down the turning off of the Na^+ influx and inhibits the turning on of the K^+ outflux; results in more of each cation inside the nerve than normal. Therefore, the inside of nerve membrane is more positive (partially depolarized)-which decreases the threshold for another action potential to occur. Sensory nerves are more readily affected by DDT than are motor nerves.

- EEG shows a diffuse low amplitude, fast frequency pattern due to partial depolarization of neurons.
- Methoxychlor, perthane, dicofol are similar to DDT in structure and mechanism.
- Methoxychlor has estrogenic effects in rats. Enhances female sexual behavior but reduces fertility
- Methoxychlor is readily metabolized and excreted.
- Mirex and kepone may have the same neurotoxic mechanism as DDT; however, mirex may also inhibit the postsynaptic binding of GABA.

Toxicity and Clinical Signs

All of these agents mainly cause tremors, salivation, ataxia, depression and sometimes vomiting. Seizures may occur in cats at low doses or in other species with very high doses. LD_{50} in most species tend to be relatively high. Absorption is variable and are typically very fat soluble.

- Potent mixed-function oxidase inducer
- Egg shell thinning - birds of prey especially aquatic predators (e.g., bald eagles, ospreys, brown pelicans)
- O'P'DDD (synonymous with TDE) and especially DDE are persistent metabolites in environment and in body
- O'P'DDD - causes thinning of the adrenal cortex in the dog; therefore used to treat Cushing's disease in the dog. Excessive use can cause Addisonian crisis. Potential problem in DDT exposed dogs
- LD_{50} rat (oral) for DDT is 113 - 2500 mg/kg & rat (iv) is 47 mg/kg
- Note in humans: Toxic signs at 10 mg/kg (oral)
- Paradichlorobenzene
  - LD_{50} oral : mouse - 3.2 g/kg, rat - 2.5 g/kg & rabbit - 2.8 g/kg.

Residues

- In addition to acute toxicoses - a primary concern, with regard to the more persistent organchlorines and their metabolites, is residues in the fats of meat and milk. Tendency to store in fat is a function of the rate of metabolism and excretion.
- Since organochlorines were used extensively in agriculture, they are often found in storage or as residues in soil on farms, near feed mills, etc., and can find their way into farm animals, usually via feed.

- Methoxychlor - eliminated fairly rapidly but still had a 30-day withdrawal at one time. More rapid dechlorination and especially oxidation versus DDT.
- DDT - concern regarding cancer, possibly unfounded. Potent mixed function oxidase inducer. DDE, DDT persistent in fat.
- For residue concerns monitor :
  - Milk fat: values may approximate body fat concentrations.
  - Fat biopsy: In cattle, fat may be taken from the tailhead, neck, and scrotum of steers. Prefer to avoid perirenal fat even at necropsy unless other fat is unavailable.
  - Can use experimentally derived data for a particular organochlorine to calculate time needed for a known concentration in body fat to fall below actionable level.

    Note: logical to consult with a veterinary toxicologist when trying to address recommendations for contaminated food animals.
  - Biological magnification—concentration in lipids of successive predators. Can sometimes result in chronic or acute (lethal) toxicoses. Most likely when aquatic systems are involved because: 1) food chains are longer permitting a greater number of bioconcentrations and 2) lipid soluble compounds are readily acquired from the environment especially sediments and the surface microlayer of natural waters. These compounds are washed into streams but are poorly soluble in the water column. Sediment concentrations should be checked.
  - Paradichlorobenzene is well absorbed, undergoes glucuronide or sulfate conjugation, and is eliminated over a period of days via the urine and bile.

Ionic Movements During Postsynaptic Potentials

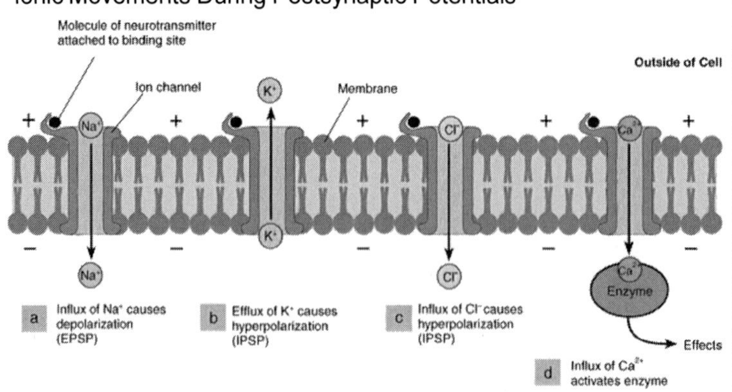

Diagnosis of Acute Toxicoses

- History of exposure, appropriate clinical signs.
- Brain analysis important for diagnosis of acute toxicosis:
  - Submit half a brain frozen
  - Other half fixed for histopathology to rule out infectious (encephalitides), degenerative, or neoplastic diseases.
- To determine sources, it may be appropriate to submit specimens for analysis such as:
  - Feed.
  - Suspect insecticidal formulation - granules, liquid, old containers, etc.
  - Gastrointestinal tract contents.
  - Hair (live animal) or skin (dead animal).
  - Liver.
- Fat or milk fat are the preferred samples to assess residue contamination.
- It is essential to avoid any cross contamination: e.g., from source material to animal or milk; or from skin or stomach contents to brain, etc.

Treatment for Acute Toxicosis

- Dermal exposure - bathe with detergent - avoid human exposure by the use of heavy-gauge rubber gloves.
- Recent oral exposure - emetics (small animals and possibly swine) (only if presented very early) and not if any likelihood of seizures is apparent: must avoid aspiration of stomach contents into lungs (as discussed with strychnine previously)

  - lavage - Usually use activated charcoal, saline cathartic.
- Monitor liver function.
- Usually seizure control is necessary for 24 hours or so, sometimes may need to medicate for longer periods of time. Suggested drug for initial control is diazepam (dogs) or, if it fails (or for other species), phenobarbital or pentobarbital. For prolonged CNS stimulation, the drug of choice is phenobarbital which may also stimulate mixed function oxidase activity to shorten half-life.

Decontamination of Residue-Contaminated Livestock

- Identify source and terminate exposure - essential.
- Determine value of animals and duration of pasturing/feeding to achieve decontamination. Assess value of animals minus costs of

decontamination versus other options. Consider costs including feed, labor, biopsy, analysis, killing and burial of highly contaminated individuals and purchase of additional animals.

- If animals must be destroyed, burial or other disposal should be approved by regulatory officials before euthanasia.
- Lactating animals tend to more rapidly eliminate insecticide residues due in part to losses in milk fat.
- Young animals sometimes metabolize/excrete significant amounts and, because of growth, dilute the residues and may therefore (sometimes) not require specific detoxification procedures.
- Placing fattened animals on pasture, so that they lean out, helps to hasten removal of the organochlorine insecticide from body fat stores. If residues are extremely high in fat, may need to monitor for neurologic effects as body fat residues are mobilized.
- The use of agents to promote metabolism or excretion such as phenobarbital, mineral oil, or repeated activated charcoal for the purposes of lowering residues in fat or milk fat are generally ineffective and not worthwhile.

Cyclodiene Organochlorine Insecticides and Lindane

Sources

Cyclodiene type: Aldrin, dieldrin, chlordane, endrin, heptachlor, ("active constituent") of toxaphene.

- Chlordane, heptachlor, aldrin used for termites.
- Aldrin used for corn root worm.
- Endrin at least in past used in "Rid-a-bird".
- Relay toxicosis possible (documented with endrin).
- Toxaphene used for animal dips, other uses.
  - Mixed isomers of chlorinated camphene containing 67 - 69% chlorine.
  - High toxicity of the cyclodiene compound 8-octachloroborane makes a very important contribution to insecticidal activity and, therefore, is referred to as the "active constituent" of toxaphene.

  Note - Lindane is also called BHC, an abbreviation for the gamma isomer of benzene hexachloride which is a misnomer. Lindane is really hexachlorocyclohexane and must not be confused with HCB. HCB is hexachlorobenzene (true aromatic ring), which was used as a fungicide and is also a significant environmental pollutant because of its extreme persistence and biological magnification, as with many but not all of the organochlorine insecticides.

- Lindane : Toxicosis is common in cats and dogs. It was never approved for cats, it is used for dogs (fleas, ticks, sarcoptic mange), also for people (Kwell) (for scabies).
- Toxicity : These cause more seizure activity and are more acutely toxic (lower LD_{50}) than the DDT type organochlorines.
- LD_{50} endrin (cats) 3 - 6 mg/kg.

Toxicodynamics Lindane

- Act by competitive inhibition of the binding of GABA at its receptor - GABA is a more widely used inhibitory transmitter in the CNS than glycine.

  Note : the effects of GABA are facilitated by benzodiazepines (such as valium) and these xenobiotics may therefore be of major benefit in treatment.
- EEG patterns - dieldrin - high amplitude - slow frequency.
- Metabolism in body and environment.
  - Aldrin-dieldrin.
  - Heptachlor - heptachlor epoxide.
  - Dieldrin and heptachlor epoxide are persistent in the body and the environment.
  - It is believed that lindane may also increase threshold by inhibiting GABA-stimulated Cl^- uptake into the neuron.
  - Lindane may have an antiestrogenic mechanism.

Clinical Signs of Cyclodiene Type OC Toxicoses

- Hypersalivation, vomition.
- Tremors, ataxia.
- Excitation or less often depression.
- Seizures, pivoting on one foot, fall over backwards.
- Possible liver failure.

Clinical Signs of Lindane Toxicoses

- Tremors
- Excitement or depression

- Seizures
- Possible cardiac arrhythmia or cardiac arrest reported in rats.
- Idiosyncratic reaction involving bone marrow depression reported in human beings exposed to lindane. Rare reports of fatal lindane-induced aplastic anemia in humans.
- Some lindane isomers are hepatotoxic and hepatocarcinogenic.

Residues

- In addition to acute toxicoses - a primary concern, with regard to the more persistent organochlorines and their metabolites, is residues in the fats of meat and milk.
- Toxaphene - comprised of chlorinated camphor extract (from pine), therefore many compounds are present. Most are rapidly eliminated. Animal uses recently banned.
- Several cyclodienes appear to be weakly mutagenic but may act as significant tumor promoters especially with regard to estrogen-responsive tumors. Most of the compounds are persistent in fat.
- For residue concerns monitor:
  - Milk fat: values may approximate body fat concentrations.
  - Fat biopsy. In cattle, fat may be taken from the tailhead, neck, and scrotum of steers. Prefer to avoid perirenal fat even at necropsy when other fat is obtainable.
  - Can use experimentally derived data for a particular organochlorine to calculate time needed for a known concentration in body fat to fall below actionable level.

    Note: Logical to consult with a veterinary toxicologist when addressing persistent residue problems in food animals.
  - Biological magnification - concentration in lipids of successive predators. Can result in chronic or acute (lethal) toxicoses (see DDT above).

Diagnosis and Treatment of Acute Toxicoses

- See Diphenyl Aliphatic Organochlorine. (DDT)
- Recovery may be complete after 3 - 6 hours to a few days of treatment.

Decontamination of Residue Contaminated Livestock

See Diphenyl Aliphatic Organochlorine. (DDT)

Key Features

- Mechanism of action: inhibition of GABA causes seizures.
- Acute toxicoses: analyze brain, stomach contents, faeces, source.
- Residue problems (fewer problems with toxaphene).
- Biological magnification.
- Diazepam, detoxification, phenobarbital, or pentobarbital for seizures.
- Residues: terminate exposure, analysis of milk fat or fat biopsy, determine if should detoxify or cull contaminated animals.

Organophosphorus and Carbamate Insecticides

An organophosphate (sometimes abbreviated **OP**) is the general name for esters of phosphoric acid. Phosphates are probably the most pervasive organophosphorus compounds. Many of the most important biochemicals are organophosphates, including DNA and RNA as well as many cofactors that are essential for life. Organophosphates are also the basis of many insecticides, herbicides, and nerve gases. Organophosphates are widely used as solvents, and plasticizers.

Organophosphates are widely employed both in natural and synthetic applications because of the ease with which organic groups can be linked together. Being a triprotic acid, phosphoric acid can form triesters whereas carboxylic acids only form monoesters. Esterification entails the attachment of organic groups to phosphorus through oxygen linkers. The precursors to such esters are alcohols. Encompassing many thousands of natural and synthetic compounds, alcohols are diverse and widespread.

$$OP(OH)_3 + ROH \rightarrow OP(OH)_2(OR) + H_2O$$

$$OP(OH)_2(OR) + R'OH \rightarrow OP(OH)(OR)(OR') + H_2O$$

$$OP(OH)(OR)(OR') + R''OH \rightarrow OP(OR)(OR')(OR'') + H_2O$$

The phosphate esters bearing OH groups are acidic and partially deprotonated in aqueous solution. For example DNA and RNA are polymers of the type $[PO_2(OR)(OR')^-]_n$. Polyphosphates also form esters. An important example of an ester of a polyphosphate is ATP, which is the monoester of triphosphoric acid ($H_5P_3O_{10}$).

Alcohols can be detached from phosphate esters by hydrolysis, which is the reverse of the above reactions. For this reason, phosphate esters are common carriers of organic groups in biosynthesis.

Structural Features of Organophosphates

Effective organophosphates have the following structural features:

- A terminal oxygen connected to phosphorus by a double bond, i.e. a phosphoryl group
- Two lipophilic groups bonded to the phosphorus
- A leaving group bonded to the phosphorus, often a halide.

Terminal Oxygen vs. Terminal Sulfur

Thiophosphoryl compounds, those bearing the P=S functionality, are much less toxic than related phosphoryl derivatives, which includes as sarin, and tetraethyl pyrophosphate. Thiophosphoryl compounds are not active inhibitors of acetylcholinesterase in either mammals or insects; in mammals, metabolism tends to remove lipophilic side groups from the phosphorus atom while in insects it tends to oxidize the compound, thus removing the terminal sulfur and replacing it with a terminal oxygen, which allows the compound to more efficiently act as an acetylcholinesterase inhibitor.

Organophosphorus (OP) insecticides are often referred to as organophosphates, which is actually a misnomer (they are not salts).

- Most are applied to surfaces of plants, animals, soils, or household floors, etc.
- Others are systemics
  - Absorbed via any route by plants or animals and distributed through the organism on which the insect pest feeds.
- The most prevalent and toxic chemical warfare agents are potent OP compounds (soman, sarin, tabun). These compounds are not used as insecticides.

Carbamate insecticides, which are derivatives of carbamic acid are used for similar surface applications.

- The original carbamate, physostigmine, is a plant alkaloid, derived from the "ordeal bean"

Both OP and carbamate groups contain members comparatively low in toxicity and others which are extremely poisonous.

Sources

Feed-Related Problems: (80% of all exposures in food animals).

- Misidentification of granular pesticides as vitamin or mineral supplements.
  - Aldicarb granules are black to grey outside; beige inside.
- Adjacent storage of feed ingredients and pesticides.
- Use of vehicles to transport pesticides prior to transporting feed.
- Accidental or excessive application to forage crops.

Other Sources

- Miscalculation of dosage during spraying, dipping, oral dosage.
- Exposure of animals to products intended for other species (e.g., cats treated with dips for dogs).
- Exposure of pets to insecticidal products applied to the home.
- Use of insecticides on stressed animals.

Host Factors

- Adult, stressed, water deprived and chilled animals more prone
- Pregnant females
- Chlorpyrifos more toxic to males than females
- Toxin factors
- Formulation used,vehicle used and droplet size
- Method of application
- Storage
- Acidic soils and acidic environment OP compounds do not degrade
- Presence of minerals in the soil increases persistence

Toxicodynamics

Acetylcholinesterase (AChE) also known as true cholinesterase is the enzyme that rapidly hydrolyzes ACh in plasma, RBCs I Neuro effector junctions.

- Red blood cells contain primarily AChE and plasma contains pseudocholinesterase. The actual physiological purposes of the enzymes located in blood are unknown.

- During its action, acetylcholinesterase is very temporarily bound to the acetyl and choline ends of the molecule until hydrolysis and release of choline and acetate occurs. Prior to the release of the acetate (which is released last), the enzyme is, for an instant, "acetylated".
- Organophosphate and carbamate insecticides competitively inhibit both acetylcholinesterases and pseudocholinesterases.
- Binding of acetylcholinesterase by a carbamate insecticide is generally followed by hydrolysis of the insecticide, but the enzyme remains temporarily carbamylated and thus inhibited. The binding, and associated inhibition, is generally reversible, but often lasts long enough to allow clinical signs and sometimes death to occur.
- The binding of acetylcholinesterase by different organophosphous inhibitors varies somewhat in affinity and reversibility. After binding, the enzyme is "phosphorylated", and thus inhibited. Much of the binding of AChE by an OP is regarded as "irreversible".
- With some of the OP compounds, after binding to acetylcholinesterase, a chemical change in the OP takes place which significantly strengthens the attachment of the phosphorus to acetylcholinesterase. This is referred to as "*aging*" of the insecticide, and it occurs to different degrees and at different rates with various OPs. After aging, treatment by oximes is not effective in reversing the binding of the OP.
- Some OPs (especially those with a -P=S moiety) require metabolic oxidation to form a -P=O before they effectively inhibit acetylcholinesterase.
- As a result of phosphorylation or carbamylation, the acetylcholinesterase enzyme ceases its normal function and acetylcholine concentrations at neuroeffector sites build up, resulting in continuous stimulation of nervous, glandular, or muscular receptors.
- Phenothiazine derivatives as well as other agents including some quaternary ammonium bases may also inhibit cholinesterases, potentiating the toxicity of the insecticide.
- Death due to OP or carbamate toxicoses is usually due to one or more of the following effects:
  - Increased respiratory tract secretions and bronchiolar constriction with hypoxia provoked by bradycardia.
  - Respiratory depression from nicotinic stimulation to the point of paralysis.

- Respiratory paralysis from CNS depression due to central effects of the insecticide (may be the primary cause of respiratory failure in some species).

Clinical Signs

3 categories of effects occur in poisoned animals: muscarinic, nicotinic, and central nervous system effects.

- Muscarinic
  - Salivation, Gastrointestinal hypermotility, pain, vomiting, and diarrhoea.
  - Lacrimation, Miosis (or mydriasis perhaps attributable to epinephrine release).
  - Dyspnea (bronchial secretion, constriction) and resultant cyanosis.
  - Micturition, Bradycardia (or tachycardia perhaps attributable to epinephrine release).
  - Death may result from hypoxia, which results from bronchial secretions, bronchoconstriction, and an erratic, slowed heartbeat.
  - Horses-colic, abdominal pain, salivation, severe diarrhoea (often watery), dehydration.
- Nicotinic
  - Stimulation of skeletal muscles
  - Twitching of facial muscles, eyelids, tongue, and eventually the general musculature, Generalized tetany.
  - Subsequent weakness and paralysis, possibly respiratory paralysis and death.
- Central nervous system
  - Vary with species: severe CNS depression common in any species.
  - Food animals-often exhibit hyperactivity, rarely if ever, seizure.
  - Dogs and cats-occasionally seizure, Hyperactive, Hyperreflexive.
  - Centrally mediated respiratory paralysis (may be lethal).
  - Cats: minimum lethal dose (oral) in cats (a highly sensitive species) of approximately 40 mg/kg.

Lesions : Non-specific ; Occasional hemorrhages in gastrointestinal tract serosa and mucosa.

Residues

- Vary with the specific compound, degree, and route of exposure.
- Generally the carbamates cause comparatively little concern in the overall environment (on a broad scale) or in animal tissues.
- The OPs tend to be much less persistent than the organochlorine insecticides.

Diagnosis

- History and appropriate clinical signs.
- Reduced whole blood cholinesterase activity may suggest exposure to an organophosphate or carbamate and, although, not a conclusive test.
- In most species, the red blood cells contribute the major fraction of the activity in total blood cholinesterase.
- In most instances, the whole blood cholinesterase values of lethally poisoned animals fall below 25% of control values.
- Brain cholinesterase is very important in assessing the probability of poisoning in dead animals (obtain as soon as possible-right away after death, freeze, ship so that specimen remains frozen).
- Testing blood or homogenized brain tissue for cholinesterase activity at several times before and during a period of laboratory incubation can be used to differentiate an OP toxicosis (minimal or no regeneration of activity) from a carbamate (substantial regeneration of activity and potentially even full toxicosis recovery to normal values).
- Internal organs (e.g., liver) of poisoned animals may contain detectable residues of organophosphorus insecticides. Also, most of the compounds (OPs and carbamates) may be found in significant concentrations in skin and subcutaneous tissue after topical exposure.
- Stomach or rumen contents are often important in confirming diagnoses after oral exposure because the insecticides are often detected in these samples (ship frozen).

Treatment

- Very early, emetics (only for very recent exposures; never when contraindicated and never when constant monitoring will not be undertaken).
- Activated charcoal (for any recent oral exposure) administered with appropriate precautions to avoid aspiration.

- Thoroughly clean with detergent all animals exposed topically-taking care to avoid exposure of human skin. Use thick rubber gloves, plastic aprons, etc.
- Atropine sulfate (generally avoid use of charged agents, such as atropine methylnitrate or glycopyrrolate, which do not effectively enter the central nervous system).
    - Atropine sulfate-dosages higher than preanesthetic doses are routinely required for acute toxicoses (OP or carbamate).
    - Small animal products may contain atropine sulfate at 0.5 or 0.54 mg/ml; large animal products may contain 2 or 15 mg/ml.
    - May want to avoid atropine sulfate altogether in horses due to gut stasis, (except with life-threatening pulmonary or cardiac effects). When used in horses, atropine is added to fluids and administered IV while ausculting the abdomen. Administration is stopped prior to a reduction (to less than normal) in gastrointestinal sounds.
    - Suggested dose cattle 0.2 - 0.5 mg/kg. One-third of dose administered IV, the remainder given SC or IM.
    - Atropine is repeated judiciously as needed; but avoid gut and rumen atony. May be required at 4 - 8-hour intervals.
    - Suggested dose SA and birds 0.2 mg/kg. Some rabbits have atropinase and may require higher dosing, begin at 1.0 mg/kg but may need to increase to 10 mg/kg.
    - In all cases, subsequent doses of atropine should depend on the reappearance and severity of clinical signs. Clinical signs to use for monitoring include degree of respiratory distress, cyanosis, and heart rate. Effects such as miosis and salivation, which are not of concern in survival, are not used as therapeutic end points for atropine administration.
- Oximes
    - 2 PAM, Pralidoxime hydrochloride, or TMB-4 act on the OP-AChE complex to free the enzyme to resume its normal function if aging has not occurred and to enhance excretion of the insecticide. Not clearly proven of any benefit in carbamate toxicoses. Based on early, but since disputed data, it is often stated that 2-PAM is contraindicated in carbamate poisoning. However, when in doubt as to whether an insecticide poisoning is due to an OP or a carbamate, but signs suggest a cholinesterase inhibitor, an oxime should be used. Oximes are usually repeated BID. Protopam is given IM or IV at 20 mg/kg BID and

continued, for days to weeks if necessary, until nicotinic signs resolve. If no response is apparent after 4 doses, the value of additional 2-PAM is in doubt and use of the drug should probably be discontinued. Cattle and horses can be dosed at 10 - 20 mg/kg.

- Topically administered organophosphorus insecticides may be absorbed into the skin and/or subcutaneous fat before systemic distribution. Thus, absorption from these sites (skin, fat) may occur over several days time, and "aging" of the insecticide on the cholinesterase enzyme may not have occurred so that oximes may still be of benefit in these cases-even days after the initial exposure.
- 2-PAM is generally of low toxicity. Overdoses can be associated with tachycardia, cardiac arrhythmias.
- The maximum shelf-life of reconstituted 2-PAM is two weeks.

- Artificial respiration may be needed to counteract respiratory paralysis. Severe bronchospasm may be responsive to theophylline therapy. Older literature, however, suggests theophylline may increase occurrence of seizures in OP toxicosis. It is essential to avoid hypoxia.
- Scopolamine maybe of value when severe CNS depression is not responsive to atropine therapy, but this is not widely accepted.
- Diphenhydramine has been recommended at 1 - 4 mg/kg per os every 6 - 8 hours to help control persistent nicotinic signs.
- Seizures may be controlled with diazepam or barbiturate anticonvulsants.
- Systemic acidosis may complicate OP or carbamate poisoning. Counteracting respiratory failure with atropine and/or assisted ventilation are recommended for respiratory acidosis. Sodium bicarbonate administered at an initial dose of 5 mg/kg IV can be used to correct metabolic acidosis. Subsequently, IV doses at 1 - 3 mEq/kg may be required. Monitor acid base status.
- Animals should be monitored for the development of chemical pneumonitis due either to aspiration of hydrocarbon solvents (when such formulations are ingested) or for aspiration of gastric contents.
- Stress of OP or carbamate toxicosis may predispose animals to secondary clinical problems: e.g., hemobartonellosis, reported in OP-poisoned cats.
- If prolonged administration of high doses of atropine is anticipated, it is best to avoid preparations containing benzyl alcohol preservatives in species/ages (e.g., cats and all neonates) susceptible to benzyl alcohol-related toxicosis.

Organophosphorus-Induced Delayed Neuropathy (OPIDN)

Sources

- This syndrome can result from single or multiple exposures.
- The appearance of clinical signs are delayed for an average of 1-2 weeks in many animals and 2-4 weeks in man.
- Most, but not all, of the implicated phosphate esters causing OPIDN are insecticides.
- Related compounds (e.g., triarylphosphates) are used in industrial applications such as hydraulic systems, as additives to high-temperature fire-resistant lubricants, and as plasticizers. This class includes triorthocresyl phosphate (TOCP).

Toxicity

- The tendency to cause OPIDN does not parallel the tendency to inhibit acetylcholinesterase. Many OPs have not been associated with OPIDN in spite of their capacity to cause acute toxicosis due to acetylcholinesterase inhibition. Other compounds with comparatively low acute toxicity with respect to cholinesterase inhibition may be potent inducers of OPIDN in the absence of any previous toxicoses. In addition, some compounds such as O-ethyl-0-4-nitro-phenylphosphonothioate (EPN) are so toxic with regard to cholinesterase inhibition that the significance of their capacity to induce OPIDN is diminished by the small number of poisoned individuals that live long enough to develop the "delayed neurotoxicity" syndrome.

If death occurs as a result of the induction of OPIDN, it is usually a result of respiratory paralysis or inability to get to water.

Susceptible Species : Chicken, duck, turkey, horse, cow, sheep, pig, dog, cat, baboon, rat, and man.

Nonsusceptible Species : Mouse, rabbit, guinea pig, hamster, and gerbil.

Clinical Signs

- Abnormal sensation in the feet and legs such as tingling and burning.
- High stepping, Weakness, ataxia.
- Ascending paralysis, may be flaccid. Gradual progression anteriorly.
- Effects may be extremely persistent or permanent after exposure terminated.

- Decreased reflex responses, Muscle atrophy.
- Severe dyspnea and absence of vocalization may be observed in cattle and pigs.
- Recovery, if any, is generally slow and often incomplete.
- Cattle: diarrhoea, posterior weakness, ataxia, stiffness, difficulty in rising, weaving back legs, wide stance. Animals often recumbent 2 - 6 days before death, although occassional sudden death noted. Animals dribble urine.
- Cattle and pigs: After a few days to several weeks, the peak of the process is reached and thereafter improvement in the functional disturbances begins.
- Cat: Cats may recover some function, probably dependent upon the extent of lesions.

Recovery

- Mild cases: very slow recovery. Recovery generally more rapid in cat than in man.
- Severe cases: no recovery.
- Occasionally can ascend to result in quadraplegia and can cause death, from respiratory paralysis but this is rare.

OP insecticides and anthelmintics implicated in delayed neuropathy.

- Tri-ortho-cresol-phosphate (TOCP), Leptofos, DFP, Fenitrothion, Cyanofenphos, Trichlornate, Trichlorfon - Insecticide and anthelmintic., Carbophenothion (Trithion), Haloxon - anthelmintic

Other compounds suggested as capable of causing delayed neurotoxicity, not OPs, are diallate and sulfallate - Carbamate herbicides.

Toxicodynamics (Postulated)

- The development of OPIDN does not correlate with inhibition of acetylcholinesterase.
- The occurrence of delayed neuropathy has a high correlation with the inhibition of an enzyme called neuropathy target esterase (NTE). Maximal inhibition of > 70% at 1 - 2 days after exposure usually is associated with the onset of delayed neuropathy 8 - 14 days later. NTE does not have an identified function in the body. Whether or how NTE inhibition actually leads to OPIDN is therefore unknown. NTE is present in peripheral nerves, lymphocytes, brain, placenta, and several other sites.

- Three mechanisms of action of these OPs have been proposed:
  - A primary toxic effect on the metabolic machinery of the nerve cell perikaryon.
  - A direct action on the axon at certain vulnerable sites without affecting axonal transport.
  - Alteration or interruption of axonal transport.
- Inhibitors of NTE can be put into 2 groups:
  - Group A (phosphates, phosphoramidates, and phosphonates) are axonopathic, can "age" and are therefore potentially neurotoxic.
  - Group B (sulphonates, phosphinates, and carbamates) are not axonopathic, will bind to esterase, do not age and can therefore be protective.
- The essential difference between these 2 groups is the ability of Group A compounds to undergo aeging. Prior administration of a compound from Group B can be protective against the delayed neurotoxic effects of subsequently administered Group A compounds.

Lesions

- Characterized as a central-peripheral distal axonopathy (axons injured first, myelin damage is secondary).
- Histopathological analysis requires longitudinal section of spinal cord and peripheral nerves (staple nerves to tongue depressor during fixation). Clumping of myelin, foamy appearance of myelin, broken axons (axonal degeneration). The distal nerves of the peripheral nervous system are affected earlier and more severely than proximal fibers "dying-back polyneuropathy".

Treatment

- No effective therapy is recognized.
- Treatment with atropine and oximes (2-PAM) minimize initial development of signs related to cholinesterase inhibition but do not prevent the development of OPIDN.

Pyrethrum (Pyrethrins) and Pyrethroids

Sources

- Pyrethrins are natural insecticides produced by certain exotic *Chrysanthemums* (sometimes called *Pyrethrum*) flowers, not by domestic horticultural varieties. Pyrethrum contains pyrethrins and cinerins.

- Pyrethroids are synthetic insecticides.
- Used in numerous formulations including aerosols, sprays, dusts, tags, dips, and shampoos. Some formulations include additional insecticides and/or insect repellants. Flea control products constitute the primary source of exposure leading to problems in small animals.

Toxicity

- Toxicity varies with the specific compound and route of administration involved.
- In general, introduction of an alpha cyano moiety (type II pyrethroids) results in an increase in toxicity.

Rat LD_{50} (mg/kg)

Type I Compounds	**Oral**	**IV**
Pyrethrin I	900	
Allethrin	680	
Tetramethrin (phthalthrin)	4,640	
Kadethrin	600	
Resmethrin	100	7
Phenothrin	10,000	> 300
Permethrin	2,000	>135
Cismethrin		5
Bromophenothrin		>30
Type II Compounds	**Oral**	**IV**
Fenpropathrin	25	1
Cypermethrin	500	6-9
Deltamethrin (decamethrin)	31	2
Fenvalerate	450	20
Fluorocyphenothrin		5-7
Fluvalinate	1,000	
Dowco 417	460	
Flucythrinate	67	
Bay-FCR	590	

Susceptible Species

Small animals, principally cats; and rodents.; Fish is extremely sensitive.

Toxicokinetics

- Rapid hydrolysis of ester linkage in digestive tract results in low oral toxicity.

- Most are rapidly metabolized by ester hydrolysis and via oxidation by liver microsomal enzymes.
- The resulting alcohol, phenol, or carboxylic acid metabolites are often conjugated with glycine, glucuronide, sulfate, and glucoside prior to excretion.
- Residues: follow label recommendations on withdrawal, usually not a problem.

Toxicodynamics

- Pyrethrins and type I pyrethroids act on sodium ion channels; decreasing peak sodium conductance, prolonging the sodium conductance, and suppressing potassium conduction. These changes result in decreases in the amplitudes of action potentials and repetitive nerve discharges. Nerve conduction block can occur.
- Type II pyrethroids (contain a cyano group) also act on sodium ion channels which is thought to account for the sensory nerve stimulation associated with paresthesias in humans (and presumably other species). A depolarization of nerve membranes without repetitive discharges occurs with decreased action potential amplitudes. Type II pyrethroids are also believed to interfere with the binding of GABA and glutamic acid at their respective nervous system's receptor sites.
- Pyrethrins and pyrethroids also inhibit various adenosine triphosphatases including the calcium-ATPase and the calcium magnesium-ATPase in nervous tissues.
- Synergists-Addition of mixed function oxidase inhibitors, such as piperonyl butoxide, N-octyl bicycloheptene dicarboxiimide MGK264, sesame oil (and/or several others) enhances toxicity in insects and mammals by prolonging the life of the intact, active form of the insecticide in the body.

Clinical Signs

- Clinical signs generally develop within hours of exposure, but may be delayed as a result of prolonged exposure from dermal absorption or grooming
- Effects on rodents classified into two syndromes: type I and type II syndromes which correlate with the chemical structures.
    - Type I syndrome: classical pyrethrins and type I pyrethroids (no alpha cyano group). Increased sensitivity to stimuli, fine muscle tremors, whole body tremors, prostration.

- Type II syndrome-alpha-cyano pyrethroids. Salivation; rodents paw, burrow, writhe, and may display clonic seizures; possible paresthesia of skin.

- In cats and dogs, clinical signs associated with toxicosis from pyrethrins and type I or type II pyrethroids may include tremors, increased salivation, ataxia, vomiting, depression, increased body temperature, hyper-excitability or hyperactivity, seizures, dyspnea, and death.
- Generally sublethally exposed animals recover within 72 hours.

Lesions

No specific gross lesions are noted. and deaths are generally rare.

Diagnosis

- History of a potentially toxic level of exposure to a pyrethrin or pyrethroid containing insecticide and the development of compatible clinical signs.

Treatment

- Topical exposure: Clean thoroughly with detergent.
- Recent oral exposure (within a few hours): (Early) emetics if not contraindicated; activated charcoal and saline cathartic.
- For severe CNS stimulation with seizures: To treat pyrethroid toxicosis in dogs, diazepam (0.2 - 2.0 mg/kg IV to effect). Or parenteral phenobarbital is recommended, induction of anesthesia with pentobarbital may be necessary.
- Cats with severe tremors due to inappropriate use of concentrated permethrin often improve after IV administration of methocarbamol at 55 - 220 mg/kg. Half the dose should be given rapidly but no faster than 2 ml/min. Administration should be discontinued briefly as the cat relaxes, then resumed until the desired effect is achieved. The maximum dose on the label (330 mg/kg) should not be exceeded.
- Atropine can reduce some clinical signs (e.g., diarrhea, hypersalivation). However, in experimental studies with lethally poisoned laboratory animals, atropine minimized excessive salivation and diarrhea without affecting the observed LD_{50}.
- Phenothiazine tranquilizers are contraindicated.

Rotenone

Sources

- Derived from roots of the *Derris* and *Lonchocupus* plant.
- Synonyms derrin, nicourine, and tubatoxin.
- More toxic than pyrethrins.
- Formulated into products for use in gardens and on dogs and cats (dips, sprays, powders). Formulations include dusts of 0.75 - 1.5% concentration, emulsifiable concentrates, wettable powders of 5% concentration, solutions (up to 57%) and resins.
- Products may be synergized with piperonyl butoxide.

Toxicity

- Highly toxic to birds and fish, may affect any species.
- Cats most often affected after deliberate use of rotenone containing products for ectoparasitism.
- Oral LD_{50} in laboratory animals range from 10 to 30 mg/kg.
- LD_{50} IP (mice) = 2.8 mg/kg.

Toxicokinetics

- Metabolized by liver, undergoes hydroxylation to form equally toxic rotenoids. Detoxification in liver by demethylation can also occur.

Toxicodynamics

- Rotenone blocks NAD-flavin electron transport in respiratory metabolism which results in blockade of nerve conduction. Specifically, interferes with the electron transport process between flavoprotein and ubiquinone (coenzyme Q). Also blocks oxidation of NADH.

Clinical Signs

- Oral exposure: Gastric irritation, Vomiting.
- Dermal exposure: Possible skin irritation and severe pulmonary irritation from inhalation of dust.
- Vomiting, lethargy, tremors, stupor, clonic, repeated convulsions, respiratory failure, dyspnea and death.
- Possible hypoglycemia.

Gross Lesions

- Pulmonary congestion, gastrointestinal tract irritation.
- Chronically fed to rats or dogs, shows passive congestion of the liver with midzonal necrosis.

Treatment

- Oral exposure: avoid fatty or oily foods as they enhance absorption.
- Minimize fraction absorbed: depending upon route of exposure and condition of patient (Clean with detergent, emetic, enterogastric lavage, activated charcoal, saline cathartic).
- Monitor blood glucose, administer glucose as needed. May not enhance survivability.
- Monitor acid-based status and, if necessary, correct metabolic acidosis with diluted bicarbonate (slow iv).
- Vitamin K3 (do not use in the horse) which activates a bypass of the rotenone sensitive site has been recommended based on theoretical (*in vitro*) rather than experimental *(in vivo*) grounds.

Amitraz

Introduction

- A formamidine pesticide.
- Used as an acaricide and a tick repellant for dogs.
- Sources: Tick-repellant collars and agricultural pesticides.

Toxicity

- The LD_{50} in rats is 800 mg/kg.
- In dogs, dermal absorption following dipping is a common route of exposure resulting in toxicosis. Ingestion by dogs of amitraz-containing collars is becoming more common as their use becomes more widespread.
- Amitraz is not approved for use in cats. Toxicosis has been reported in cats following administration of the liquid preparation in the external ear canal.
- Puppies up to 3 - 4 months old seem to be especially sensitive to amitraz.

Toxicodynamics

- Centrally, amitraz exerts toxic effects by acting as an alpha-2 adrenergic agonist, which are reversible by yohimbine.
- α-2 adrenergic stimulation results in vasodilation, bradycardia, hypotension, coma, and decreased insulin release culminating in hyperglycemia.
- In addition, in the periphery both alpha-1 and alpha-2 receptors are stimulated. The effects at α-1 receptors sometimes result in hypertension.
- Amitraz also inhibits monoamine oxidase.

Clinical Signs : vomiting, sedation, depression, disorientation, ataxia, gastrointestinal hypomotility, bradycardia, hypotension, hypothermia, hyperglycemia, and seizures. Signs of CNS depression such as depression, ataxia, or coma may be due to coincidental xylene toxicosis. Clinical signs usually begin within hours of exposure. Bradycardia and hypotension appear to be due to the compound's central alpha-2 adrenergic effects and are reversible with yohimbine.

Diagnosis

- History of exposure and the clinical signs.

Treatment

- Thoroughly wash with liquid dish detergent if dermal exposure has occurred.
- If a collar has been eaten, induce vomiting and/or remove collar via endoscopy. Administer activated charcoal.
- If solid or liquid preparations without xylene or other solvents have been ingested, give food mixed with activated charcoal then induce vomiting, if not contraindicated by bradycardia, hypotension, ataxia and/or weakness.
- Because hypotension may increase the severity of myocardial ischemia and thus arrhythmias, and because Amitraz may cause marked gut stasis and colic, atropine is contraindicated as a treatment for bradycardia.
- Ingestion of amitraz dip is unusual and is usually coincidental with toxicosis from dermal exposure. The presence of xylene in the formulation may make the wisdom of inducing vomiting or performing gastric lavage questionable.

- Yohimbine, 0.1 mg/kg IV antagonizes the alpha-2 adrenergic effects (bradycardia, hypotension, sedation, GI hypomotility), regardless of the route or amount of exposure. Repeat as needed.
- Fluids (IV) should be administered only to hypotensive animals and with care.
- Fluids are contraindicated with marked bradycardia or hypertension.

Herbicides

A herbicide is used to kill unwanted plants. Selective herbicides kill specific targets while leaving the desired crop relatively unharmed. Some of these act by interfering with the growth of the weed and are often synthetic "imitations" of plant hormones.

Herbicides used to clear waste ground, industrial sites, railways and railway embankments are non-selective and kill all plant material with which they come into contact. Some plants produce natural herbicides, such as the genus *Juglans* (walnuts). They are applied in total vegetation control (TVC) programs for maintenance of highways and railroads. Smaller quantities are used in forestry, pasture systems, and management of areas set aside as wildlife habitat. Herbicides are widely used in agriculture and in landscape turf management. In the world they account for about 70% of all agricultural pesticide use.

Classification of herbicides : Herbicides can be classified based on activity, use, chemical family, mode of action and type of vegetation controlled.

Based on Activity

- *Contact* herbicides destroy only the plant tissue in contact with the chemical. Generally, these are the fastest acting herbicides. They are less effective on perennial plants, which are able to regrow from rhizhomes, roots or tubers.
- *Systemic* herbicides are translocated through the plant, either from foliar application down to the roots, or from soil application up to the leaves. They are capable of controlling perennial plants and may be slower acting but ultimately more effective than contact herbicides.

Based on Use

- *Soil-applied* herbicides are applied to the soil and are taken up by the roots and/or hypocotyl of the target plant. The following two categories are examples of soil-applied herbicides.

- *Pre-plant incorporated* herbicides are soil applied prior to planting and mechanically incorporated into the soil. The objective for incorporation is to prevent dissipation through photo decomposition and/or volatility.
- *Pre-emergent herbicides* are applied to the soil before the crop emerges and prevent germination or early growth of weed seeds.
- *Post-emergent herbicides* are applied after the crop has emerged.

Mechanism of Action : The Main Mechanisms of Action are

- Acetyl coenzyme A carboxylase (ACCase) is part of the first step of lipid synthesis. And cell membrane production in the meristems of the grass plant. The ACCases of grasses are sensitive to these herbicides, are inhibited by these agents whereas the ACCases of dicot plants are not.
- Acetolactate synthase (ALS) enzyme (also known as acetohydroxyacid synthase, or AHAS) is the first step in the synthesis of the branched-chain amino acids (valine, leucine, and isoleucine). These herbicides slowly starve affected plants of these amino acids by inhibiting ALS, which eventually leads to inhibition of DNA synthesis. They affect grasses and dicots alike. The ALS inhibitor family includes sulfonylureas, imidazolinones, triazolopyrimidines,pyrimidinyl xybenzoates, and sulfonylamino carbonyl triazolinones. ALS is a biological pathway that exists only in plants and not in animals thus making the ALS-inhibitors among the safest herbicides.
- The inhibition of enolpyruvylshikimate 3-phosphate synthase enzyme EPSPS, which is used in the synthesis of the amino acids tryptophan, phenylalanine and tyrosine. They affect grasses and dicots alike. Glyphosate (Roundup) is a systemic EPSPS inhibitor but inactivated by soil contact.
- Synthetic auxin inaugurated the era of organic herbicides., based on study of the plant growth regulator auxin. Synthetic auxins mimic this plant hormone. They have several points of action on the cell membrane, and are effective in the control of dicot plants. 2,4-D is a synthetic auxin herbicide.
- Photosystem II inhibitors reduce electron flow from water to $NADPH2^+$ at the photochemical step in photosynthesis. They bind to the Qb site on the D1 protein, and prevent quinone from binding to this site. Therefore, this group of compounds cause electrons to accumulate on chlorophyll molecules. As a consequence, oxidation reactions in excess of those normally tolerated by the cell occur, and the plant dies. The triazine herbicides (including atrazine) and urea derivatives (diuron) are photosystem II inhibitors.

2, 4-D

Sources

- Phenoxyacetic acid (chlorinated) derivatives, such as 2,4-D (2,4-dichlorophenoxyacetic acid), 2,4,5-T (2,4,5-trichlorophenoxyacetic acid), silvex, MCPP, MCPA, and others may possibly be involved.
- 2,4,5-T was contaminated with very toxic chlorinated dibenzodioxins, especially 2,3,7,8 tetrachlorodibenzodioxin, but these are not encountered in 2,4-D. Dibenzodioxins were the toxic contaminant found in the defoliant Agent Orange, which was a 50/50 combination of 2,4-D and 2,4,5-T.

Toxicity

- 2,4-D
  - LD_{50} dog 100 mg/kg (oral).
  - Lethal to dogs at 25 mg/kg/day for 6 days.
  - Oral LD_{50} rat 375 - 1,200 mg/kg.
  - Toxicity observed in calves at 200 mg/kg, swine 100 mg/kg.
- 2,4,5-T
  - Oral LD_{50} dog approximately 100 mg/kg.
  - Oral LD_{50} rat 500 mg/kg, guinea pigs 381 mg/kg.
- MCPA
  - Oral LD_{50} rat 612 - 1,200 mg/kg.
- Dicamba (a benzoic acid herbicide with some toxic effects similar to the phenoxy herbicides).
  - Oral LD_{50} 757 - 1414 mg/kg.
- Phenoxyherbicides may cause an increased palatability of some types of poisonous plants due to abnormal plant carbohydrate metabolism. Phenoxy herbicides can also increase the concentration of nitrates and cyanogenic glycosides in some plants.

Susceptible Species

- Canids are predisposed as compared to other species possibly due to their poor ability to excrete organic acids in the urine.
- In practice, dogs do seem to eat inordinate amounts of phenoxy-herbicide treated grass.

Toxicokinetics

- 2,4-D salts or esters are readily released in the gastric acid and rapidly absorbed due to protonation (addition of hydrogen ion) of the free anion in the gastric acid.
- Most of the herbicide is excreted in the urine as the unchanged acid. 2,4,5-T may undergo enterohepatic circulation.

Toxicodynamics

- 2,4-D has a direct effect on muscle membranes causing increased irritability and rigidity followed by paralysis.

Clinical Signs

Dogs

- Often the only signs seen in the field from moderately toxic doses of phenoxy herbicides are related to gastrointestinal effects like vomiting and diarrhoea, sometimes bloody.
- Serious toxicosis more often occurs after exposure to concentrates or pools of sprays, or when dogs are present and heavily exposed during spraying, muscular effects may predominate:
- Hesitation to move, rigidity of skeletal muscles, ataxia, weakness especially in the rear legs.
- Neurologic signs including seizures occur only with highly toxic doses.
- Chronic spasms and coma. Opisthotonus occasionally occurs.
    - The most sensitive effect of 2,4-D toxicosis in the dog is found by use of the electromyogram. Greatly increased insertional activity (harmonic response upon insertion of the needle electrode) occurs at doses well below those causing notable clinical effects. This is an indication of a primary muscle effect of 2,4-D. At much higher doses, nerve degeneration which is at least partially reversible **may** also occur. This may be largely a result of damage to the nerve at the neuromuscular junction.
- Additional effects, which may occasionally occur in dogs, include: oral ulcer, small intestine mucosal damage, renal tubular degeneration and focal hepatic necrosis.

Ruminants

- Clinical signs include anorexia, depression, bloat, rumen atony, weakness, and diarrhea. Oral mucosal ulceration may be noted.

Swine

- Diarrhoea, ataxia, depression, vomiting, and weakness.

Lesions

- Congestion of kidney, hyperemia of lymph nodes, and congested friable liver may be seen on postmortem examination.
- Rumen stasis commonly observed.
- Clinical pathological changes include elevation of CDK, SGOT, LDH.

Prognosis : Most animals should be expected to make an uneventful recovery.

Treatment

- Usually there is an oral exposure from drinking or eating the herbicide or from eating heavily treated grass. Grooming of 2,4-D from the body by the animal may prolong exposure.
- Therefore the use of activated charcoal and a saline cathartic for very recent exposures is indicated, along with a bath in a detergent.
- Ion-trapping of 2,4-D may enhance the removal from the tissues and promote its excretion in the urine. Fluids containing 1 - 2 mEq/kg bicarbonate are therefore indicated, if normal renal function is present.
- A bland diet and good nursing care should be provided.

Paraquat

Sources

- Paraquat is a dipyridyl herbicide which is applied at low application rates such as 1/2 lb/acre which is generally low enough that animals exposed to treated fields are not at risk of acute toxicosis.
- Problems arise, however, as a result of exposure to the concentrate or from ingestion of solutions of the chemical, not yet applied.
- Paraquat is a nonselective herbicide, causing a fast acting, contact kill on treated plants.
- It is also used as a desiccant to remove the herbage prior to the harvest of soybeans, potatoes, melons and fruit from trees, as well as for other similar applications.
- Paraquat can be used on aquatic weeds and it apparently has a low toxicity to fish.

- Forage would possibly serve as a source of toxic amounts of paraquat if treated at extremely high rates since solutions as strong as 20% are sometimes prepared.
- Paraquat has been used for malicious poisoning of dogs.

Toxickinetics

- Paraquat accumulates in the lungs until about 10 times the concentration of other tissues is reached.
- About 20% of orally ingested paraquat is absorbed. Even less is absorbed when applied topically.
- Most of the paraquat is excreted unchanged in the urine although some is metabolized and approximately 15% of the absorbed paraquat leaves in the feces. Passage of paraquat in milk is low (0.015%).

Toxicodynamics

- Paraquat is a very reactive compound, and the compound readily accepts an electron to become a paraquat free radical.
- When the paraquat free radical is reoxidized by loss of the electron it previously had accepted, a superoxide free radical is formed instead.
- This superoxide free radical is unstable and spontaneously breaks down to the reactive, singlet oxygen.
- Singlet oxygen, in turn, reacts with lipid membranes to form lipid hydroperoxides.
- Lipid peroxidation then continues in the lung in the same manner as it does in the liver after initiation by carbon tetrachloride, leading to membrane destruction and dysfunction with subsequent cell death.

Toxicity

The oral LD_{50} values in various species are

Species	Oral LD_{50} (mg/kg)	Dermal LD_{50} (mg/kg)
Rat	100	80 - 90
Cat	35	
Dog	25 - 50	
Turkey	290	500
Rabbit	50 - 150	350
Sheep	50 - 75	
Pig	25 - 50	
Man	4 - 40	
Cattle	35 - 50	

- Paraquat binds tightly to clay soils and, while such binding tends to decrease the availability and therefore the toxicity of a range of pesticides, it also tends to enhance the persistence of the chemical.
- Paraquat not bound to soil photodegrades rapidly. For example, approximately 50% is degraded in sunlight within 3 weeks.
- Diquat differs from paraquat in that the former does not cause significant pulmonary problems and, instead, tends to cause cerebral hemorrhage, lethargy, coma, and renal failure.

Clinical Signs

- Apparently dogs and cattle have been poisoned more often than other domestic species
- Because of the time involved in the toxification of paraquat in the body, there is a delay after exposure of several hours up to 3 days prior to the onset of signs.
- If large amounts of paraquat are ingested, acute clinical signs may be seen, including excitation, ataxia, diarrhea, respiratory distress, and convulsions.
- Surfaces contacted by paraquat may be irritated or even ulcerated.
- In dogs, the onset of clinical signs is typically 1 - 3 days after exposure.
- Initial signs in dogs include vomiting and depression, as well as dehydration.
- Respiratory signs usually begin 2 - 7 days after the exposure and include tachypnea, dyspnea, moist rales and cyanosis. Gasping and death can occur within 8 days.
- Pneumomediastinum occasionally occurs as a result of the respiratory distress.
- The most troubling aspect of paraquat toxicosis is the progressive pulmonary damage that may continue to develop over a period of 7 or as many as 21 days.
- Initial pulmonary effects are dose dependent. Some animals die from pulmonary edema, while others survive only to develop severe pulmonary fibrosis a week or more thereafter.
- Paraquat toxicosis in cattle may first be noticed 1 - 3 days after exposure (ingestion). Anorexia, depression and diarrhea may occur and respiratory signs are somewhat less prevalent than in dogs.

Lesions

- Dark congested and hemorrhagic lungs with multiple areas of atelectasis.
- Bronchioles and alveoli may be dilated, and bullous emphysema may be present.
- In chronically affected animals, the lungs may be shrunken and fibrotic.
- There is also intraalveolar hemorrhage and edema.
- Necrosis is seen in the bronchiolar and alveolar epithelium, especially in the Type I alveolar pneumocytes.
- Progressive fibrosis in alveolar and interstitial tissues may result in significant pulmonary insufficiency.
- Paraquat toxicosis can also cause renal proximal tubular degeneration and focal centrizonal hepatic degeneration.

Diagnosis

- Analysis of the suspected source with detection of potentially toxic amounts.
- Analysis of urine may confirm exposure rather than necessarily establishing a diagnosis. With appropriate history and clinical signs and lesions, however, a diagnosis can be made.
- It has been suggested that lung or even muscle may be worth analyzing in selected cases.
- Because of rapid excretion, urine may be analyzed in many cases but would be of most value for only the first 2 days or so after exposure.

Treatment

- Rapid removal and adsorption of the ingested paraquat is the most important aspect of treatment.
- Because of the high affinity of paraquat for clays, it is widely known that bentonite or Fuller's earth is the preferred adsorbent for the herbicide.
- When these agents are not immediately available, however, it would be preferable to use activated charcoal immediately rather than waiting until the clay is available. Oral administration of ground clay kitty litter may serve as a worthwhile absorbent.

- A saline (magnesium or sodium sulfate) cathartic or an osmotic (sorbitol) cathartic should be given in every case, when animals are presented after recent exposure (i.e., last 12 hours or so).
- Forced diuresis and peritoneal dialysis may be used in selected cases, but care must be taken to avoid aggravating pulmonary edema.
- Agents which have been shown to be of benefit in paraquat toxicosis experimentally include niacin, riboflavin, ascorbic acid, superoxide dismutase (enzyme) (one form of superoxide dismutase is also known as orgotein = Pallosein ®), and N-acetyl-cysteine (mucomyst).
- Oxygen is contraindicated due to the possibility of aggravating oxidative injury to the lung.
- Clients should be made aware, early on, of the possibly grave prognosis in many cases. Some animals will, however, recover and detoxification efforts are worthwhile.

Polychlorinated Biphenyls (PCBS) and Polybrominated Biphenyls (PBBS)

Sources

Transformers, other electrical insulators (especially fluids), building materials, old lubricants.

- Polychlorinated biphenyls (PCBs) are organic compounds which are widely distributed in the environment. Polybrominated biphenyls (PBBs) are similar compounds which are less widespread, but still constitute a chemical hazard.
- Commercially, PCBs and PBBs consist of mixtures of several major and many minor components, the major ones being biphenyl compounds with varying degrees of chlorination or bromination, in some 210 possible halogenation patterns.
- The minor components are contaminants such as brominated naphthalenes and halogenated dibenzofurans or dibenzodioxins.
- These organic compounds are highly stable, nonflammable, lowly volatile, resistant to acids and bases, insoluble in water, and have a high dielectric constant. These characteristics make them useful in heat exchangers and dielectric fluids, hydraulic and lubricating fluids, plasticizers, printing inks, paints, adhesives, duplicating paper, flame retardants, and extenders for pesticides.

- Although, the production of PCBs and PBBs was halted prior to 1979, after the potential toxicity of polyhalogenated biphenyls was realized, many PCB and PBB containing products are still in use.
- It is estimated that over 400,000 tons of PCBs have been lost to the environment since 1932.
- Most of these compounds are highly lipophilic, largely resistant to microbial breakdown and biotransformation, and only slightly photodegradable; characteristics which have resulted in intensive bioaccumulation. Persistence depends on the degree and pattern of halogenation. They persist in food chains, aquatic sediments, landfills, and other biological and physical reservoirs. Fish and fish-eating wildlife are the primary biological magnifiers.
- Contaminated feedstuffs are responsible for most exposures of domestic animals. This contamination is often a result of utilizing fishmeal or recycled animal or paper products in the feed; leakage of lubricants from processing machinery; dissolution of compounds from paints and sealants on Soils, water and feed troughs, or storage tanks; availability of insulation or flaking paint in degenerated animal housing; and occasionally from an accidental mixing of PCBs or PBBs in feed or other products offered to livestock.

Toxicokinetics

- All species of animals, whether clinically affected or not, can accumulate PCBs and PBBs in their tissues.
- Cattle have been shown to excrete up to 76 ppb PCBs in their milk when fed PCB containing paper products as 30% of their diet. Several studies have reported transmission *in utero* or through the milk to feti or nursing offspring of contaminated dams. The fetal fat of cows fed PCBs at 200 mg/day contained 130.6 ppm PCBs as opposed to 0.65 ppm in that of control cows.
- In addition, PCBs were still detected in high amounts 6 months after cessation of the test feed.
- Dermal application of PCBs also results in extremely rapid absorption., Species differences exist with regard to relative susceptibility to PCBs and PBBs.
- Among domestic animals, the ranch mink appears to be the most susceptible with a dietary level of only 1 ppm PCB causing decreased litter size and viability of offspring.

- Swine appear to be somewhat tolerant clinically, but high doses elicit effects.

Toxicodynamics

- The mechanism of action of even the most studied components of PCB and PBB mixtures are not completely understood.
- In mammals, birds, and fish, most halogenated biphenyls are inducers of hepatic mixed-function oxidases, but the potencies and specificities vary widely. Generally, PBBs appear more potent than comparable PCBs in inducing these enzymes. In contrast, some congeners depress P450 activity.
- Toxicity of PCBs and dioxins depends on the chlorination pattern.
- PCBs with chlorines to the outside (flat = coplanar molecules which are therefore similar to 2,3,7,8,-TCDD) bind to the arylhydrocarbon hydroxylase receptor and are translocated into the nucleus where they initiate transcription of a number of proteins - including some P450 enzymes (e.g., "arylhydrocarbon hydroxylase" = Ah) → liver enlarges. Generally, these are also result in chronic weight loss, skin damage (chloracne in people, scaly, scabby lesions in animals), birth defects (crossed bills in birds), and anti-estrogenicity (altered sexuality, sexual function, low milk production).
- PCBs and dioxins with chlorines to the inside (large chlorines interfere with one another causing the molecule to twist the two rings are no longer flat via the same plane, therefore = noncoplanar) tend to be associated with antithyroid, antidopaminergic, and/or estrogenic effects. Their acute toxicity is generally lower than with the coplanar molecules. However, their chronic effects may be significant (some think that they may contribute to decrements in intelligence in children via effects on thyroid during development - partial cretinism - and inhibition of dopamine synthesis/concentrations in the brain).
- Higher doses of the lower halogenated compounds may induce hepatic dysfunction with subsequent abnormalities in heme synthesis that result in accumulation of large quantities of dermatitis-inducing porphyrin.
- Some of these compounds are also known to be acnegenic, and capable of producing hyperkeratosis and hyperpigmentation of the skin in various species.
- Some studies have shown the metabolism of endogenous substances such as steroids and estradiols to be enhanced in liver and skin, but

inhibited in the adrenals. A variety of reproductive effects have been seen in numerous species.

- Effects on the immune system are unclear. PCBs have been shown to potentiate duck hepatitis virus in ducklings, induce septicemia in sows, increase disease susceptibility in fish, and reduce the response of guinea pigs to tetanus toxoid. Gestating sows fed PBBs at 200 ppm of the diet showed a decreased lymphocytic response to mitogen stimulation, however, bacteriocidal activity was not consistently altered. In one study, however, lactating cows exhibited normal immune competence until tissue concentrations exceeded 1000 mg/kg at which time they became moribund.

Clinical Signs

- The toxic response to PCBs differs depending on species, age, sex, and dose with young animals and, often, females being more susceptible.
- Relatively high concentrations of PCBs or PBBs can accumulate in animal tissues without expression of acute effects or lesions. Nevertheless, chronic biochemical and physiologic changes occur with dietary exposure to feedstuffs containing less than 1 ppm.

Swine: With low level feeding, the usual signs are depressed weight gain and anorexia. Intermittent exposure appears to be more detrimental than constant and/or gradually increasing exposure. In addition, a dose of PCBs administered over time produces more severe effects than the same dose administered acutely.

- Depression, septicemia, mummification of feti, and an increase in stillbirths may occur in swine. Sows fed 20 ppm PCB during gestation and nursing, farrowed and weaned about half as many pigs as control sows.

Cattle: acute signs of toxicosis do not appear until dietary concentrations approach 5,000 ppm.

- Clinical signs include decreased milk production, anorexia, lacrimation, salivation, dehydration, diarrhea, alopecia, hyperkeratosis, weight loss and terminal recumbency.
- Many of these, especially hyperkeratosis, are also observed in animals suffering from "X disease" which affects cattle, sheep, and swine. This is now known to be caused by highly chlorinated naphthalenes which are frequent contaminants of PCBs.

Lesions

- Necropsy findings in swine and primates characteristically include gastric irritation and hyperemia. With higher exposures, mucoid hyperplasia and ulceration of the stomach may be present.
- Reproductive effects in cattle include abortions, embryonal resorption, and decreased fertility. Prepartum exposure to PBBs significantly increases fetal birth weight and the subsequent incidence of dystocia. Cows fed 250 mg per day for 180 or 202 days had a 100% incidence of dystocia. In addition, offspring exposed to PBBs *in utero* had significant conception difficulties at puberty.
- Necropsy findings in cattle may include dehydration, marked emaciation, fetal death with cotyledonary necrosis and hemorrhage, greatly enlarged pale kidneys, and dermal hyperkeratosis.
- Occasional findings include mucosal edema and ulcerations of the gastrointestinal tract, especially the abomasum, a thickened gall bladder wall, and thymic atrophy.
- Gross lesions are rarely present at dietary concentrations below 5000 ppm, so that necropsy may fail to indicate actual PCB or PBB poisoning. However, varying amounts of liver hypertrophy occur with either low level chronic exposure or high level acute exposure. The enlargement is not usually severe and is characterized histologically by scattered areas of glycogen depletion, dilatation of sinusoids, fatty degeneration, and very rarely, at higher exposures, centrilobular necrosis.

Effects in Birds

- In birds, PCBs and PBBs initiate clinical signs and lesions somewhat different than those of mammals. "Chick Edema" is now known to be caused by PCBs and their chlorinated naphthalene and dibenzodioxin contaminants. Primary signs and lesions include decreased body weight, anorexia, ascites, subcutaneous edema, dermatitis, hydropericardium, enlarged kidneys, centrilobular hepatic necrosis, splenic atrophy, and occasional enteritis with intestinal hemorrhage. A toxic plant (*Crotalaria*) may cause similar lesions.
- A diet containing 10-20 ppm PCBs or PBBs may cause adverse reproductive effects including decreased comb weight in cockerels, decreased fertility and egg production in hens, teratogenesis, reduced hatchability of eggs, and reduced chick viability.
- PCBs have been associated with abnormal sea gull wing development.

Diagnosis

Diagnosis is aimed at detecting PCBs or PBBs in milk fat, body fat, fresh liver samples, feed or other suspected sources. Specimens of milk should be collected in clean (acetone rinsed) glass jars with caps lined with aluminum foil. Tissues may be shipped frozen in (acetone rinsed) aluminum foil. Analysis is usually by gas chromatography with electron capture detection.

Treatment and Control

- There is no specific treatment for PCB or PBB toxicosis. Various agents such as activated charcoal, phenobarbital, vitamin A, vitamin D, and vitamin E, and thyroprotein have been administered without significantly affecting the rate of elimination from the body fat.
- In guinea pigs, ascorbic acid had some therapeutic potential based on its inducement of mixed function oxidases.
- The major goal in control is to discover and eliminate the source of contamination.
- The residue level must be determined in order to calculate the estimated clearance time, and thereby decide whether to decontaminate or destroy the animal.
- The long-term residue problems and potential for permanent effects often makes treatment in livestock uneconomical.

Pentachlorophenol

Sources

- Also referred to as penta and "PCP" although the latter term should be avoided due to its street use as a term denoting phencyclidine, which is also known as "angel dust".
- Pentachlorophenol was, until recently, the most commonly employed chemical in wood preservation. It was principally applied in hydrocarbon solvents as pentachlorophenol itself, although some sodium pentachlorophenate, which is water solubilized has also been used. Pressure-treated often meant "penta-treated", but at the present time, pressure-treated usually means treated with CCA (copper chromated arsenic).
- Pentachlorophenol is still sometimes used in light oils for brush-on application to wood, often used on natural, outdoor wood surfaces. Should never be applied indoors.

- "Penta"-treated feed and water troughs, fencing, and barn boards have been sources of contamination of livestock.
- Pentachlorophenol pressure-treated wood would sometimes "bleed" when it was relatively new. Its application under pressure would heavily soak the wood. Generally 11 g of penta was applied per board foot.
- Light solvent-based products may sometimes crystalize on wood surfaces and become airborn or sublime into sufficiently warm, enclosed surroundings.
- Miscellaneous other applications involve the herbicidal, fungicidal, insecticidal, bacteriocidal and molluscacidal (biocidal) properties of pentachlorophenol.
- Has been used in treatment of leather and in paper (to control mildew), in rug shampoos and for mothproofing of fabrics.
- Most wood is at least surface treated with a wood preservative to prevent mildew during shipping.
- Many other commonly used wood preservatives are also highly toxic. They may contain creosote (a phenolic), and the previously mentioned copper chromated arsenic (which causes effects most like arsenic toxicosis), among other possibilities. Such toxicants have a different spectrum of effects than those of pentachlorophenol.

Toxicity

- In all species evaluated, including domestic animals, the acute oral or dermal LD_{50} is 10-200 mg/kg.
- The multiple exposure lethal dose is 50-70 mg/kg. Minimal toxic daily doses of 20-35 mg/kg in calves.
- Young swine have died following exposure to oily, freshly treated wood used in farrowing crates or farrowing houses.
- Toxic to fish at 30 - 300 ppb and fish kills have resulted from spills into lakes and streams, primarily after a rain has flushed pentachlorophenol from an area used in wood treatment into the body of water.
- LC_{50} in the feed of birds is 3400-5200 ppm.
- Rats tolerate feed containing 1000 ppm (approx. 50 mg/kg) for 90 days but develop moderate hepatocellular necrosis and interstitial fibrosis. The no-effect feed concentration in rats was 25-50 ppm in the diet (1.5 - 3.0 mg/kg).

Toxicokinetics

- Rapid absorption from the skin, digestive tract and lung. Peak blood concentrations are reached within a few hours of ingestion.
- With a constant level of intake, blood concentrations generally plateau in five days.
- Most pentachlorophenol is in the plasma, with only small amounts in red blood cells.
- The highest tissue concentrations are in liver and kidney.
- Eliminated in the urine of all species tested and has a half-life of 1.5-2 days.
- Metabolites include tetrachlorohydroquinone and glucuronide conjugates, although some free pentachlorophenol is eliminated in the urine.

Toxicodynamics

- The acute toxicity of pentachlorophenol-containing products is primarily a result of the pentachlorophenol itself, which uncouples oxidative phosphorylation. Uncoupling of oxidative phosphorylation by pentachlorophenol appears to be due to the chlorophenate ion. By "uncoupling" the transfer of electrons down the cytochromes from the actual mitochondrial production of ATP, there is rapid utilization of the body's energy stores.
- It has also been suggested that there are inhibitory effects on enzymes, such as cellular kinases, dehydrogenases and reductases.

Clinical Signs

- When cows received technical grade penta, they became unthrifty after 8 weeks and, at 160 days, had dry scaly skin, diarrhea, urethritis, cystitis and a normocytic, normochromic anemia.
- With respiratory exposure, pain in the respiratory tract is accompanied by sneezing and coughing. Acclimated humans will tolerate up to 2.4 mg/m^3.
  - Mild toxicoses: weakness. Anorexia and lethargy.
  - Moderate toxicoses: rapid respiratory rate, hyperpyrexia (106-108 ^oF) and possible hyperglycemia, and glycosuria. Diaphoresis (sweating) in capable species.

- Lethal toxicoses: The above listed signs, plus cardiac and skeletal muscular collapse and death.
- Rapid onset of rigor mortis.
- Renal damage may result in proteinuria and increased blood urea nitrogen.

❒ Chronic toxicoses.

- Anemia.
- Dependent upon contaminants and may include weight loss, poor growth, dry scaly skin, diarrhea, and urethritis/cystitis.

Lesions

❒ Local irritation of areas contacted by the pentachlorophenol.

❒ Pulmonary edema and congestion.

❒ Hepatic enlargement, centrilobular degeneration and fatty change.

❒ Renal tubular hydropic and fatty change.

❒ Reduction in splenic white pulp (nonspecific change reflecting stress, similar to lesions of acute viral infection).

❒ Bile duct hyperplasia, and no other hepatic changes noted.

- Villous hyperplasia of the mucosa of the urinary bladder (severe).
- Hyperkeratosis of the skin (probably largely dependent upon contaminant concentrations).

Diagnosis

❒ A background blood pentachlorophenol determination in control animals revealed levels of 130 ppb.

❒ Clinical signs of acute lethal toxicoses occur with blood concentrations of 100 ppm and tissue of 200 ppm.

Treatment

❒ *Terminate exposure :* May include the use of bedding materials to remove animals from surfaces bleeding penta and resulting in dermal exposure; avoidance of contact of feed with penta-treated surfaces; control of interior temperature to reduce volatilization from warm areas; consider increased ventilation or removal of animals if extremely high concentrations or toxic effects are already present.

❒ Bathe off any exposed surfaces with a dish detergent.

- For early ingestions, the use of an emetic, activated charcoal and a cathartic are likely to be of value. For higher doses, lavage, including enterogastric or rumen lavage, may be appropriate depending upon the species and time factors involved.
- Correct acidoses if present with bicarbonate in fluids.
- Correct dehydration and promote excretion of pentachlorophenol and conjugates by the administration of fluids.
- Maintain positive energy balance to combat energy losses due to the biochemical effects of pentachlorophenol and to allow hepatic conjugation of the pesticide.
- Minimize stress and control any environmental conditions which may result in physiological increases in body temperature, stressors these have previously been shown to increase the likelihood of acute toxicoses with other uncouplers of oxidative phosphorylation.

Rodenticides

Rodenticides are a category of pest control chemicals intended to kill rodents.

Single feed baits are chemicals sufficiently dangerous that the first dose is sufficient to kill.

Rodents are difficult to kill with poisons because their feeding habits reflect their place as scavengers. They will eat a small bit of something and wait, and if they don't get sick, they continue. An effective rodenticide must be tasteless and odorless in lethal concentrations, and have a delayed effect. The redencticides are classified into different categories based on their mechanism of action as follows.

Anti-coagulant rodenticides	Non-anticoagulant rodenticides
1st generation: Warfarin and congeners Pindone, diphacinone, coumafuryl, chloroacinone, diphenadione, naphthylindandione (multiple feed)	a) Zinc phosphide - lung edema and haemorrhages b) Bromethalin - CNS depression and paralysis, death with in seconds. c) Cholecalciferol - hypercalcemia. d) ANTU - Lung edema
2nd generation: Bromadialone, brodifacoum (single feed)	

Anticoagulant Rodenticides

Today's anticoagulants are structurally related to coumarin or a similar prototype compound, indanedione. Other commercial rodenticides, notably sodium fluoroacetate (compound 1080®), zinc phosphide, strychnine, cholecalciferol (vitamin D3) and bromethalin operate by completely different mechanisms and present separate, specific problems for diagnosis and treatment.

Sources

Anticoagulant rodenticides are used extensively by the lay public and professional exterminators.

First Generation Anticoagulant Rodenticides

Warfarin

- There are a multitude of commercial warfarin-based anticoagulant rodenticides available for rodent control. These vary widely in concentration and formulations from 0.025% baits (most baits) to 1.0% throw-packs are encountered. Baits are often tan in color and may be mixed with grain. Pharmaceutical preparations (2 - 10 mg tablets) for use in cardiac patients may be a source of accidental exposure to pets from the household medicine cabinet. The chemical name of warfarin is 3(alpha-phenyl-beta-acetylethyl)-4 hydroxycoumarin. All warfarin-containing products should have the "4-hydroxycoumarin" chemical suffix included under the "active ingredient" on the package label.

Indanediones

- Indanedione-containing anticoagulant rodenticides also vary in concentration between products and formulations. Products range from 0.025% bait to 5.0% powder. Pharmaceutical preparations include tablets containing up to 50 mg active ingredient. Indanedione-containing products should contain the chemical suffix "1,3'indanedione" or "1,3(2H)-dione" listed under "active ingredient". Examples of generic names include: pindone, chlorphacinone, valone, anisindone (pharmaceutical), phenindione (pharmaceutical) and difethialone (pharmaceutical and rodenticide).

Second Generation Anticoagulant Rodenticides

- This group of anticoagulants was developed in the 1970s to answer the problems that existed with the use of the older, first generation anticoagulants.

- The basic coumarin or indanedione nucleus was retained to give the anticoagulant properties, but chemical structures were selected for increased potency (single lethal feeding potential), and efficacy against resistant rodents. These include the coumarin-based generics brodifacoum, difenacoum, and bromadiolone, and the indanedione diphacinone (sometimes called diphinadione). These are among the most widely used and most toxic anticoagulants.
- All of today's anticoagulant rodenticides have in common the basic coumarin or the structurally similar indanedione nuclei.

Warfarin

Toxicity and Susceptible Species

- The anticoagulant rodenticides are a potential hazard for all mammals, birds, and possibly other species. The susceptibility varies among animal species and the toxicity of the compounds also varies. Dogs and cats are most frequently involved, with occasional problems encountered in swine, ruminants, horses, pet birds, rodents and rabbits.
- Secondary toxicity
  - Although consumption of warfarin-poisoned rodents or birds by carnivores does not appear to present a likely hazard for the predator, consumption of tissues from diphacinone-poisoned animals has caused secondary poisoning in eagles, rats, dogs, and mink. Secondary toxicity may rarely occur with other second-generation anticoagulants.

LD_{50} Values for Warfarin Toxicity

Species	Toxic Level Single Dose	Toxic Level Repeated Doses
Rats	50 - 100 mg/kg	1 mg/kg x 5 days
Dogs	5 - 50 mg/kg	5 mg/kg x 5 - 15 days
Cats	5 - 50 mg/kg	1 mg/kg x 5 days
Swine*	3 mg/kg	0.05 mg/kg x 7 days
Ruminants		200 mg/kg x 12 days
Poultry	50% of BW of feed containing 0.1 mg/kg	

**Note that swine are particularly sensitive.*

LD$_{50}$ Values for Various Indanediones

Generic	Rat	Mouse	Dog	Cat	Pig	Rabbit	Duck	Human
Diphacinone	1.5	340	3	15	150	35		5 (LDLO)
Chlorphacinone	2.1	1				50	100	
Pindone	280		5 (LDLO)			150		50 (LDLO)

LD$_{50}$ Values for Brodifacoum

Species	LD$_{50}$ (mg/kg)	Species	LD$_{50}$ (mg/kg)
Dog	0.25 - 3.6	Guinea pig	2.8
Cat	25	Rat, Mouse	0.27 - 0.50
Sheep	25 - 33	Mink	9.2
Pig	0.5 - 2.0	Mallard duck	2.7 - 4.6
Rabbit	0.2 - 0.29	Harrier hawk	10

Toxicokinetics

- Absorption of warfarin is rather complete but occurs slowly, with peak plasma levels seen after 6 - 12 hours. Most of the warfarin is bound to plasma protein, but high concentrations are also found in the liver, spleen, and kidney.
- Metabolism of the coumarins occurs in the liver and involves mixed function oxidase enzymes. Inactive hydroxylated metabolites have been found in the urine. The acute toxicity of the coumarins is reduced when phenobarbital has been given to induce the hepatic enzymes. Vitamin K does not appear to enhance the rate of disappearance of the anticoagulant.
- The anticoagulant rodenticides are eliminated at various rates, depending on the compound and the amount ingested. The compound may accumulate with time, as in the case of an animal ingesting small amounts over several days. The half-life of warfarin in dog plasma is 14.5 hours. The half-life of diphacinone is 15-20 days in humans, which compares to a mean of 48 hours for warfarin in humans. The half-life of brodifacoum is yet to be reliably determined, but it is assumed to be at least as bioaccumulative and persistent as diphacinone. These differences in residual half-lives have very important implications when considering treatment of poisoned animals.

Pre-disposing Factors

- Animal factors: *1)* a high dietary fat intake [fatty acids displace the plasma protein bound anticoagulant increasing the free (active) fraction in the plasma so that more reaches the liver]; *2)* prolonged oral antibiotic therapy (decreased synthesis of vitamin K by intestinal bacteria); *3)* biliary obstruction and liver disease which presumably reduces metabolism and excretion of the anticoagulant and reduces clotting factor synthesizing ability.
- Plasma proteins (albumin) play a significant role in the patient's response to an anticoagulant. Warfarin is over 90% bound in canine plasma. The plasma proteins therefore constitute a great reservoir for warfarin. Warfarin cannot be excreted as long as it is in the tissues or bound to plasma proteins.
- Like fatty acids, certain xenobiotics displace warfarin from the albumin and shunt it down a concentration gradient into the tissue (liver), unless the tissue is already equilibrated, then the warfarin will be free to be excreted in the urine. Xenobiotics known to displace warfarin from albumin in the blood, include oxyphenbutazone, phenylbutazone (also decreases platelet integrity), diphenylhydantoin, sulfonamides, and adrenocorticosteroids.
- Uremia also causes decreased binding of the anticoagulant to serum proteins and may slow down excretion of the unbound fraction.
- Aspirin interferes with platelet function. Other xenobiotics generally contraindicated include promazine-type tranquilizers, local anesthetics, nitrofurans, antihistamines, anabolic steroids and epinephrine.
- Although evidence is very limited, there is some reason for concern regarding transmission of anticoagulants to young, perhaps via the milk. Because neonates tend to be hypoprothrombinemic, they may be particularly susceptible to anticoagulant exposure.

Toxicodynamics

- Interference with normal blood clotting as a result of reduced concentrations of clotting factors II (prothrombin), VII, IX, and X, due to competitive inhibition of the enzyme vitamin K epoxide-reductase.
- There does not appear to be any direct hepatotoxic damage from warfarin. Hypoxia and anemia, however, can lead to hepatic necrosis.

Clinical Signs

- Although signs have been observed within 1 day of ingestion, there is usually a lag period of 3 - 5 days between exposure and appearance of clinical signs.
- Onset of death may be acute, without the presence of other clinical signs. This is most common when hemorrhage occurs in the cerebral vasculature, abdominal cavity, pericardial sac, mediastinum, or thorax. Outward signs of hemorrhage may not exist in these instances.
- More often, the animal may be initially only depressed, anorexic, and anemic. Pale mucous membranes, dyspnea (due to hypoxia or pulmonary hemorrhage), hematemesis, epistaxis, and bloody or "tarry" feces are common soon thereafter. The animal may be febrile and display nonlocalized abdominal pain. Scleral, intraocular, conjunctival, nasal, oral, urogenital, and subcutaneous hemorrhage may be noted.
- Staggering or ataxia can be observed with severe blood loss., the heart rate may be irregular, and the pulse weak, extensive external hematomata may occur at pressure points or traumatized areas.
- Swollen, tender joints are common, especially in pigs and abortions have been noted in cattle.
- Animals experiencing prolonged toxicosis may be icteric from breakdown of impounded blood.

Lesions

- Generalized hemorrhage, especially in the thoracic or abdominal cavities, gut, mediastinal space, periarticular space, periarticular tissues, subcutaneous tissues, and subdural space.
- The heart is often flaccid and hemorrhagic.
- Centrilobular hepatic necrosis may result from anemia and hypoxia.

Diagnosis

- History of exposure
- Clinical signs may vary, but there should be an indication of hemorrhage or swellings.
- Laboratory evaluation of clotting parameters:
  - An elevated prothrombin time (PT) shows up first (24 - 48 hours postingestion) due to the involvement of factor VII (which has the

shortest half-life [6.2 hr] of the K-dependent clotting factors [II, VII, IX, and X]). This is followed soon thereafter by an elevated activated partial thromboplastin time (APTT). Platelet count will generally be in the normal to low-normal range.

- Consult your local hospital if you need help. Send in a citrated blood sample (bright blue stopper) from a "normal" dog to help with the interpretation.
- Clotting parameter times are suggestive if prolonged beyond 25% of the normal value.

❒ Chemical detection of specific anticoagulants in biological fluids, vomitus, or baits.

- Antemortem or postmortem sample of choice is whole blood (refrigerate).
- Another postmortem sample of choice is liver. Specimens should be wrapped in foil, well identified, sealed in plastic, and frozen during storage and shipment.

Differential Diagnosis

❒ Poor response to vitamin K1 therapy is helpful in ruling out anticoagulant toxicosis, provided that the animal is not anemic or in liver failure in addition to being poisoned by an anticoagulant.

❒ Autoimmune thrombocytopenia (AITP):

- Initial presentation: petechial to ecchymotic hemorrhages on mucous membranes, sclera, skin are characteristic; due to lack of platelets.
- Platelet numbers will be low (generally below 20,000) unless there is a functional platelet disorder, then numbers may be normal.
- Otterhound, Foxhound, Basset Hound are predisposed.

❒ DIC (disseminated intravascular coagulation).

- Important to identify a primary disease such as neoplasia, pancreatitis, heat stroke, sepsis, chronic active hepatitis, etc. Involves a careful history and physical workup or necropsy.
- Hematology to confirm: AT III, fibrinogen, plasminogen are decreased.
- Fibrin degradation products (fibrin split products) are present in blood; kits are available to test in clinics.

❒ Hereditary diseases (not common).

- Von Willebrand's disease
  - Hemorrhage is often less severe than with anticoagulant toxicosis.
  - Deficiency of a key component (von Willebrand factor) of the coagulation factor VIII, which is itself functional. The defect affects platelet function.
  - Analysis for factor VIII-C and factor VIII-RAg.
  - Scottish Terriers and Doberman Pinschers are predisposed.
- Hemophilia A
  - Factor VIII deficiency
  - Irish Setter, French Bulldog, Cairn Terrier, Greyhound, Poodles, others - more common
  - Intrinsic pathway is defective in coagulation elevated APTT

❒ Liver disease

- All coagulation factors except factor VII are synthesized in the liver.
- Portal hypertension may cause a backup and redistribution of platelets to the spleen, resulting in a deficiency in the circulation.
- Lack of bile secretion into the gut. Required for absorption of fat-soluble vitamin K. Biliary function tests indicate obstruction.

Treatment

If patient is presented with clinical complications:

❒ Correct low PCV and/or hypovolemia and provide clotting factors as needed using transfusion of fresh whole blood.

❒ Handle affected animals with care; sedate (promazine contraindicated) if necessary.

- 10 - 20 ml of fresh, whole blood/kg BW, IV; first 25% of the dose relatively fast, and the rest by slow drip.

❒ Vitamin K1 (phytonadione, phylloquinone) is the most effective form of the various forms of the vitamin. It is similar to the natural form of the vitamin and works rapidly (begins to reverse the situation in about 30 minutes provided the animal is not anemic and/or hypoxic). Oral vitamin K is faster acting and more effective than the parenteral form. It is absorbed from the GI tract and transported directly to the liver via the portal vein. It should be given with food to enhance its absorption. Use the oral form unless contraindicated (e.g., concurrent administration of activated charcoal, GI hemorrhage, severe depression, etc.). When the injectable form is required use the smallest possible needle and carefully wrap the leg to prevent hemorrhage.

- Dogs: 3 - 5 mg/kg (lower dose in larger animals), SQ or IM. IV administration may cause anaphylaxis; if you use the IV route, be sure the product is approved for this route and administer over 20 minutes with continuous monitoring; dose may be divided into 2 daily doses if preferred.
- Cats: 15 - 25 mg, total dose, SQ or IM.

❒ Recommended oral doses of vitamin K for dogs and cats range from 0.25 - 2.5 mg/kg/day for warfarin toxicosis and 2.5 - 5 mg/kg/day for long-acting rodenticide toxicosis.

- Pigs: 2 - 5 mg/kg (lower dose in larger animals), SQ/IM. Vitamin K3 (menadione sodium bisulfite), feed-grade, should be added to all swine rations at 20 g/ton of feed as a good preventative management tool because of the common idiopathic, vitamin K-responsive coagulopathy of swine.
- Horses: Vitamin K1 at not over 2 mg/kg, SQ/IM; use aseptic techniques for injection. Do not use vitamin K3 (menadione) in Equidae. Deaths have occurred from use of injectable menadione at manufacturer's recommended dosages. Mechanism of toxicity is unknown, but acute renal failure is observed.
- Ruminants: Vitamin K1 at 0.5 - 1.5 mg/kg, SQ/IM, not more than 10 ml/injection site. Vitamin K3 is reportedly of little or no value.

❒ Duration of therapy.

❒ Warfarin.

- Daily administration is recommended for 10 - 14 days, depending on the amount ingested and severity of the symptomatology.

❒ Bromadiolone.

- Daily administration for 21 days.

❒ Diphacinone, brodifacoum (and others).

- Suggested daily administration for 30 days.
- Follow in 5 - 7 days after end of treatment period with a prothrombin time (in severe cases, very young, or debilitated patients, continued vitamin K therapy may sometimes be necessary).

- Pasture and green forages provide some vitamin K and may lessen the need somewhat for prolonged treatment of anticoagulant-exposed herbivores.

If dyspnea continues, a thoracic radiograph may be indicated. Thoracocentesis to remove extravasated blood may be indicated to save the patient's life, but extreme caution must be exercised to prevent further hemorrhage.

- Oxygen may be beneficial in severely dyspneic animals.
- Keep patient warm and still until stabilized. Minimal rates of balanced electrolyte solutions may be used if needed for extra fluids and only after sufficient clotting factors (generally whole blood) are on board.
- Once stable, the patient can be sent home and dosed with oral form of vitamin K1. Client education is very important to ensure that the medication is continued as directed.
- Avoid elective surgery.
- Avoid protein bound xenobiotics as much as possible. Contraindicated xenobiotics during recovery period include corticosteroids, sulfa s, antihistamines, phenylbutazone, epinephrine, and aspirin.

Instructions to the owner

- Avoiding fatty foods, table scraps, etc.
- Restricting exercise for duration of therapy.
- Strict attention to daily medication, even if patient looks and acts normal. Clinical relapses have occurred with premature withdrawal of medication.

If patient is presented asymptomatic within several hours of a suspected or confirmed exposure:

- Induce emesis if within 3 hours of ingestion with apomorphine (dog), syrup of ipecac, or xylazine (cat), or 3% H_2O_2 (either species). Do not induce emesis if patient is depressed or recumbent or if other contraindications are present.
- Activated or superactivated charcoal.
- Osmotic cathartic (sorbitol). Alternatively, a saline cathartic may be administered after being mixed with at least 5 times as much water. Administer via stomach tube or orally. Effective for as long as bait is in the gut.

- Decision to begin vitamin K therapy will depend on the situation, i.e., amount ingested, effectiveness of emesis procedure, time since ingestion. In cases of suspected low dose exposures (i.e., < 1/8 of the LD_{50}), may elect (after emetic and activated charcoal, etc.) to give an injection of vitamin K1, and send patient home with instructions to observe the animal closely for 10 - 30 days, depending upon the compound involved.
  - Vitamin K3 has the disadvantage of not being as effective as vitamin K1. Do not use vitamin K3 alone in symptomatic or highly exposed small animals, use vitamin K1.
- Adverse effects related to vitamin K1 therapy generally stem from IV administration. Anaphylactoid reactions occur quite often, including cutaneous manifestations such as urticaria. Large doses (10 mg/kg) of vitamin K1 have been associated with Heinz body anemia and hemolysis.

Alpha-Naphthyl Thiourea (ANTU)

Sources

- Alpha-naphthyl thiourea is a fine gray insoluble powder possessing almost no odor or taste.
- The compound is extremely stable and does not deteriorate on prolonged storage.
- It finds primary use as a rodenticide, though rarely used at present and in doses less than 100 mg/kg has been found to be toxic only to the rat, cats, dogs, mice and pigs.
- Usually baits are prepared by including 2% ANTU in cereals, meats or bread mashes.
- Baits containing ANTU are readily accepted by animals, but they are able to develop a tolerance towards the substance.

Toxicity

Dogs are the domestic species most often poisoned with ANTU. The LD_{50} is influenced by species and age. Comparative LD_{50} of ANTU in mature animals are presented in the following table.

Species	Route of Administration	LD, mg/kg Body Weight
Wild rat	Oral	6.9 + .05
Dog	Oral	38
Mouse	Oral	19
Guinea pig	Oral	143
Cat	Oral	75 - 100
Pig	Oral	25 - 50

Toxicodynamics

- ANTU kills by producing a marked hydrothorax and pulmonary edema. The animal literally drowns in its own fluids.
- The accumulation of fluids is due to an increase in the permeability of capillaries in the lungs. When lymph flow from the lungs was monitored following the administration of ANTU to dogs, increase in the flow was noted within 90 minutes following dosing. At the eighth hour after dosing, the lymph flow had increased to 80 times its original value. The exact mechanism resulting in increased capillary permeability has not been determined.
- Reaction of ANTU with sulfhydryl groups may be a necessary part of the mechanism of toxic action, since it has been reported that sulfhydryl group blocking agents are effective antidotes in rats in some experimental conditions.

Clinical Signs

- Vomiting is one of the first signs noted, occurring a few minutes to a few hours following ingestion of ANTU.
- Breathing becomes rapid (short, jerky inspirations) and a shallow hacking cough may be noted. Moist rales can be detected in the lung fields.
- The extremities are cold to the touch and the visible mucous membranes appear cyanotic. The peripheral pulse is almost imperceptible while the cardiac impulse is accelerated and weak.
- Normal or subnormal temperature, with animal continuing to vomit as the disease progresses and the vomitus may consist entirely of blood.
- Watery fluid diarrhea becomes hemorrhagic if the patient survives the acute symptoms.
- The affected animal remains standing or sits on its haunches to relieve thoracic pressure. As the animals become weaker, they assume a position of sternal recumbency.
- In the terminal stages, the lungs are congested or filled with fluid and fluid may escape from the mouth.
- The animal becomes comatose and fails to respond to external stimuli. Most deaths occur in 2 - 4 hours after symptoms appear. If the animal survives for 12 hours after ANTU exposure, the prognosis becomes more favorable.

Lesions

- The most apparent change noted at necropsy is hydrothorax. The thoracic cavity is often completely filled with a clear, colorless fluid. Severe edema of the lungs is a consistent finding and, in some instances, fluid will actually flow from the trachea when the lungs are removed from their cavity.
- The poison is moderately irritating to the stomach and intestines, and catarrhal inflammation is usually present in these organs.
- In many instances, the kidneys assume a blood red color as a result of intense hyperemia or congestion.

Diagnosis : Since chemical tests for ANTU are usually inconclusive, diagnosis is based on history, characteristic clinical signs and necropsy findings.

Treatment

- Emetics such as apomorphine (in the dog) may be of value if animals are presented early in the course of the poisoning and if the ingestion of baits containing ANTU is suspected.
- Because of the seriousness of ANTU toxicosis, measures to eliminate the gastrointestinal tract contents should be followed as soon as possible after exposure.
- Activated charcoal may possibly be of value in the lavage solutions and should be left in the lumen thereafter. If a thorough enterogastric lavage is not performed, then a saline cathartic should also be administered.
- Mineral oil fats can enhance absorption of ANTU and should be avoided.
- Although silicone aerosols may prevent foaming of excessive bronchial fluids, there is no specific treatment for ANTU poisoning.
- Experimental evidence indicates that providing thiol groups may reduce mortality. Potential thiol-containing compounds include N-amyl mercaptan, N-acetyl cysteine, or thyacetyl cysteine.
- Atropine has not been helpful in controlling the pulmonary edema. The prognosis for animals suffering from clinically significant ANTU poisoning is poor.

Cholecalciferol Based Rodenticides

Sources

- Cholecalciferol (Vitamin D3)-containing rodenticides are marketed as an acute single feeding or chronic (multiple feeding) rodenticide.

- Cholecalciferol is present at 0.075% concentration in final bait formulations. Cholecalciferol naturally exists in animals as a precursor of active vitamin D. Its intrinsic biological activity, however, is low.
- Advertised as having no bait shyness, and reported effective against anticoagulant-resistant rodents. Rodent death is delayed for 2-5 days. After lethal dose is consumed all feeding stops.
- Cod liver oil is another source of Vitamin D as well as Vitamin A.
- Vitamin D2 (ergocalciferol) is the plant form of Vitamin D. It is not utilized by poultry and only poorly utilized by swine).

Toxicity

- Based upon clinical reports, toxicoses have occurred in dogs from the ingestion of cholecalciferol at 0.5 - 3 mg/kg body weight.
- Acute oral LD_{50} in dogs of technical material in oil has been reported to be 85 mg/kg. This has lead to an underestimate of the actual hazard of the rodenticide products for this species.
- 40 IU vitamin D = 1 mcg. Thus, 1 IU of vitamin D3 = 0.025 mcg of cholecalciferol.

Toxicodynamics

- Calcium homeostasis is under the control of: 1) parathyroid hormone (PTH), 2) calcitonin, and 3) vitamin D metabolites. Calcium concentration of the blood is composed of "diffusible calcium" including the citrate bound and free calcium ion (ionic calcium) fraction (40%), and a "nondiffusible" protein-bound fraction (30 - 50%).
  - Parathyroid hormone (PTH) is secreted by the chief cells of the parathyroid gland. Parathyroid hormone feedback system is relatively simple, controlled primarily by serum calcium ion concentration (magnesium ion has lesser effects). As serum calcium levels rise, PTH levels decline. Parathyroid hormone has its primary effects on the bone, kidney, and to a lesser degree the intestine. PTH acts on bone to mobilize calcium (from skeletal reserves) into the extracellular fluid (increased osteoclasic and osteocytic activity. Prolonged PTH levels results in increased osteoclast numbers). PTH exerts a rapid effect on the proximal renal tubules resulting in decreased phosphate reabsorption. PTH also enhances distal convoluted tubule reabsorption of calcium. Finally, increased intestinal absorption of calcium occurs as a result of PTH influence.

- Calcitonin (CT) is secreted by thyroid parafollicular (C) cells. PTH and CT have antagonistic effects on bone reabsorption, but synergistic effects on renal tubular reabsorption of phosphorous. Blockade of osteoclastic and osteocytic bone reabsorption occurs as a result of calcitonin activity.
- Cholecalciferol (vitamin D3) is synthesized in the epidermis under the influence of sunlight from its precursor, 7-dehydrocholesterol. Vitamin D binding protein transports cholecalciferol from the skin into the blood. Vitamin D3 from dietary sources is absorbed by facilitated diffusion and becomes bound to alpha-2-globulin in blood. Cholecalciferol is then enzymatically (calciferol-25-hydroxylase) converted to 25, hydroxycholecalciferol (25-OH-D3) in the liver. Then 25-OH-D3 is transported to the kidney, where further metabolism (by 25-OH-D3-1 hydroxylase) to 1,25 dihydroxycholecalciferol (1,25-(OH)2-D3) occurs. The conversion of 25-OH-D3 to 1,25-(OH)2-D3 is rate-limiting, and partially explains the delay in biological activity of dietary vitamin D3.
- In the liver, 1,25-(OH)2-D3 can also be converted by 24-hydroxylase to 24,25 dihydroxycholecalciferol (24,25-(OH)2-D3). The 24,25-(OH)2-D3 is less active and is preferentially formed when high serum calcium levels exist. Vitamin D metabolites increase serum calcium concentration in the following ways:

1. Vitamin D and its active metabolites function to increase the absorption of calcium and phosphorus from the intestines. The major target tissue for 1,25-(OH)2-D3 is the small intestine where it increases the active transcellular transport of calcium and phosphorus.
2. The absorptive capacity of the intestine for calcium is a direct function of the amount of calcium binding protein (CaBP) present. Synthesis of CaBP is stimulated by vitamin D metabolites.
3. The active metabolites of cholecalciferol also act on bone. Vitamin D (in the presence of PTH) is required for osteoclastic resorption and calcium mobilization from bone. Cholecalciferol, 25-OH-D3 and 1,25-(OH)2-D3 stimulate osteoclastic proliferation and resorption of bone. On a per weight basis 1,25-(OH)2-D3 is 100 times more potent in stimulating bone resorption than is 25-OH-D3.

- Active metabolites of vitamin D also stimulate the retention of calcium by increasing its renal distal tubular reabsorption.

Clinical Signs

- Clinical signs most commonly associated with cholecalciferol-induced hypercalcemia can be divided into neurologic, cardiovascular, gastrointestinal, and especially renal.
- Clinical signs generally develop within 18 - 36 hours postexposure and include: anorexia, lethargy, nausea, weakness, vomiting (+ blood), diarrhea (+ blood), polyuria, polydipsia, and rarely neurological disturbances (e.g., seizures). Clinical signs become more severe as serum calcium levels increase.
- Hypercalcemia can result in ECG changes including shortened Q-T interval and prolonged P-R interval. Vasoconstriction and hypertension may occur.
- Effects on the kidney include an interference with the ability of the collecting tubules to reabsorb water. Hypercalcemia reduces the concentration of cAMP in cells that normally respond to antidiuretic hormone (nephrogenic diabetes insipidus). Hypercalcemia and hypercalciuria also cause decreased sodium-chloride reabsorption leading to a degree of medullary washout. Clinically, polyuria and hyposthenuria are observed. In dogs with induced hypercalcemia, vasoconstriction of glomerular afferent arterioles occurs with a resultant decrease in GFR.
- Death is thought to result from hypercalcemia, calcification of tissues, renal and heart failure.

Clinical Pathology

- The most profound alteration in serum chemistry is an elevated serum calcium (more than 11.5 mg/dl in adult). Elevations in serum phosphorous occurred at 12 hours postingestion and preceded serum calcium rise (occurred 24 hours postingestion). Increased BUN and creatinine are also seen.
- Urine specific gravity may be in the hyposthenuric range (1.002 - 1.006). Proteinuria and glycosuria may be seen.

  Note - Adjusted calcium values (adjusted for protein binding by albumin) may need to be considered.

  Corrected calcium = Ca (mg/dl) - albumin (gm/dl) + 3.5. Alternatively, ionized calcium concentrations can be determined directly by many laboratories.

- Condition must be distinguished from normally occurring (physiologic) juvenile hypercalcemia; therefore, a baseline serum calcium determination is generally indicated as soon after ingestion as possible.

Lesions

- Morphological changes seen in dogs given vitamin D experimentally included: roughened, red, raised plaques in aorta or pulmonary artery. Histopathologically, these were characterized by intimal proliferation, subintimal edema, and hemosiderin deposition. Thyroid glands were grossly enlarged and paler than normal, microscopic changes included hypertrophy and hyperplasia of parafollicular cells.
- Kidneys with red and gray cortical surfaces. Calcium deposition was random. Degeneration of renal tubular epithelium was evident microscopically. Mild glomerular degeneration was observed. Mineralization occurred in the basement membrane of tubules, especially the ascending loop of Henle, collecting and distal convoluted tubules. This can be a critical problem since renal tubular epithelium regeneration requires an intact basement membrane.
- Calcification and necrosis of intramural coronary arteries, gastric mucosa, intestinal wall, parietal pleura, terminal pulmonary airways, thyroid, pancreas, and urinary bladder was observed. Myocardial degeneration, necrosis, and mineralization may occur.

Diagnosis

- Based upon exposure history, clinical signs, development of hypercalcemia, and if death occurs, lesions.
- Differential diagnoses include hypercalcemia secondary to paraneoplastic syndrome (most commonly observed with lymphosarcoma), juvenile hypercalcemia, and hyperparathyroidism.

Treatment

Current recommendations for the control of hypercalcemia are as follows (treatment should be followed in order):

- If patient has recently (< 3 hours) consumed cholecalciferol bait, emesis should be induced.
- Activated charcoal and a saline cathartic are administered depending upon the likelihood of the presence of unabsorbed bait in the digestive

tract. Also, repeated administration may be of value in counteracting enterohepatic recirculation of vitamin D and its active metabolites.

- Determine baseline serum calcium levels as soon as the animal is presented if a potentially toxic dose was digested. Continue monitoring serum calcium levels approximately every 24 hours to determine if further therapy is required. If therapy is required, it is continued until, when it is withdrawn, serum calcium levels are found to remain normal.
- Fluid therapy consists of IV normal saline and furosemide (5 mg/kg given IV followed by 2.5 - 4.5 mg/kg TID to QID per os) as a diuretic. Thiazide diuretics should not be used because they decrease urinary excretion of calcium and may contribute to or cause hypercalcemia. Saline is preferred over other fluids, because of enhancement of calcium elimination in the urine.
- Patient should be placed on a low calcium diet, and sunlight should be avoided.
- Cortisone should be administered (2 - 3 mg/kg). Corticosteroids have several beneficial effects including inhibition of osteoclast-activating factors (OAF) action on bone. In addition, cortisone directly inhibits release of OAF and depresses PG 2 mediated release of OAF. Corticosteroids also exert a hypercalciuric effect and cause decreased intestinal absorption of calcium.
- Calcitonin (salmon calcitonin) has been used in the treatment of hypercalcemia. This is to be given in microgram quantities (4 - 6 IU/kg) SQ every 2 - 3 hours initially until serum calcium levels stabilize. Therapy should be individualized according to need. Long-term calcitonin administration (weeks) at increased doses may be required. Foreign protein reactions are possible necessitating therapeutic administration of epinephrine and possibly other agents as well as discontinuation of further use of calcitonin.
- Pamidronate, a second generation biphosphonate, blocks dissolution of hydroxyapatite and decreases conversion of calcifidiol to calcifitriol. It has a long half life *in vivo*. It can be used instead of calcitonin. Although very expensive, e.g., $300 for one dose for a 25 kg dog, only one to a few treatments may be needed.
- Treatment with diuretics and corticosteroids should continue until the animal's serum calcium concentrations have stabilized in the normal range. Often treatment should continue for 2 weeks, followed by removal of therapy, and retesting of serum calcium levels after 24 hours. Continue

1-week-long regimens of diuretic/corticosteroid until serum calcium remains normal after their withdrawal (check serum Ca^{++} at 24, 48, and 72 hours after final therapy). Monitor serum calciums and BUN as needed throughout therapy.

Zinc Phosphide and Aluminum Phosphide

Sources

- Zinc phosphide is a dull, grayish-black powder used mainly as a rodenticide and for killing moles.
- Zinc phosphide, or occasionally aluminum phosphide, may be used in baits of bread, buns, soaked wheat, damp rolled oats, or sugar at concentrations of 2 - 5%.
- Aluminum phosphide is used as a grain fumigant for insect and rodent control and in dusts for insect control.
- Zinc phosphide is unstable in water or acid, but is stable for about 2 weeks under average climatic conditions. Can be stable for long time periods if kept dry.
- Aluminum phosphide degrades more readily than zinc phosphide.
- Either compounds degrade to reactive (toxic) phosphine gas which accounts for much of the toxicity and smells like garlic or rotten fish.

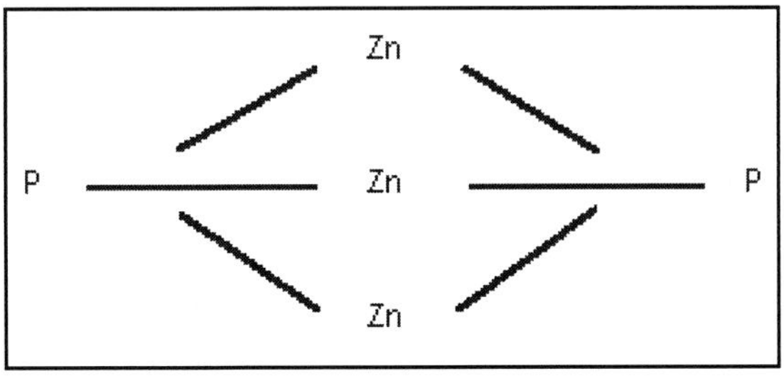

Structure of zinc phosphide

Toxicity

- Lethal doses in cattle, sheep, pigs, goats, dogs, cats between 20-50 mg/kg.
- Animals poisoned by feeding directly on bait or relay toxicosis associated with eating tissues of zinc phosphide-poisoned animals.

Toxicodynamics

- Food in the stomach increases HCl production which greatly increases the breakdown to toxic phosphine (PH_3) gas which induces serious acute effects due to enteric and pulmonary irritation.

$$Zn_3P_2 + 6H_2O \rightarrow 3Zn(OH)_2 + 2PH_3.$$

- CNS effects are due to an unknown mechanism but acidosis and hypocalcemia may occur.
- Both phosphine and intact zinc phosphide are absorbed from the GI tract. The phosphine is believed to cause the majority of acute signs, while the intact phosphide may cause hepatic and renal damage later.

Clinical Signs

- Zinc phosphide causes emesis frequently in nonrodent species and, because of this effect, fatal poisoning is not a consistent sequel to ingestion. A few preparations have added tartar emetic to increase vomiting.
- Onset of clinical signs usually occurs from 15 minutes to 4 hours after ingestion, but may be delayed for up to 18 hours.
- Large doses may cause death within 3 - 5 hours.
- Severely affected animals rarely live longer than 48 hours.
- The vomitus of zinc phosphide-poisoned animals often contains dark blood.
- Dogs may show lateral recumbency with whole body tremors and salivation. May proceed into "running fits" and repeated jerking of the head. Terminal exhaustion may occur.
    - Anorexia, lethargy, and rapid deep breathing which often becomes wheezy or "clicky" sounding.
    - Abdominal pain, ataxia, weakness, and recumbency may follow.
    - Acidosis is prominent, and there may be hypocalcemia, terminal hypoxia, gasping, and struggling.
    - Hyperesthesia and sometimes seizures may be seen, and in some dogs these may closely resemble strychnine convulsions.
    - Hepatic and renal damage often may be detected 5 - 14 days later.
    - Acetylene (garlic, rotten fish) odor on breath.
- Abdominal pain, colic in horses, and bloat in cattle.

Lesions

- Opening the stomach will reveal a characteristic acetylene odor and possibly evidence of gastritis
- Nonspecific postmortem findings.
- The lungs are often markedly congested and may have interlobular edema, pleural effusion, subpleural hemorrhages also noted.
- Acutely affected animals have extreme congestion of the liver and kidney.
- Myocardial degeneration sometimes may occur.
- Pale yellow mottling of liver may appear in subacute cases.
- On histopathology, there is fatty change and congestion of the liver and kidneys. Also, there may be renal tubular degeneration, hyaline change, and necrosis.

Diagnosis

- Tentative diagnosis based on compatible clinical signs, an acetylene odor to the breath, and opportunity for or, better, evidence of exposure to zinc phosphide. Phosphine gas rapidly dissipates.
- Frozen vomitus or gastric lavage fluid may be submitted in air-tight containers keeping the samples frozen as an attempt to obtain confirmation (phosphine gas identified for zinc or aluminum phosphide analyses).
- Rapid freezing (and care to maintain the frozen state in transit) of stomach contents, liver, and kidney increases the probability that laboratory analysis for phosphine gas may turn out to be worthwhile. However, with phosphine method, false negatives may be encountered.
- In some cases, concentrations of zinc in serum, liver, and kidney may be elevated but these assays are more difficult to interpret. Because of the use of zinc stearate to coat rubber, serum samples for analysis of zinc must be drawn in all glass or all plastic syringes (no rubber), and all glass or all plastic vials (no rubber stoppers) must be used for transport.

Treatment

- The gastrointestinal contents should be evacuated by emesis in suitable species following administration of aluminum plus magnesium hydroxide gel ; empirically recommended, rather than oral bicarbonate to decrease phosphine release.

- Activated charcoal orally, preferably mixed with sorbitol.
- Respiratory failure may necessitate administration of 100% humidified oxygen or possibly artificial respiration via a ventilator with positive and expiratory pressure (PEEP).
- Metabolic acidosis is corrected by IV administration of sodium bicarbonate (slow, in fluids).
- Fluids may be administered IV and corticosteroids may be needed to help alleviate shock.
- B-vitamins and dextrose may be used for possible hepatic injury along with appropriate dietary therapy.
- Seizures may be controlled with diazepam or phenobarbital or, if it fails, anesthesia induced with pentobarbital.

Metaldehyde

Sources

- Molluscicide - slug and snail baits - polymer of acetaldehyde. Occasional baits contains cereals: increases palatability.
  - Pellets. Snarol, Buggetta.
  - Liquid. Dead-line (sticky liquid).
  - Bait usually 3.5% metaldehyde.
  - Some products contain arsenic or carbamate (insecticidal compounds) which are usually of less toxicologic importance than the metaldehyde present.
  - Poisoning - coastal areas and south (especially in California).
- Used as a fuel in small heaters.
- Incidence in the early 1970's in California:
  - 4.5 cases/month/small animal practice - Sacramento area.
  - Some emergency clinics averaged 20 - 30 cases/week.

Susceptible Species

Dogs, cats, sheep, humans, others.

Toxicity

- Toxic oral dose of metaldehyde for most species is from 60 - 500 mg/kg.
- Minimum oral lethal dose metaldehyde.

- Dog: 100 mg/kg.
- Horse: 60 - 360 mg/kg.
- Cow: 200 mg/kg.

- Reported LD50
  - Dog: LD50 oral: 100 - 1000 mg/kg.
  - Cat: LD50 oral: 207 mg/kg.
  - Guinea pig: LD50 oral: 175 mg/kg.
  - Mouse: LD50 oral: 200 mg/kg.
  - Rat: LD50 oral: 227 mg/kg.
  - Rabbit: LD50 oral: 290 mg/kg.
- 3 - 4 ounces of most pelleted baits would be toxic to average size dog, sheep.

Toxicokinetics

- Acetaldehyde liberated by gastric hydrolysis of metaldehyde.
- Acetaldehyde - milder odor than formaldehyde.

Toxicodynamics

- Precise mechanism of action in mammals unknown.
- Acidosis presumably results from the subsequent metabolism of acetaldehyde and from other effects (tremors, seizures, exertion).
- Acetaldehyde may or may not directly cause the problems occurring in metaldehyde toxicosis.
  - Acetaldehyde not detected in tissue or serum from metaldehyde poisoned dogs.
- Brain concentration of 5-HT (5-hydroxytryptamine = serotonin) and noradrenaline are often inversely related to the prevalence of seizures.
  - A decrease in brain 5-HT and noradrenalin occurs in metaldehyde-poisoned animals.
  - Intraperitoneal administration of acetaldehyde to mice did not result in significant depression of 5-HT.
- An increase in monoamine oxidase (MAO) activity occurs during metaldehyde toxicosis in mice. However, MAO activity was unrelated to survivability of mice in this study. Conversely, MAO activity is decreased in acetaldehyde-poisoned mice.

- Decreases in the important inhibitory neurotransmitter gamma amino butyric acid (GABA) also occur in metaldehyde poisoned animals (mice). As GABA levels decreased so did survival rates.

Clinical Signs

- Cattle
  - Salivation, ataxia, hyperpnea, tremors, convulsions (convulsions may start at posterior end and progress forward). These may pitch cattle forward on their muzzles if severe. Frothy diarrhea sometimes occurs. Cyanosis. Loss of "blink" reflex and blindness. May overreact to external stimuli.
- Sheep and Goats
  - "CNS signs tremors fore and hind limbs, ataxia, convulsions, nystagmus, cyanosis, liver damage (pale and friable) in goats and sheep
  - Uncommon cause of poisoning.
- Horses
  - Colic
  - Mild leg tremors, hyperesthesia, diarrhea, sweating, hyperpnea (severely fluted nostrils)
  - Tachycardia, clonic spasms, incoordination, extended head, convulsive spasms
  - Violent muscle spasms and ventroflexion of the spinal column just before death.
- Dogs
  - Often eat all the snail bait available to them
  - Onset of signs - almost immediate up to 3 hours
  - Sequence
    - Increased heart rate, anxiety, nystagmus.
    - Mydriasis, hyperpnea, panting, hypersalivation (may be frothy) stiff legs, ataxia.
    - May be rapidly followed by muscle tremors, then vomiting, hyperesthesia, continuous convulsions, cyanosis, acidosis, diarrhea, dehydration, hyperthermia (to 108° F).

- Convulsions more continuous than in strychnine poisoning. Also, external stimuli do not have the marked effect as seen in strychnine toxicosis.
- Later stages may have depression followed by narcosis.
- If death occurs, it is usually from respiratory failure and takes place from 4 - 24 hours after exposure. If animal survives this period, it may succumb to liver failure within 2 to 3 days.

❐ Possible to have temporary blindness (which may last weeks) with normal pupillary reflexes.

❐ Feline (toxicosis not reported frequently)
- Similar to canine except nystagmus may be more prevalent.
- Depression, dyspnea, convulsions, tachycardia.

❐ Birds
- Poisoning reported in ducks and geese.
- Lethal dose ducks 300 mg/kg.
- Signs include ataxia, opisthostonus, dyspnea, polypnea, tremors.

Lesions

❐ Cattle
- Blood may fail to clot.
- Dark, congested lungs.
- Petechia in airways, throughout body.
- Sometimes enteritis and massive endocardial hemorrhages.

❐ Horse
- Lesions not diagnostic (not sufficiently specific).
- Epicardial hemorrhage.
- Moderate pulmonary congestion.
- Swollen red liver.
- Slight hyperemia of upper gastrointestinal mucosa.

❐ Birds
- Engorged vessels in mesentery and intestinal serosa.
- Petechiation gizzard.
- Lungs congested, bloody fluid in air sacs.
- Swollen hepatocytes with coagulative degeneration.

- Dogs
  - Nonspecific lesions
    - Hepatic, renal, pulmonary congestion, subendocardial, subepicardial hemorrhages.
    - Gastrointestinal hemorrhages.
- Any species
  - Acetaldehyde odor in stomach/gastrointestinal tract may help in diagnosis.

Diagnosis

- Acetaldehyde in stomach content, lavage washings, tissues: Submit frozen. Freeze rapidly. Acetaldehyde smells similar to formaldehyde.
- Metaldehyde in baits can be analytically detected.
- Metaldehyde in liver, urine, and plasma. Urinary excretion is low.

Treatment

- *Seizure control* : Diazepam 2 - 5 mg/kg IV to effect may be preferred over barbiturates because barbiturates compete with an enzyme that degrades acetaldehyde. Phenobarbital or pentobarbital may be required for unresponsive cases.
- *Horses* : Xylazine with acepromazine has been recommended.
- Artificial respiration.
- Enterogastric lavage, activated charcoal.
- *Severe cases* : Gas anesthesia, fluids with bicarbonate.
- Fluid therapy to control dehydration, acidosis, electrolyte imbalances.

Fluoroacetate - 1080

Sources

- Primarily used in commercial rodent control (e.g. by Pest Control Operators in very controlled conditions). Not legally found in rodenticides for use in homes in the USA.
  - Tasteless, odorless, colorless; dyed black.
  - Relay toxicosis - especially in dogs, possible in other species.
- Coyote control

- Large bait stations - used in past; now illegal.
- Occasional experimental coyote control permits.
- Toxic collars (various forms) on sacrificial sheep - on market now.
- Single lethal dose baits - proposed and studied but not marketed.

- Used for control of ground squirrels and rabbits in some countries.
- Still in use as a widely available rodenticide in some Latin American and other countries of the world. Sometimes products are smuggled into the USA from Mexico.
- Characteristic lag period after ingestion, may limit the development of bait shyness.
- Fluoroacetic acid is the toxic principle in several poisonous plant species from South Africa, Australia, and Brazil (see front index).

Fluoracetate is an important toxic metabolite of some fluorinated ethanes that might be inhaled, e.g.: 1,2-difluoroethane, 1-chloro-2-fluoroethane, 1-chloro-1,2-difluorethane, and 1-bromo-2-fluoroethane of fluoroethylnitrosoureas. The enzyme involved in bioactivation is likely to be cytochrome P450 2E1.

Toxicity

- Oral lethal doses (LD50)
  - Canine and feline 0.05 - 1.0 mg/kg of b.w.
  - Rodent 0.2 - 8 mg/kg.
- Oral lethal doses
  - Cattle: 0.15 - 0.62 mg/kg.
  - Sheep: 0.25 - 0.50 mg/kg.
  - Goat: 0.30 - 0.70 mg/kg.
  - Horse: 0.50 - 1.75 mg/kg.
  - Pig: 0.30 - 0.40 mg/kg.
  - Fowl: 10 - 30 mg/kg.

Toxicodynamics

Classical Theory

(Lethal synthesis) : Fluoroacetate + Acetyl-Co-A → Fluoroacetyl-Co-A + Oxalacetate → Fluorocitrate

Inhibits Aconitase (Kreb's cycle inhibited, energy depleted), which results in accumulation of citric and lactic acids.

- Kun's hypothesis (not widely accepted).
  - Fluorocitrate is formed as shown above and is the active (toxic) metabolite.
  - Primary mechanism is not primarily due to inhibition of aconitase - but is due to inhibition of citrate transport across the inner mitochondrial membrane.
- Relay toxicoses possible. Occurs especially when canids consume poisoned rodents.

Clinical Signs

- Affects CNS and heart.
- Effects and signs vary with species.
- Latent period 1/2 to several hours.
- Cardiotoxic: cattle, horse, rabbit.
- Neurotoxic: dog, guinea pig.
- Both: pig, cat, monkey, sheep.
- Dogs
  - Anxiety.
  - Running in a straight line or around the perimeter of an enclosure.
  - Wild barking.
  - Vomiting. Vomiting generally occurs too late to save animal's life.
  - Hyperthermia.
  - Repeated defecation, urination - tenesmus (persistent).
  - Seizures which are largely tetanic; increase in frequency and severity with time. Later, as animal becomes exhausted seizures become weaker but even more frequent. Paddling occurs during seizures.
  - Breathing ceases before heart stops.
  - Death occurs within 2 - 12 hours after ingestion. Death may occur during seizures or from subsequent respiratory paralysis.
- Cats
  - Excitation or depression, vocalization.
  - Ropey salivation, possible evacuation of bowels, possibly diarrhea.
  - Arrhythmia common.
  - Generally do not display "running fits".

- Ruminants, herbivores
  - Cardiac signs primarily noted : Arrhythmia, rapid weak pulse, ventricular fibrillation. Stagger, tremble, collapse, grind teeth, terminal seizures.
- Horses
  - Tremble, sweat. May die from ventricular fibrillation.
- Swine and sheep
  - Cardiac and nervous syndromes.

Clinical Pathology

- Hyperglycemia (poor utilization - Kreb's cycle inhibited).
- Lactic acidosis.

Lesions

- Empty stomach, colon, urinary bladder.
- Cyanosis.
- Rapid rigor mortis.
- Congestion - liver, kidney.
- Heart- diastole with subepicardial hemorrhage (nonspecific lesion).
- Sheep that died acutely from fluoroacetate toxicosis had degeneration and necrosis of individual or small groups of myocardial fibers.
- Cerebral edema and lymphocytic infiltration of the Virchow-Robin space have been described.

Diagnosis

- Signs
  - History of exposure, negative tests for other agents help to rule out other causes.
- Analysis of
  - Baits, stomach contents, vomitus, liver, kidney. Few labs perform analyses; analysis difficult; best lab at present is the State Diagnostic Laboratory in Fargo, North Dakota.

False negatives at any lab, especially at inexperienced lab.

Differential Diagnosis in 1080 Poisoning

- Initial considerations.
  - Lead-running fits, convulsions, vomiting, but usually much slower onset.

- Hypomagnesemia, hypocalcemia, brain injury.
- Cardioglycoside toxicosis, Japanese yew (*Taxus* spp.) poisoning.
- Strychnine, organochlorine insecticide or methylxanthine toxicosis.

Treatment

- Do not use an emetic unless it is very early, no signs are observed, and the animal will be constantly monitored in case of seizures. Perform enterogastric lavage if there is any likelihood of continued absorption.
- activated charcoal + saline cathartic.
- Most symptomatic treatments (when used alone) are not reliably effective after severe signs develop. Treatment often fails but can permit some animals to survive.
- Barbiturates (pentobarbital to control presenting seizures followed by a prophylactic dose of Phenobarbital and additional pentobarbital, repeat as needed) (Tourtellotte and Coon, 1950).
- Solutions containing 50% alcohol and 5% acetic acid have been given orally at 8.8 ml/kg. In almost all cases, this therapy is ineffective. Moreover, combined therapy with ethanol and barbiturates was associated with prolonged (days) anesthesia and a high incidence of pneumonia.
- Barbiturates alone are therefore preferred over barbiturates with ethanol and acetic acid. Barbiturates are far better than ethanol and acetic acid alone.
- Calcium gluconate has been recommended to control tetany (0.2 - 0.5 ml/kg of 5% solution, IV, slowly in fluids).
- Monacetin (glyceryl monoacetate) at 0.55 gm/kg, IM. Apparently, the theory is to provide an available source of acetate to compete with fluoroacetate and thereby increase the production of citrate.
  - Short shelf-life.
  - May be difficult to obtain.
  - Not very effective unless dose of 1080 is near or less than the LD50<.
  - Antiarrhythmics may be of value in appropriate species; apparently these have not been tested for efficacy in 1080 poisoning.

Chapter 7

MYCOTOXICOLOGY

Introduction

The word mycotoxin is derived from myco, meaning mold and toxin, a poison. A great number of mold metabolites have been identified as mycotoxins. Thus mycotoxins are secondary fungal metabolites (i.e., metabolites not essential to the normal growth and reproduction of the fungus) which cause pathologic, physiologic, and/or biochemical lesions in other species (may include animals, plants, other microbes, etc.).

Mycotoxicosis - Poisoning of a biological system by a mycotoxin.

Mycotoxins are defined as toxic metabolites released by moulds under certain conditions conducive for their growth. Acute or chronic toxicoses can result from exposure to feed or bedding contaminated with toxins that may be produced during growth of various saprophytic or phytopathogenic fungi or molds on cereals, hay, straw, pastures, or any other fodder. A few principles characterize mycotoxic diseases:

1) The cause may not be immediately identified
2) They are not transmissible from one animal to another
3) Treatment with drugs or antibiotics has little effect on the course of the disease
4) Outbreaks are usually seasonal because particular climatic sequences may favor fungal growth and toxin production
5) Study indicates specific association with a particular feed.

There are various types of mycotoxins and are classified as follows:

i) Based on the causative organism:

Aflatoxins - *Aspergillus flavus, A. parasiticus.*

Rubratoxins - *Penicillium rubrum, P.purpurogenum.*

T-2 toxins - *Fusarium sp. F.gramaenareum and F. roseum.*

Ergotoxins – *Claviceps purpurea and C. paspali.*

ii) Based on the system they affect

Hepatotoxic	Nephrotoxic	Musculoskeletal system	Oestrogenic	Histaminergic
Afla & rubra toxins	Ochratoxins T-2 / citrinin	Ergotoxins (F-2 toxin)	Zearalenone & ergotoxins	Slaframine

General list of various Mycotoxins affecting various species of live organisms

- Aflatoxins B1, B2, G1, G2, M1, M2, Q1, and aflatoxicol.
- Sterigmatocystins
- Versicolorins
- Aspertoxins
- Autocystins
- Sterigmatin
- Bipolarin
- Averufarin
- Curvularin

- Rubratoxins A and B - Hepatotoxic
- Sporodesmin - Hepatoxic
- Penicillic acid - Hepatoxic

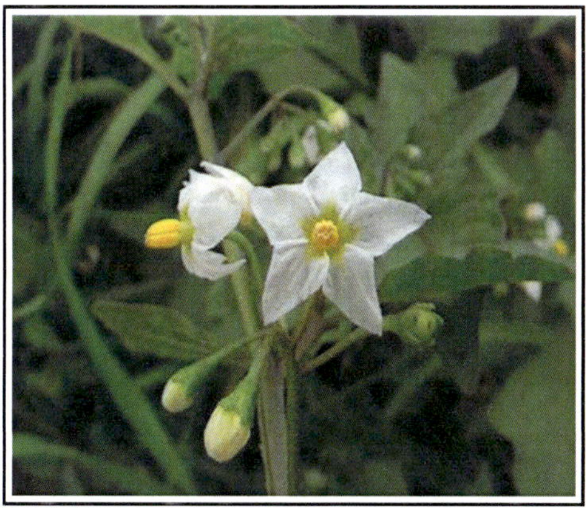

Picture showing the leaves and flowers of *Solanum nigrum* plant

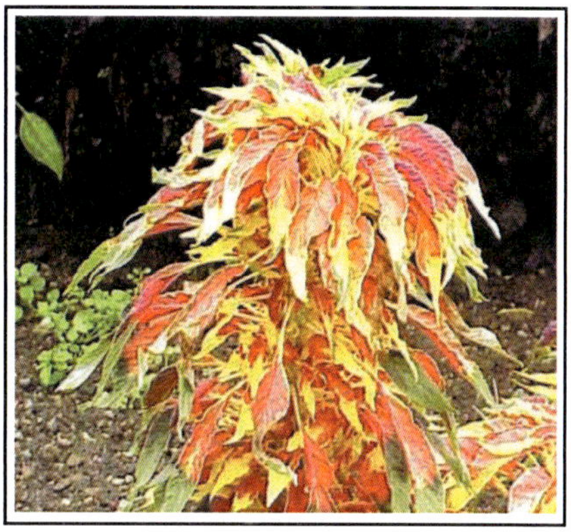

→

Amaranthus retroflexus L. 1, lower stem and roots; 2, upper stem with leaves and flower clusters; 3, flower; 4, seed. Annual, reproducing by seeds. Taproot shallow, reddish. Stems erect, up to 6 feet (1.8 m) high, rough, branching freely if not crowded. Leaves dull green, usually at least 6 inches (15 cm) long when mature, ovate to lanceolate. Flowers green, small, in thick, stiff, paniclelike terminal spikes with many short, crowded lateral branches. Bracts much longer than sepals and utricles. Sepals longer than utricle, curved, rounded, often with small notch at end. Seeds shiny black, lens-shaped, ovate, notched at the narrow end, about 1mm in diameter. Found in cultivated fields, yards, fence rows, and other waste places. Other species, such as smooth pigweed and Powell amaranth, are similar to redroot pigweed in morphology and weedy habits, and may often be found in the same area. Redroot pigweed is also commonly known as rough pigweed.

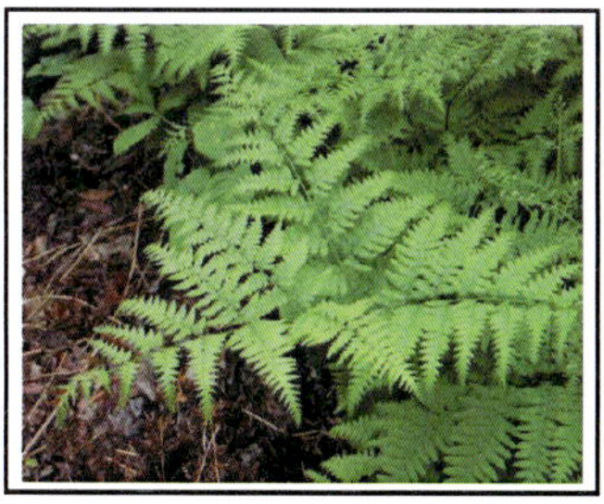

Pteridium Aquilinum (Bracken Fern)

Picture :Oleander (*Nerium indicum*) - The narrow leathery leaves, the colorful flowers, and the hairy seed and slender seed pod (lower right) are characteristic of this deadly plant →

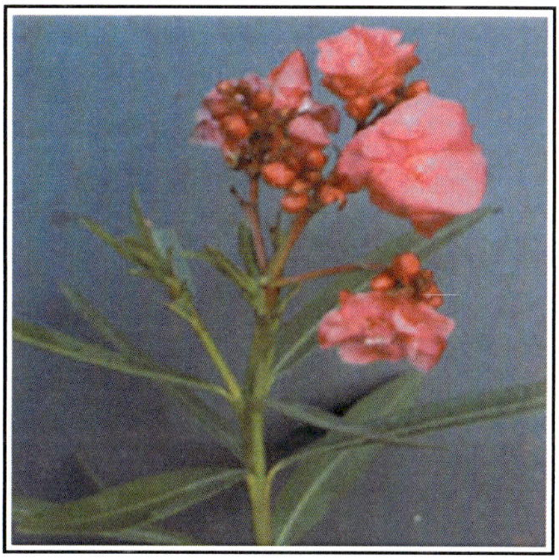

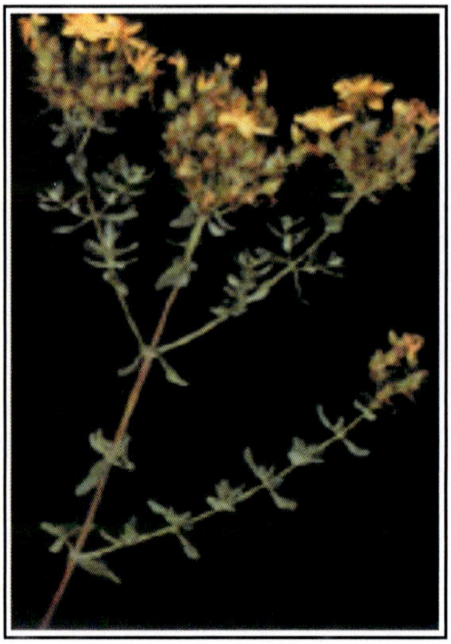

Hypericum perforatum

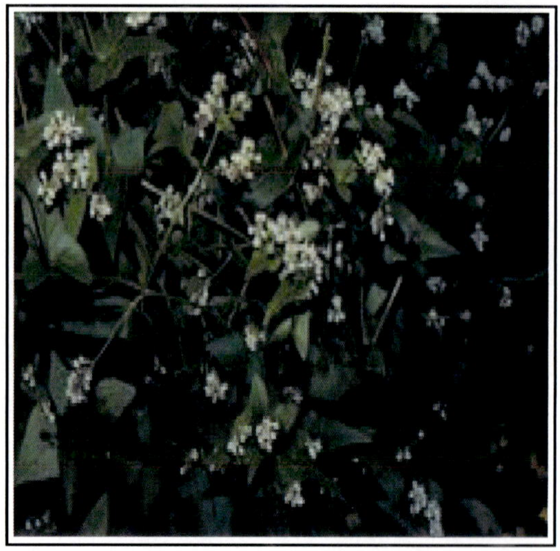

Fagopyrum esculentum

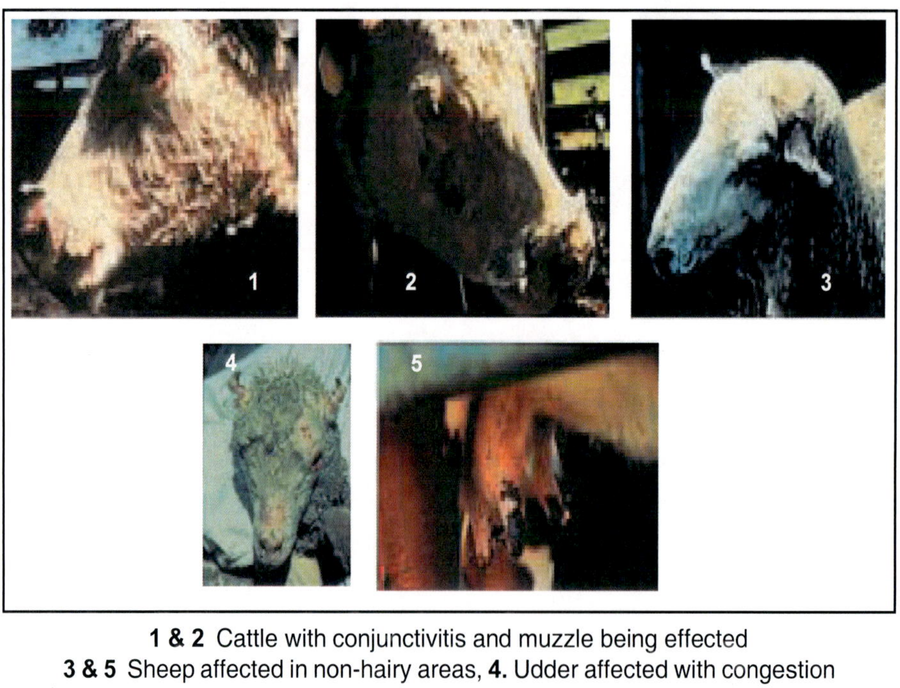

1 & 2 Cattle with conjunctivitis and muzzle being effected
3 & 5 Sheep affected in non-hairy areas, **4.** Udder affected with congestion

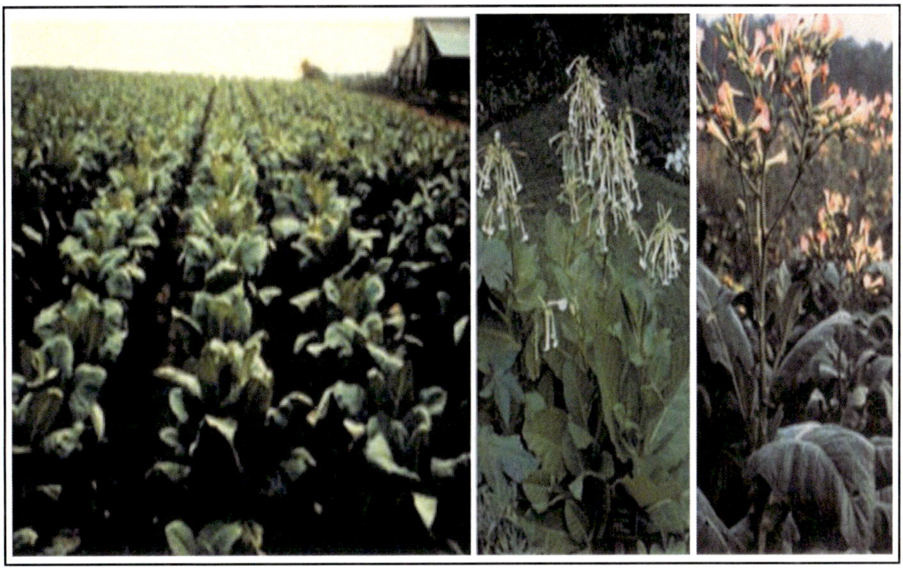

Picture showing the leaves and flowers of *Nicotiana tobaccum*

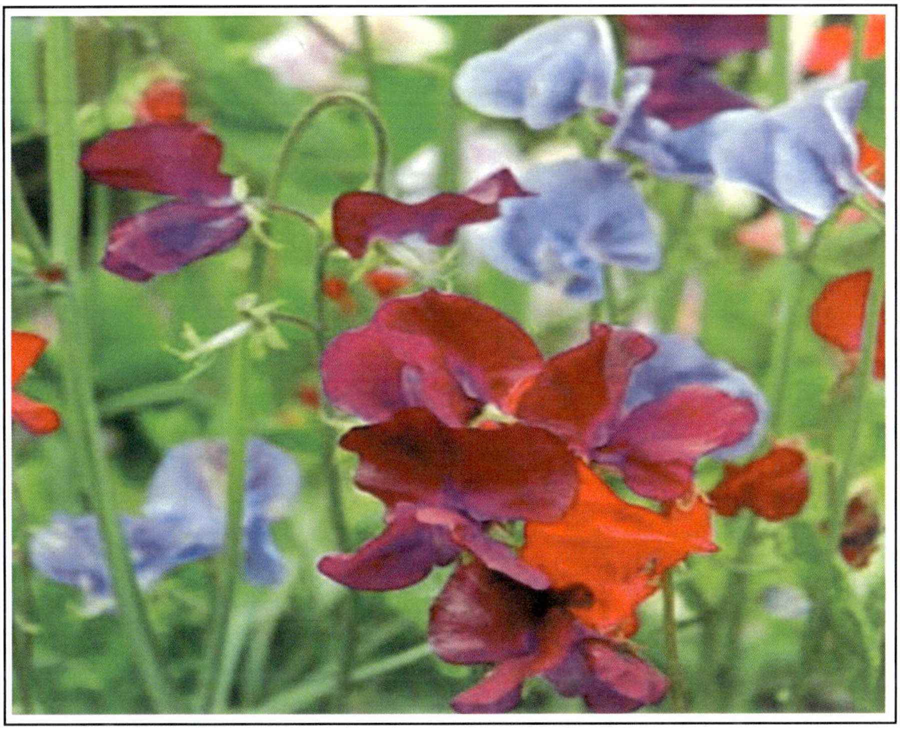

Picture showing the flowers and stems of *Lathrus odoratus*

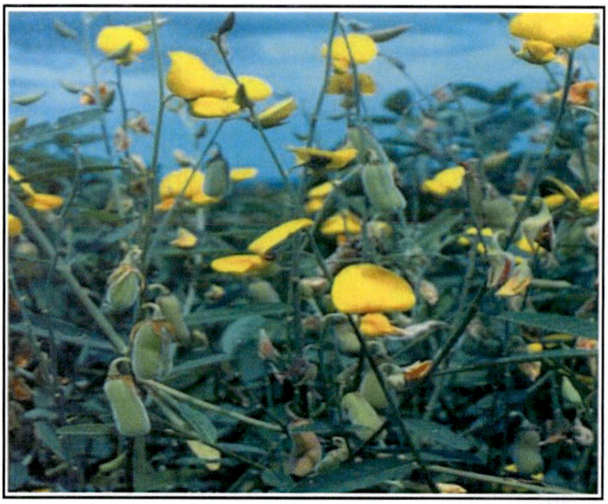

Picture showing the flowers and stems of *Crotalaria juncea*

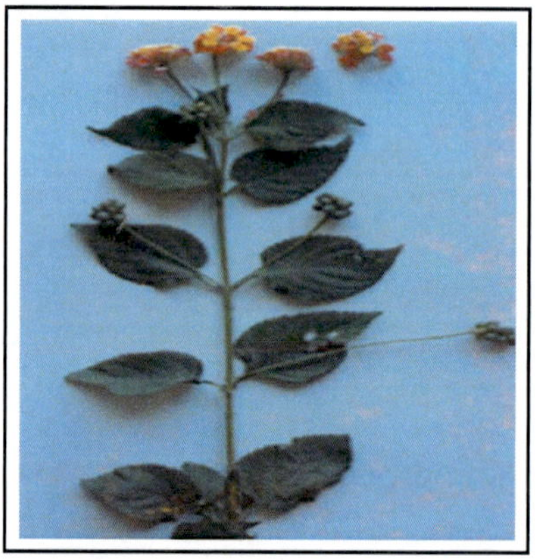

Picture : *Lantana* - The oval, toothed, and veiny leaves; the square prickly stems; the terminal flower clusters; and the black berries are characteristic of this attractive ornamental shrub.

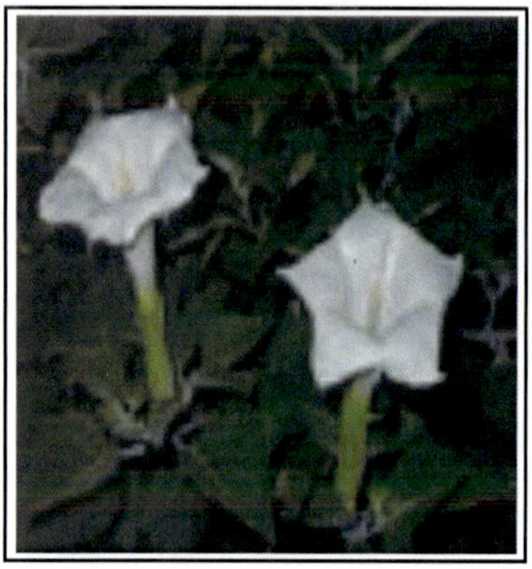

Picture :*Datura stramonium* - L. 1, upper portion of plant; 2, flower; 3, seed pod; 4, seed. Annual, reproducing by seed. Roots thick, shallow, extensively branched. Stems smooth, thick, erect, branching widely in upper part, 2 to 4 feet (0.6 to 1.2 m) tall. Leaves alternate, large, course, smooth, ovate, with irregularly toothed edges and a distinctive rank odor. Flowers large, funnel-shaped, white to pinkish, 2 to 5 inches (5 to 12.5 cm) long, borne singly on short stalks in the axils of the branches. Seed pod about 1 inch (2.5 cm) in diameter, egg-shaped, covered with short, sharp spines. Seed dark brown to black, kidney-shaped, flattened, surface irregular and pitted. Found in cultivated crops on rich land and especially in old feedlots. This plant contains poisonous materials.

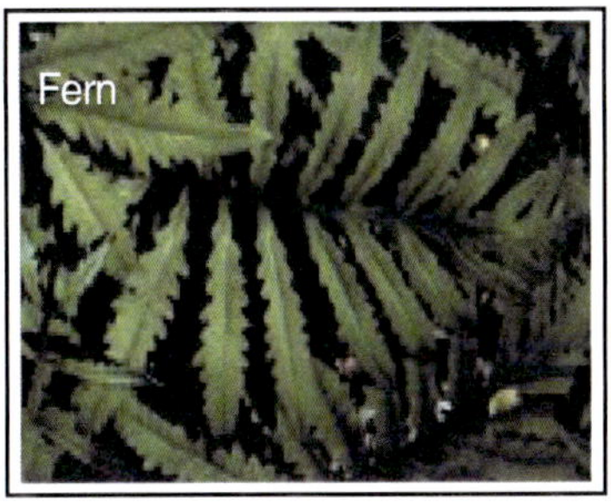

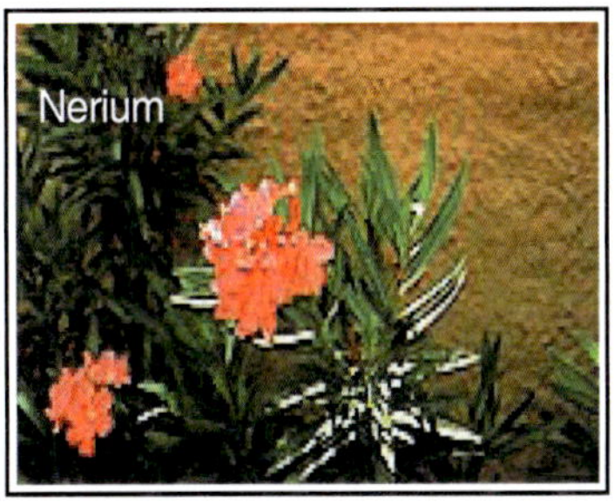

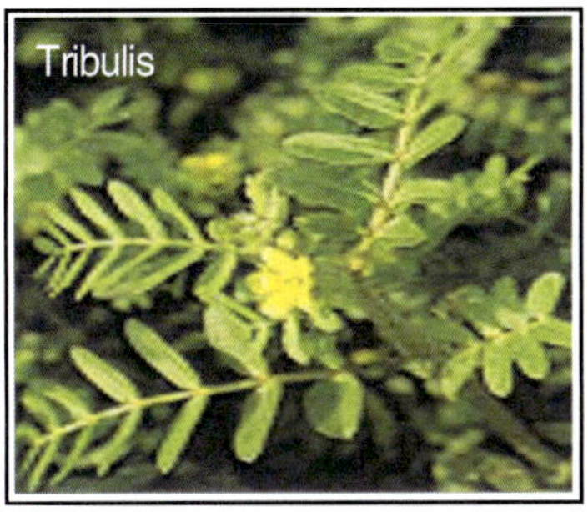

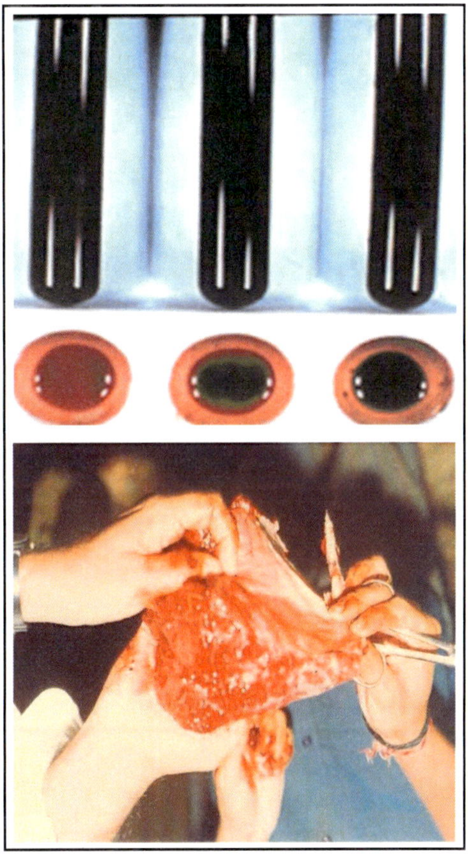

Diagnosis of Poisoning

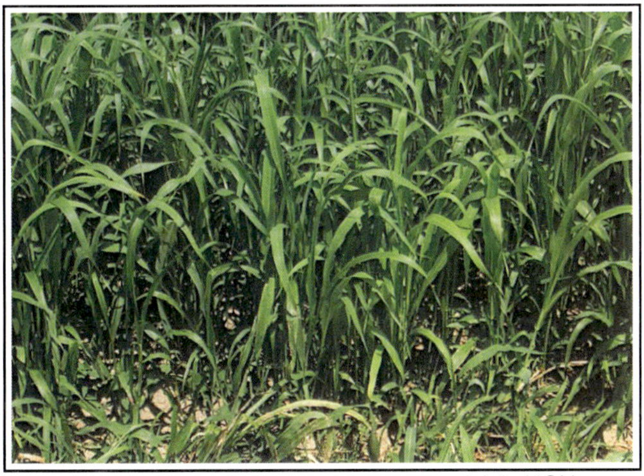

Picture showing the immature *Sorghum vulgare* crop rich in HCN concentrations

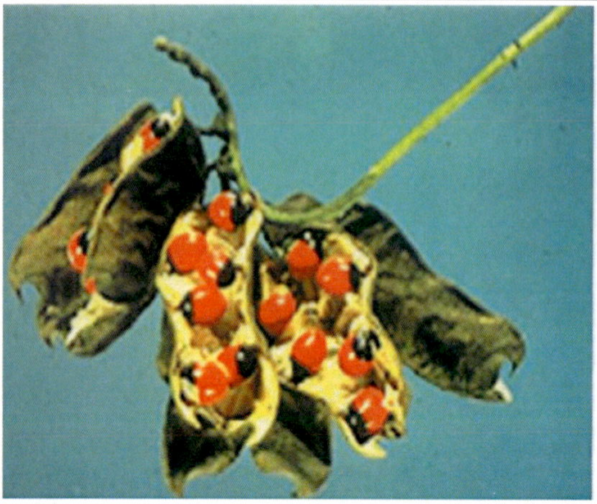

Abrus Precatorius

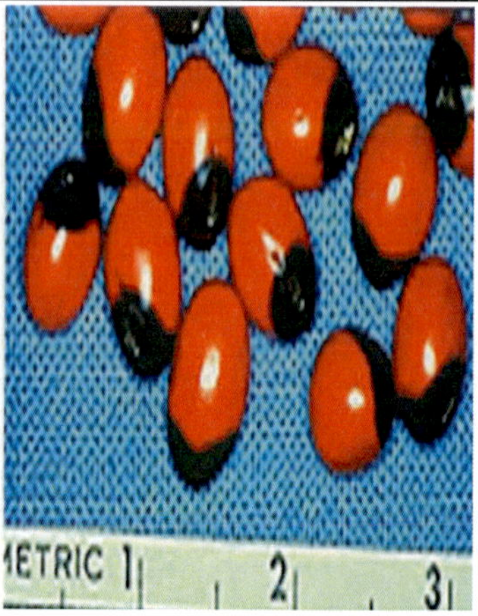

Picture showing the seeds of *Abrus precatorius*

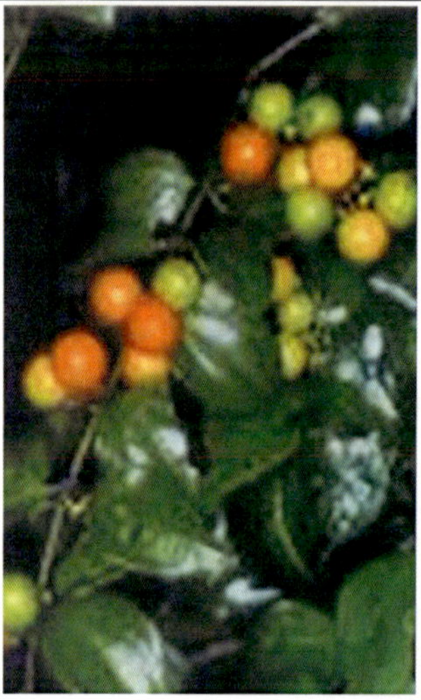

Picture showing the leaves and fruits of *Strychnus nuxvomca*

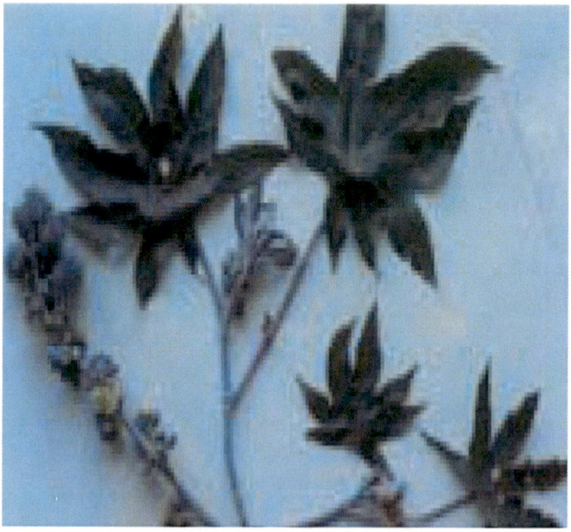

Picture showing the seeds and flowers of Ricinus communis

- ❒ Ochratoxin series, especially ochratoxin A - Nephrotoxic, carcinogenic, immunosuppressive
- ❒ Citrinin
- ❒ Citreoviridin
- ❒ Luteoskyrin
- ❒ Ergot alkaloids
  - Ergotamine
  - Ergonovine
  - Others
- ❒ Tremorgens
  - Penitrem A
  - Roquefortine
  - Paspaline
  - Paspalanine
  - Paspalitrems A and B
  - Verruculogen
  - Fumitremorgen
  - Fumigaclavine
- ❒ Slaframine
- ❒ Patulin
- ❒ Fusarium toxins
  - Trichothecenes
    - ° T-2 toxin
    - ° Diacetoxyscirpenol (DAS)
    - ° Deoxynivalenol (Vomitoxin) (DON)
    - ° Verrucarins
    - ° Roridins
    - ° Satratoxins
    - ° (30+ others)
  - Zearalenone and zearalenol
  - Butenolide
  - Moniliformin
  - Fusaric acid
  - Fusarin A-D
  - Unidentified refusal factors
  - Fumonisins

Conditions Predisposing to Mycotoxin Production

1. Moisture

Field fungi - Invade developing and mature seed grain while still on the plant. The optimal moisture content for growth is 22% - 25%.

Storage fungi - Invade seed grain after harvest while in storage. Optimal moisture for growth is 13% - 18%.

Advanced decay fungi - Generally require moisture of 22% - 25% but rarely develop and grow on seed grain in the field.

2. Temperature

Generally molds grow readily between 20 °C and 30 °C. But optimal temperature ranges from below 0 °C to above 60 °C. Temperature variations affect the growth rate of the mold and also the type and amount of toxins produced.

3. Aeration

Molds are aerobic organisms, but a significant difference in oxygen requirements exist between types of molds.

4. Substrate Availability

Molds can either be parasitic or saprophytic in nutrient requirements.

5. Host Stress

Important for field fungi. Environmental stress, insect damage, and plant disease encourage colonization, growth, and toxin production by fungi.

Many factors contribute to the occurrence of mycotoxicoses in livestock. For example, modern harvesting methods in which corn is handled at higher moisture concentrations combined with damage occurring in harvesting machinery increases the number of kernels in which molds can get started. Also the feeding of ground rations prevents the animals from sorting out and avoiding damaged kernels.

Our present knowledge of many of these and numerous other known mycotoxins is extremely limited. In many instances, no surveys of the frequencies of occurrence have been done. In other instances, the compounds have been investigated in some detail but surveys have not revealed sufficiently. Frequent occurrence in the developing countries for these toxins to be of major concern to veterinarians. For example, T-2 toxin and diacetoxyscirpenol have been studied in some detail but are only rarely encountered in the india and other developing countries. T-2 toxin, however, was apparently responsible for severe outbreaks of mycotoxicosis in humans and animals in the asian countries including india,Russia and has caused occasional outbreaks of toxicosis in the western countries. Similarly the nephrotoxic mycotoxin, ochratoxin A, although not often a major problem in the western countries has caused severe problems in poultry in the Asiatic countries including india.

Constraints in detection of Mycotoxicosis:

- The identified toxin is consumed along with related mold metabolites and possibly other unidentified mycotoxins.
- Mold damaged, stressed grains may be of lower nutrient value and altered palatability.
- The toxin(s) is (are) unevenly distributed in the diet.
- The concentration(s) is (are) generally so variable that **multiple** samples are required to estimate concentration(s) present.
- If sufficient moisture and appropriate temperatures occur during transit, additional mold growth and toxin production may occur.
- Stresses such as infectious agents, reproduction, lactation, crowding, temperature variation, etc., overlap and interact with effects of mycotoxins.

Confirmation of diagnosis of Mycotoxic disease requires a combination of information. Detection of fungal spores alone, even at high concentrations, is not sufficient for diagnosis, fungal spores or even mold growth may be present without formation of mycotoxins. Especially important in diagnosis is the presence of a disease documented to be caused by a known mycotoxin, combined with detection of the mycotoxin in either feedstuffs or animal tissues. Sometimes more than one mycotoxin may be present in feedstuffs, and their different toxicologic properties may cause clinical signs and lesions that are not consistent with those seen when animals are dosed experimentally with pure, single mycotoxins. Several mycotoxins are immunosuppressive, which may allow viruses, bacteria, or parasites to create a secondary disease that is more obvious than the primary. In reaching a diagnosis of mycotoxicosis characterized by reduced feed intake, reproductive failure, or increased infectious disease due to immunosuppression, differential diagnoses must be carefully established and eliminated by a combination of thorough clinical and historical evaluation, examination of production records, and close attention to appropriate diagnostic testing. There are no specific antidotes for mycotoxins, removal of the source of the toxin (ie; the moldy feedstuff) eliminates further exposure. If financial circumstances do not allow for disposal of the moldy feed, it can be blended with unspoiled feed just before feeding to reduce the toxin concentration or fed to less susceptible species. When contaminated feed is blended with good feed, care must be taken to prevent further mold growth by the toxigenic contaminants. This may be accomplished by thorough drying or by addition of organic acids (eg, propionic acid) to prevent mold growth.

Sample Collection

Much of the error in detecting mycotoxins in feed results from sampling (or subsampling) rather than from analytical methodology. Samples can be taken at various stages—from growing crops or during transport or storage. Whenever possible, samples should be taken after particulate size has been reduced (Ex: by shelling or grinding) and soon after blending has occurred (as in harvesting, loading, or grinding). Sampling is most effective if small samples are taken at periodic, predetermined intervals from a moving stream of grain or feed. These individual stream samples should be combined and mixed thoroughly, after which a subsample of 10 lb (4.5 kg) should be taken.

Probe sampling is acceptable when grain has been recently blended but is less reliable because different microenvironments within the storage facility may cause areas of mold or mycotoxin concentration. A suggested method of probe sampling is to sample at 5 locations, each 1 ft (30 cm) from the periphery of a bin, plus once in the center. This should be done for each 6 ft (2 m) of bin depth. Thus, taller bins would require more samples, and the total weight should be >10kg.

Dry samples are preferable for transport and storage. Samples should be dried at 176-194°F (80-90°C) for >3 hr to reduce moisture to 12-13%. If mold studies are to be done, drying at 140°F (60°C) for 6-12 hr should preserve fungal activity.

Containers should be appropriate for the nature of the sample. For dried samples, paper or cloth bags are recommended. Plastic bags should be avoided unless grain is dried thoroughly. Plastic bags are useful for high-moisture samples only if refrigeration, freezing, or chemicals are used to retard mold growth during transport and storage. Once a sample has been cooled or frozen, warming may induce condensation and allow mold growth.

Aflatoxins

Sources

- Aflatoxins are secondary mold metabolites produced by some strains of *Aspergillus flavus* and *A. parasiticus*.
- Chemically they are polycyclic furan compounds possessing intense blue or green fluorescence under long wave UV light.
- Although at least 13 aflatoxins have been identified, 4 (B1, B2, G and G2) are most common.
- Under suitable conditions for growth i.e moisture and temperature they grow on the peanuts, corn, walnuts, almonds, cottonseed and grain sorghum are more susceptible to *A. flavus* than soyabeans, wheat, rye and oats.
- *A. flavus* may grow on corn in the field as well as in storage.
- Sometimes "high moisture" corn may not be high enough in moisture to ensile. Consequently, fungal growth and toxin production may occur instead.

Factors Affecting Sensitivity

- Species : Sensitivity to aflatoxin.
- Most sensitive -------------------------- Least sensitive.
  - Ducklings, trout, dogs, pigs, cattle, sheep, chickens. Piglets, pregnant sows, feeder pigs-calves-horses, finishing hogs, lambs, dairy cows (residues in milk possible), feeder cattle, mature sheep.
- Duration
- Dosage
- Age : young animals are generally more sensitive than adults
- Nutrition
- Sex

Maximum dietary permissible concentration as per international standards

- 20 ppb maximum allowable for corn destined for human consumption, for interstate transport, or to be fed to dairy cattle or immature animals.
- 100 ppb - Approved for corn destined for consumption by breeding cattle, breeding swine, and mature poultry.
- 200 ppb - Approved for corn intended for finishing swine

- 300 ppb - Approved for corn intended for finishing cattle
- Individual states can act at levels below the above levels if they deam it necessary.
- Limit in milk.
    - 0.5 ppb of aflatoxin M1 = the actionable level in milk.
    - Milk is routinely monitored for aflatoxin M1 by spot checking followed by trace back to the source farm(s).
- Aflatoxin M1 is the principal aflatoxin residue in meat and milk. It retains only a limited amount of the toxic potential of parent compound.

Properties

- Lipid soluble
- Heat resistant
- Hydrophobic
- Unstable in U-v radiation
- B1>G1 & M1(twice greater)
- B1>B2 & G2 (four & eight folds)

Chemistry

- Polycyclic furan compounds
- Coumarin Nucleus with reactive bifuran system on one side and either a pentenone (B series) or lactone (G series)
- Total 18 compounds
- B1 & B2
- G1 & G2

LD_{50} Values

- Horse, sheep, goat : 2 mg/Kg
- poultry & swine : 2 mg/Kg
- Cattle : 0.5-2 mg/kg
- Dog : 0.5-1mg/kg
- Ducks : 0.3-0.6mg/kg
- Rabbits : 0.3-0.5mg/kg

Toxicokinetics

- Rapid absorption from GIT
- Bound to serum albumin

- Metabolites - water soluble conjugates or Lipid soluble - liver - excretion - urine & bile (enterohepatic circulation)
- B1 7metabolites (q1, p1, b2a, m1, aflatoxicol)
- M1 is more toxic,carcinogenic & excreted in milk
- M1, M2, p1, q1 & aflatoxicol

Toxicodynamics

- Aflatoxins are potent hepatotoxins and hepatocarcinogens.
- React with and modify the DNA template to interfere with RNA transcription or may specifically inhibit RNA polymerase which would also impair transcription.
- Increase the rate of RNA breakdown by alteration of lysosomal membranes resulting in the release of ribonuclease from lysosomes.
- Stimulate the alkylation of RNA by stimulation of RNA methylase.
- As a result of a reduction in the active forms of RNA, protein synthesis is secondarily impaired.
- Effects include hemorrhage, immunosuppression, stunting and liver damage.

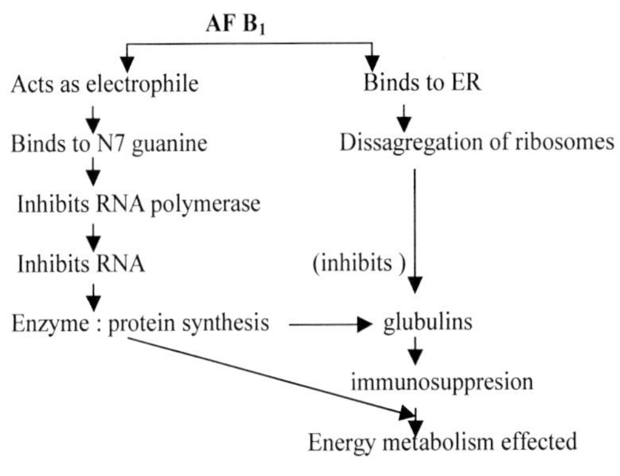

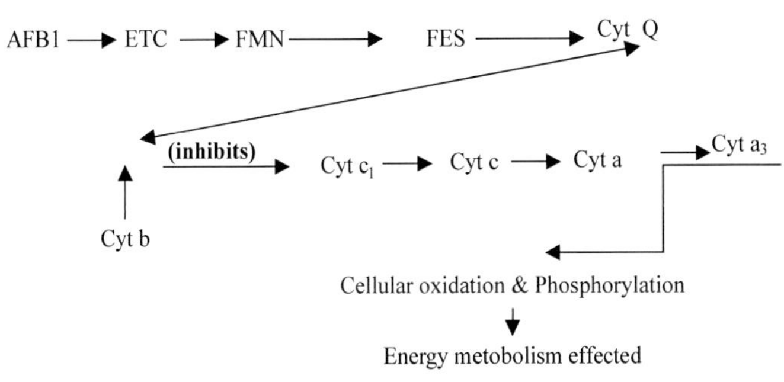

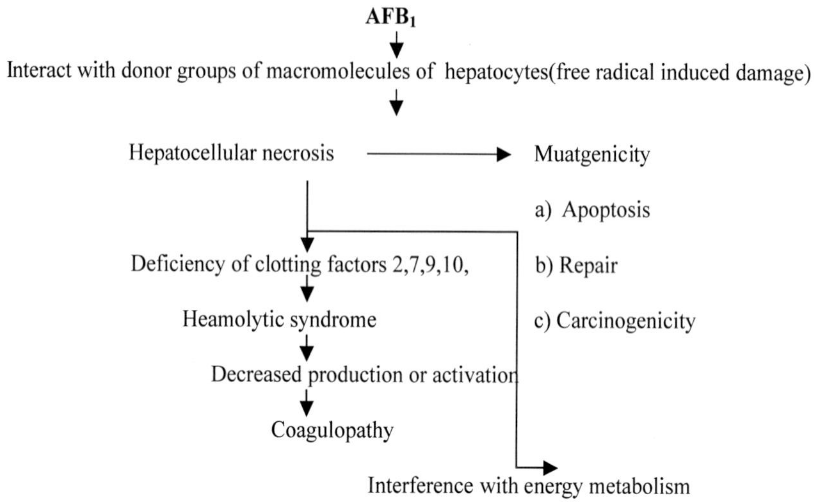

Clinical Signs

Acute

- Hepatopathy, sudden death or anorexia, depression, dyspnoea, coughing, nasal discharge, anaemia, epistaxis, bloody faeces, haematemesis, possible convulsions and death.

Sub- Acute

- Jaundice, hypoprothrombinemia, haematomas and haemorrhagic enteritis.

Chronic

- Decreased feed efficiency, decreased productivity and weight gain, rough hair coat, anaemia, enlarged abdomen, mild jaundice, depression and anorexia.
- Abortions, teratogenecity, immunosuppresion, hepatic tumours may occur.

Lesions

- Wide spread heamorhages
- Icterus
- Gastroenteritis
- Hepatic necrosis
- Massive centrilobular necrosis,fibrosis of bile duct

- Enlarged liver
- Hydrothorax
- Ascites
- Oedema of Gall bladder wall
- Pericellular cirrhosis
- Histopathologic hepatic lesions.
    - Biliary hyperplasia.
    - Hepatocellular swelling.
    - Hepatic lipidosis proceeding to vacuolation.
- Thymic involution.

Diagnosis

Based on

- Case history
- Clinical signs
- PM lesions
- Laboratory examination of suspected samples
- Detection of Aflatoxin M1 in milk & urine,liver, kidney
- Serum liver enzymes AST, ALT, ALP, ornithine carbamyl transferase, isocitric dehydrogenase elevated
- Reduced prothrombin activity
- Decreased albumin and A/G ratio
- Hyperbilerubinemia
- Detection of toxins in the feed by thin layer chromatography (TLC), High performance liquid chromatography (HPLC), radio immunoassay (RIA), Enzyme linked immunosorbent assay (ELISA)

Differential Diagnosis

- Warfarin (haemorrhages)
- Coal tar (mottling of liver)
- Copper poisoning (haemoglobinuria, hemolysis)
- Pyrrozolidine alkaloids (present in plants)
- CCL_4
- Blue-green algae, crotalaria are hepatotoxic

Treatment

- Eliminate the source
- No specific treatment
- Avoidance of contaminated feed
- NovaSil ®Hydrated sodium calcium alumino silicate (HSCAS) adsorb aflatoxins @5kg / ton of feed
- Treatment of grains with anhydrous NH_3,H_2O_2,Chlorine,O_3 but efficacy not been established
- Feeding easily digestible and low fat diet containing adequate protein
- Change to aflatoxin-free ration.
- Increase dietary protein.
- Vitamin B_{12} and Vitamin K
- Supportive measures with multi vitamins Like E & K
- Supplementation of selenium
- Stanzolol (2 mg / kg) IM decreases hepatic necrosis
- Oxytetracycline (10mg / kg) I/M decreases hepatic necrosis.
- Never administer oxytetracycline and stanzolol combination, they are mutually antagonistic.
- Activated charcoal 6.7 mg / Kg intra ruminal as 30% W/V slurry in M/15, pH_7 Phosphate buffer.
- Along with charcoal, stanzolol/oxytetracycline (any one may be given)
- Glutathione (GSH) Precursors Cysteine,methionine @2.2mg/kg intraperitoneal.

Control Measures

Use of Contaminated Feedstuffs

- Feed affected foodstuff to less susceptible species and/or ages
- Dilute with clean feed.
- Ammoniation of corn to reduce aflatoxin
- Hazards include:
    - Inhalation of mold spores and aflatoxin.
    - Ammonia lung-eye-skin irritation.
    - Ammonia vapor combustible.
    - Treated corn may cake up in equipment and not flow. Persons should not enter ammonia treatment bins "to help".

Avoidance of Mycotoxins

- Dry feed ingredients at less than 14% moisture.
- Aerate regularly during storage to prevent condensation
- Harvest not more than one week after maturity
- Clean and decontaminate storage bins with Clorox ®/water 1:9.
- Repair storage bins to avoid leakage
- Clean the feeding system-feeders, augers, mixers, etc.
- Be sure that they:
    - Do submit appropriate samples for mycotoxin analyses when toxins are suspected.
    - Do have necropsies performed to establish that lesions compatible with specific mycotoxin poisonings are present.

Rubratoxins

Sources

- Rubratoxins A and B are produced by *P. rubrum* and *P. purpurogenum*. Both are common soil fungi.
- Sources of exposure - Cereal grains-primarily corn. The natural distribution of rubratoxin is not well established.

Chemistry

- Occurs in Two forms
- Rubrotoxin A & B
- RBTA : Pencillium rubrum
- RBTB : Pencillium purpurogenum
- Toxicity is due to presence of unsaturated lactone ring

Properties

- Insoluble in oil & water
- Soluble in alchohol and esters
- Stable at room temperature
- Rubratoxin B is major toxin LD_{50} Value 400-450mg/kg
- Potentiates Aflatoxicosis in mouldy feeds
- Dog, cat, goat & horse Susceptible

Toxicity

- LD_{50} values of rubratoxin range from 0.27 to over 5 mg/kg when given parenterally but were 400 to 450 when given orally to rats. The LD_{50} in chicken feed was 83 ppm.
- Males and females (rats) are equally susceptible; but neonate rats are 49 times as susceptible as adults.
- At sufficient doses, chronic dosing causes same effects; but animals getting subclinical doses had no lesions suggesting effective detoxification.
- Chicks.
  - 500 ppm rubratoxins (80% B) in diet was required to affect growth rate.
  - Dose of over 1,000 ppm in diet caused atrophy of liver and bursa of *Fabricius*.
  - (These levels not known to occur in nature.)

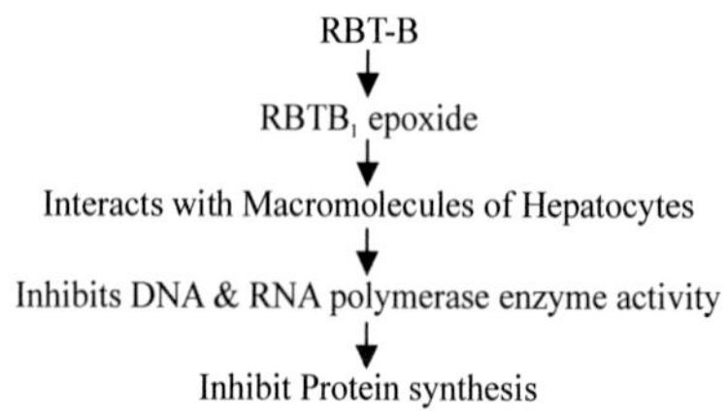

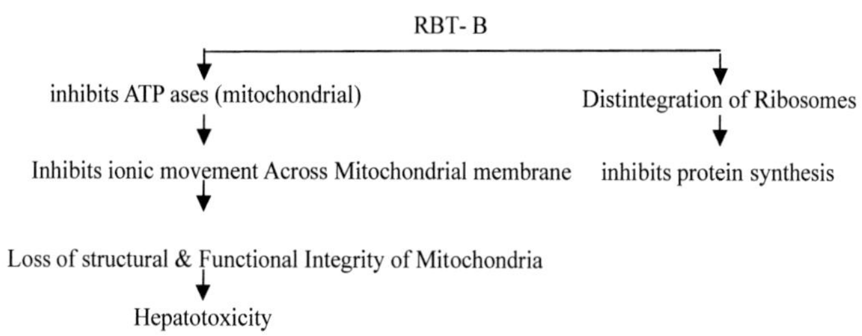

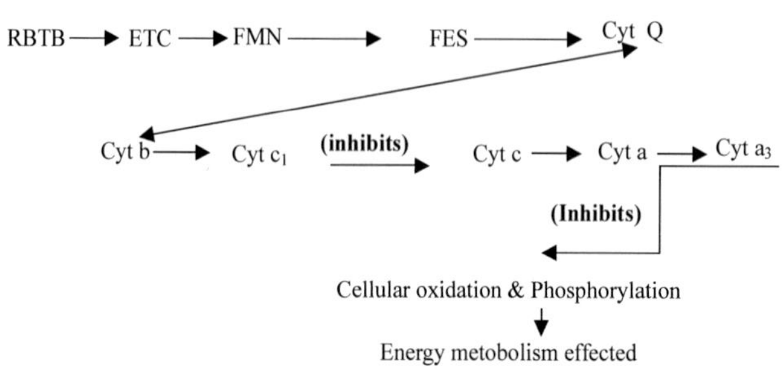

Toxicokinetics

- Under go metabolism in liver
- Undergoes enterohepatic cycle
- Undergo glucoranide and sulphate conjugation
- Excreted in bile, urine, feaces.

Toxicoydnamics

Clinical Signs

- Signs related to hepatotoxicity
- Anroxia
- Dehydration
- Depression
- Jaundice
- Diarrhoea
- Weight loss
- Swine : head pressing& colic
- Horse : Incordination.

Lesions

- Hemorrhages in various organs
- Damage to liver and spleen
- Renal damage
- Horse : brain hemorrhage
- Early midzonal hepatic necrosis
- Later extending to massive necrosis and replacement with hemorrhage with chronic doses.

Diagnosis

Based on

- Case history
- Clinical signs
- PM lesions
- Laboratory examination of suspected samples

- Detection of toxins in the feed by thin layer chromatography (TLC), High performance liquid chromatography(HPLC),radia immunoassay (RIA), Enzyme linked immunosorbent assay (ELISA)

Treatment

- Eliminate the source
- No specific treatment
- Avoidance of contaminated feed
- NovaSil ®Hydrated sodium calcium alumino silicate (HSCAS) adsorb aflatoxins @5kg /ton of feed
- Treatment of grains with anhydrous NH_3,H_2O_2,Chlorine,O_3 but efficacy not been established
- Feeding easily digestible and low fat diet containing adequate protein
- Change to aflatoxin-free ration.
- Increase dietary protein.
- Supportive measures with multi vitamins Like E
- Supplementation of selenium
- Stanzolol (2 mg / kg) IM decreases hepatic necrosis
  - Never administer oxytetracycline and stanzolol combination, they are mutually antagonistic.
  - Activated charcoal 6.7 mg / Kg intra ruminal as 30% W/V slurry in M/15, pH_7 Phosphate buffer.
  - Along with charcoal, stanzolol/oxytetracycline (any one may be given)
- Glutathione (GSH) Precursors Cysteine,methionine @2.2mg/kg intraperitoneal.

Control Measures

Same control measures are to be followed as intended for aflatoxicosis

Ochratoxins

Ochratoxins comprise a series of related metabolites (at least 7 in all) isolated from several species of *Aspergillus* and *Penicillium* molds. Ochratoxins A, B, C, D, and their methyl and ethyl esters have been isolated. Ochratoxin A is thus far believed to be the most toxic and most common of the ochratoxins.

Sources

- Ochratoxin is primarily a contaminant of feed grains and cereals. The toxin occurs in barley, sorghum and especially wheat. It has also been found in corn, dried beans, rye, oats, mixed feeds, and peanuts.
- Ochratoxin A is presumed to be the cause of porcine nephropathy seen in Denmark, Sweden, and the USA.
- Production by *Penicillium viridicatum* occurs at temperatures as low as 4 °C and with a moisture content of the affected grain of 18.5 to 40.4%.
- Concentrations reported in Denmark were as high as 27.5 ppm in barley.
- During the porcine nephropathy epidemic in Denmark, over 50% of the barley had 0.2 ppm; and 0.2 ppm can cause experimental nephropathy in pigs.
- Has often been detected in Swedish barley and oats as well as in Japanese rice.
- Detected in concentrations (1.0 to 2.7 ppm) believed to be toxic to swine and cattle.
- Occurrence generally tends to be sporadic.

Susceptible Species

Potentially hazardous to livestock. Toxicity has been demonstrated in swine, ducklings, chickens, turkeys, and dogs.

Toxicity

- Synergistic or additive effects with aflatoxin, citrinin or penicillic acid (other mycotoxins) (see below).
- The toxicity of ochratoxin A is approximately equal to that of ochratoxin C, although ochratoxin A is much more commonly encountered. Ochratoxin B is several times less toxic.

Species	Ochratoxin A Oral LD_{50} mg/kg
Chicken	2 to 4
Turkey poult	6
Japanese quail	16.5
Rat	22 to 30
Mouse	22 to 58

- *Swine are very sensitive.* Doses of 1 to 3 mg/kg in swine caused considerable gastrointestinal and lymphoid damage.

- In swine, ochratoxin A at 1 or 2 mg/kg BW caused toxicosis, and death occurred within 5 to 6 days.
- Also in swine, dietary concentrations of 1 ppm for 3 months caused polydipsia and reduced growth rate and feed conversion in addition to impaired renal function.
- In swine microscopically detectable renal lesions were induced by as little as 0.2 ppm of ochratoxin in the diet.
- **Cattle are reportedly** extremely **resistant** to ochratoxin A, **but calves are sensitive** until the rumen is developed. Thirty-day-old calves given 0.1 to 0.5 mg/kg/day for 30 days displayed polyuria, CNS depression, decreased weight gain, urine of low specific gravity and dehydration.
- In calves, an approximate lethal dose is between 11 and 25 mg/kg BW while doses of 0.1 to 0.5 mg/kg produced only polyuria.
- A dose of 3 mg/kg BW **in dogs** produced acute toxicosis.
- In dogs, doses of 0.2 to 0.4 mg/kg caused clinical signs to develop over 10 to 14 days, while no clinical signs developed during 21 days of dosing at 0.1 mg/kg.
- In rats, average doses of 210 and 70 ìg/kg (5 days/week) for 2 years caused decreased weight gains on the order of 12% less than controls and decreased urine concentrating ability, decreased kidney weights and renal tubular epithelial damage.
- Ochratoxin A has been shown to be teratogenic in rodents.
- **Chickens are very sensitive**. Decreased growth and enlarged kidneys occurred in chickens fed ochratoxin A at 1 ppm in the diet.

Factors Affecting Toxicity

- Moisture content >16%
- RH > 85%
- Temparature 12-25^{0}c
- Species : swine & poultry more susceptible
- Swine Mould nephrosis or Mycotoxic nephropathy
- Ruminants least susceptible.

Chemistry

- Isocoumarin compounds
- Synthesized from phenyl alanine
- Nine ochratoxins present A is more toxic

Interactions with Other Mycotoxins

- Ochratoxin may prevent fatty liver resulting from alfatoxin exposure (poultry). In the same study, however, the combination of ochratoxin and aflatoxin caused greater inhibition of growth when compared to aflatoxin alone.
- Doses of ochratoxin alone and penicillic acid alone, neither of which were lethal, caused 100% deaths when given simultaneously.

Toxicokinetics

- Ochratoxins bind to serum albumin (protein bound).
- The only metabolic reaction of ochratoxin A so far identified, is hydrolysis by carboxypeptidase A to break an amide bond. The reaction produces ochratoxin-alpha, which is much less toxic than the present compound. This reaction is especially prevalent in ruminant protozoa, and it is estimated that it allows cattle to tolerate up to 12 ppm of ochratoxin A in their feed.
- Ochratoxin A is believed to be hydrolyzed to a significant degree in the functional rumen.
- In spite of the ruminal destruction of some of the ingested ochratoxin, large doses reportedly result in some ochratoxin excretion in milk and may be associated with renal failure in cattle (see below).
- Ochratoxin A binds strongly to the proximal tubules of the kidney. Animals especially(Pigs) exposed to ochratoxin A accumulate the toxin in the kidney, liver and muscle (in decreasing order)
- The approximate half-life of ochratoxin A in swine tissues is 3 to 5 days, and little or no ochratoxin can be detected in kidney 30 days after exposure is terminated.
- Crosses placental barrier fetal blood concentrations are 100 to 400 times lower than maternal blood concentration.

Toxicodynamics

- Inhibits protein synthesis by competition with phenylalanine in the phenylalanine-tRNA synthetase reaction.
- The kidney and spleen were more sensitive than the liver with regard to ochratoxin-induced protein synthesis inhibition.
- Acts as immunosuppressant causing decreased immunoglobulin production

- Inhibits bovine carboxypeptidase A
- Inhibits several aspects of mitochondrial respiration
- Causes increased glycogen deposition in the cytoplasm of hepatocytes, which is a sensitive indicator of ochratoxicosis.
- Increases hepatic glycogen content at low doses, while high doses of the toxin cause decreased hepatic glycogen
- Causes a loss of collagen in the large intestine resulting in breakage and loss of integrity in the affected gut.
- Decreases carotenoid pigmentation of chickens which will reduce the yellow color from the fat of chickens causing decreased marketability
- Effects coagulation factors V, VIII, and X in chickens causing multifactorial coagulopathy
- Associated with urinary tract cancers and is weakly mutagenic.
- Ochratoxin A is a potent teratogen causing neonatal deformties like malformations, fetal death, and occasional brain necrosis.

Clinical Signs

- Acute exposure to ochratoxin A generally causes anorexia, polydipsia, dehydration and depression. Continued intake of toxic levels causes reductions in rate of gain and feed efficiency. Diarrhea may occur.
- Primary clinical signs include:
  - Polydipsia
  - Polyurea
  - Dilute urine
  - Reduced gain and feed efficiency
  - Cattle may be similarly, but much less commonly affected as compared to swine.
- In turkeys, one bite of ochratoxin containing feed causes immediate feed refusal, although this does not occur similarly in the chicken.
- In poultry, reduced egg production and egg shell quality may be seen.

Lesions

Lesions vary with duration of the exposure

- Carcass is dehydrated
- Enteritis
- Gastric and intestinal hyperemia

- Pale, swollen kidneys
- Few lesions except for greyish white kidneys that are firm, and may have cystic dilation at the cut cortical surface
- Potential urinary tract tumors
- Microscopic lesions in the acute form may include:
  - Proximal tubular (especially the P3 segment) necrosis and dilation
  - Focal areas of intestinal mucosal damage in the lower intestine
  - Prolonged exposure of animals to low levels of ochratoxin A causes a primary problem of nephropathy
  - Exposure to high doses of ochratoxin A causes nephrosis, enteritis, lymphoid necrosis and hepatic necrosis.
  - A similar nephropathy in cattle fed ochratoxin-contaminated feedstuffs was also reported.
  - Birds may have visceral gout and nephrosis.

Clinical Pathological Findings and Lesions

- Acute toxicosis
  - Clinical pathology.
  - Increased PCV and hemoglobin.
  - Increased blood urea nitrogen, total protein, and the activities of lactic dehydrogenase, isocitric dehydrogenase & aspartate aminotransferase.
  - Increasingly dilute urine, with increased urine glucose and protein, and increased urinary enzymes such as leucine aminopeptidase.
  - Lesions vary with the dose and duration of exposure.
- Microscopic findings in the chronic form may include:
  - Mild degenerative changes in the tubular epithelium of the kidneys with prominent dilated tubules and interstitial fibrosis, and tubular atrophy. Basement membranes may be thickened and sclerosis of the glomeruli may be seen. The tubular epithelial nuclei become enlarged and nuclei become enlarged and necrotic. Thickened basement membranes may occur and dilated tubules with flat tubular epithelial cells may be seen.
  - Birds may have urate crystals and nephrosis with more chronic effects than in the acute form. Other lesions encountered experimentally were mentioned with regard to Mechanisms of Action (above).

Diagnosis

- Change of feed prior to the onset of illness.
- Feed may be moldy but this can be difficult to recognize due to differences between different areas of the feed and due to inability to recognize mold damaged feed after milling.
- Polydipsia, polyuria.
- Appropriate lesions, especially in the kidneys.
- Poor egg production with poor, stained, or rubbery shells in chickens.
- Detection of ochratoxin in the feed in toxic concentrations.
- Detection of ochratoxin-alpha in kidney, liver and skeletal muscle.
- Urine and faeces may also be analyzed for ochratoxin.

Treatment

- No specific antidote is avialable
- Activated charcoal reduces absorption but not useful in case of chronic exposure
- Symptomatic therapy
- In acutely exposed animals, such as dogs, appropriate measures to evacuate the gastrointestinal tract may be used with adsorbents and saline cathartics as indicated to remove ochratoxin containing feedstuffs.
- Supportive therapy should be similar to that for other causes of renal failure
- Care & management.

Trichothecene Mycotoxins

Introduction

Trichothecene mycotoxins: (12,13 epoxytrichothecenes) comprise a group of over 50 compounds of widely varying toxicity that are produced primarily by field fungi of the genus *Fusarium*.

Sources

- Trichothecenes tend to be produced in toxic concentrations in years of wet weather when harvests are delayed and prolonged.
- Trichothecenes known to cause problems in farm animals include: deoxynivalenol (vomitoxin), nivalenol, T-2 toxin, diacetoxyscirpenol

(DAS), macrocyclic trichothecenes (roridin A verrucarin A satratoxins), as well as others. Deoxynivalenol appears to be the most significant member of the group despite its comparatively low toxicity. T-2 toxin has caused widespread epidemics in human beings in the Soviet Union and, as with DAS, is an occasional cause of outbreaks of important toxicoses in animals.

- Deoxynivalenol is produced by *Fusarium* fungi, especially *F. roseum* (*Giberella zeae, F. graminearium*) with corn (*Zea mays*) and sometimes wheat (*Triticum* spp.) as well as other small grains being the most important sources of exposure to livestock.
  - Mild temperatures tend to encourage mold growth and cool temperatures increase toxin production by *F. roseum*. Therefore fluctuating warm to cool temperatures in the presence of high grain moisture concentrations increase the likelihood of deoxynivalenol and zearalenone poisoning. These toxins arise especially as a result of field infection, but occasionally improper storage can greatly magnify the problems.
- T-2 toxin is produced especially by *F. sporotrichioides*.
- Undulating temperatures on the cold side tend to be associated with contamination of cereal grains with T-2 toxin and diacetoxyscirpenol. Thus, T-2 toxin and diacetoxyscirpenol occur especially during years of delayed harvests when grains are left in the field over the winter and temperatures are highly fluctuant. These toxins, along with deoxynivalenol and zearalenone, were detected in specimens of the alleged chemical warfare agent, yellow rain. T-2 toxin may occur in corn but the highest concentrations generally occur in small grains such as barley and wheat. Forages are sometimes contaminated.
- Macrocyclic trichothecene toxins in plant tissues of the *Baccharis* genus cause severe toxicoses in herbivores in Brazil.
- Macrocyclics also are sometimes produced by *Stachybotrys atra* in wet forages and/or straw as well as in rain-damaged building materials and water-soaked air ducts. All these sources have resulted in clinical poisoning problems.

Toxicity

- Experimentally, 4 ppm deoxynivalenol has caused a 2% reduction in feed intake while at 40 ppm a 90% reduction was observed. In the field, however, concentrations of DON associated with feed refusal may be as low as 1 ppm

- T-2 Toxin and DAS are far more acutely toxic than deoxynivalenol, T-2 and DAS infrequently cause major outbreaks of serious toxicosis in livestock and poultry.

Toxicodynamics

- Trichothecenes are potent inhibitors of peptidyl transferase a ribosomal enzyme that is essential for protein synthesis. Thus, the trichothecenes inhibit protein synthesis.
- Trichothecenes also inhibit uptake of amino acids.
- Trichothecenes promote uptake of calcium and this is believed to trigger apoptosis.

Clinical Signs

- Deoxynivalenol (DON, Vomitoxin):
    - Swine appear to be most susceptible, but cattle, horses, dogs and poultry are all reported to be susceptible.
    - Though not among the more acutely toxic trichothecenes, deoxynivalenol, has caused great economic loss to the livestock industry.
    - The predominant sign associated with contaminated feed is reduced feed intake (or occasionally feed refusal) and decreased rate of gain.
    - Other signs may include soft stools, diarrhea, failure to thrive, and a predisposition to other disease entities and poor nutrition.
    - Vomiting is infrequently seen therefore the name vomitoxin seems inappropriate.
    - Animals may develop a resistance to deoxynivalenol and make compensatory gains.
    - Although a mild thickening of the squamous mucosa of the stomach has been noted experimentally, specific lesions may not be found.
- T-2 Toxin, Diacetoxyscirpenol (DAS), and Macrocyclic Trichothecenes.
    - Problems involving T-2 toxin, DAS, and macrocyclic trichothecenes occur mainly in cattle, hogs and poultry, and occasionally in horses, dogs, cats, and humans.
    - Signs most often would include:
        - Increased incidence of infection.

- ° Reduced feed intake or feed refusal.
- ° Vomiting and diarrhea.
- ° Necrosis of skin and oral mucosal damage.

• Less often one may see:

- ° Hemorrhage and necrosis of GI mucosa (high doses).
- ° Destruction of hemopoietic tissue and lymphoid necrosis (high doses).
- ° Meningeal hemorrhage (massive doses).
- ° Shock and death (massive doses).

Reproductive Effects

- At doses toxic to the dam, embryo toxicity and fetotoxicity, and possible abortion may occur.
- Testicular damage in males may occur with highly toxic levels of exposure.
- *Stachybotrys atia*, cause of stachbotryotoxicosis is a black mold that produces macrocyclic trichothecenes. These toxins in straw have poisoned horses and farm workers. When the mold grows in water-damaged homes or air ducts people become chronically affected.

Dermal Effects of Trichothecene Mycotoxins

- Only the more potent trichothecene mycotoxins are known for their effects on the skin. The local cytotoxic effects of these compounds may produce lesions on the snout, muzzle, lips and tongue. T-2 toxin, diacetoxyscirpenol and other trichothecenes, especially the macrocyclic toxins which have been recognized primarily in Europe, have dermal effects although other effects are more toxicologically important. The trichothecene believed to be of greatest importance, deoxynivalenol, also called vomitoxin, is less potent in most respects and is not known for any significant dermal effects.
- Stachbotryotoxicosis results from macrocyclic trichothecenes in Europe, especially in the eastern countries. The most severe outbreaks have occurred in large animals and are a result of contact with contaminated forages. Persons handling the affected forages have also experienced dermal and respiratory irritation. Affected animals experience the effects of the cytotoxic properties of the trichothecenes present. Perioral, pharyngeal and gastrointestinal irritation all result.

- Similar perioral, pharyngeal and gastrointestinal effects are seen with T-2 toxin and diacetoxyscirpenol.
- In calves dosed with T-2 toxin orally for up to 6 weeks, atrophy of the thymus was a consistent finding. Clotting disorders and reproductive problems have also been reported with T-2 toxin but the former have not been readily reproduced experimentally.

Diagnosis

- When a history includes feed refusal and failure to thrive, several mycotoxins should be included in the differential diagnosis.
- When mycotoxins are suspected, feed should be submitted for a mycotoxin screen.
- It may be wisest to submit some of the worst looking feed to account for "the worst case exposure" and a separate sample collected as to represent the balance of the feed on hand (a composite from several locations) to represent the feed as a whole. Ship at least 3 kg of each frozen or at a moisture concentration of 3% or less to the lab via priority mail or some even faster method.
- Testing for the presence of the trichothecene mycotoxins in feed is the most important means of arriving at a definitive diagnosis. Specific quantitative assays are available for a limited number of trichothecenes at most diagnostic laboratories. Agri-Screen ELISA tests for DON and T-2 toxin are available.
- These mycotoxins are not found at very high concentrations in tissues, although stomach contents may contain detectable levels if the animals were eating prior to death.

Treatment

- There are no specific antidotes for trichothecene mycotoxins, therefore, supportive and symptomatic treatment are indicated.
- Questionable feed should be removed and replaced by good quality feed with additional protein supplementation.
- Stress should be reduced to a minimum.

Prevention

- These mycotoxicoses are best controlled by proper grain handling and avoidance of questionable feeds.

- When necessary, analyses may be performed on feed, however, a negative test result does not preclude the presence of mycotoxins in some other areas of the bulk feed.
- Test animals can also be fed suspected grain and monitored for feed refusal and other signs of trichothecene mycotoxicoses.

Zearalenone and Zearalenol

Introduction

- Zearalenone
  - This estrogen-like toxin and its relatives such as zearalenol cause subacute poisoning, as a rule, but do not cause death losses, and probably do not greatly predispose to either nutritional or infectious disorders. Zearalenone and its derivatives are the only known mycotoxins whose effects are primarily estrogenic in nature and swine are among the most sensitive domestic animals to this toxin. A 3-dimensional model of the zearalenone molecule can be used to demonstrate the similar configuration of this toxin to estradiol. As a result, zearalenone can occupy and stimulate estrogenic receptors.
- Zearalenol
  - α-Zearalenol is associated with natural zearalenone occurrence and may have 3 times the estrogenic activity of zearalenone. It is not, however, routinely included in mycotoxin screens by analytical laboratories. Although zearalenone and a-zearalenol may occur as products of other species of *Fusarium* and may coexist with T-2 toxin and other mycotoxins, they are produced primarily by *F. roseum* and coexist (as far as we know at present) primarily with deoxynivalenol (vomitoxin). In the field, estrogenic effects may occur in swine fed rations in which only a few parts per million of zearalenone are present. In these instances the diagnosis is usually confirmed when normal reproductive function occurs after withdrawal of the contaminated feed. Of course efforts to rule out infectious agents, in the case of infertility and/or abortion should not await the results of mycotoxin assays. In swine, estrogens are luteotropic and would be expected to maintain pregnancy.

Sources

- Zearalenone is produced by species of *Fusarium*, primarily *F. roseum*.
  - Corn, wheat, other grains, and occasionally forages may be contaminated by zearalenone.

- Very high concentrations up to approximately 20 ppm have been found in wheat.

Susceptible Species

Swine, cattle, sheep; whereas chickens appear to be largely resistant.

Effects of Zearalenone

Swine (Most Susceptible)

- In prepubertal gilts.
  - Swelling and edema of vulva.
  - Vaginal and rectal prolapse.
  - Uterine enlargement, edema.
  - Atrophy of ovaries.
  - Enlargement of mammary glands.
  - Thin catarrhal exudate from vulva.
  - Differential diagnosis-normal estrus, injury to external genitalia.
- ❐ In young boars.
  - Atrophy of testes.
  - Zearalenone in prepubertal boars may reduce libido and plasma testosterone.
- ❐ In castrated or prepubertal males.
  - Enlargement of mammary glands.
  - Preputial enlargement.
- ❐ In sows.
  - Anestrus or nymphomania dependent on stage of animal's estrous cycle when first exposed.
  - Reduced litter size due to fetal resorption (mummification) and/or implantation failure when dietary zearalenone is present at 7 - 10 days postmating.
  - Weak or stillborn pigs. Piglets occasionally exhibit swollen vulvas at or shortly after birth (juvenile hyperestrogenism) whether this is from exposure *in utero* and/or through the dam's milk is currently under investigation.
  - Pseudopregnancy.

- Field observations of zearalenone-caused abortions are now thought to be largely erroneous since estrogens are luteotropic in swine. Instead, it is suspected that implantation failure followed by pseudopregnancy leads to a diagnosis of abortion. Other etiologies (different mycotoxins, viruses, etc.) should be considered more likely to account for most late-term abortions.
- Encephalomyocarditis (EMC) virus.
- Other mycotoxins.

Cattle

- In cattle, ruminal metabolism may alter toxicity; may be associated with precocious udder development in heifers and reduced fertility in breeding animals.
- Most animals exposed to zearalenone for brief periods of time will probably recover normal reproductive function. However, at least in females, severe toxicosis may be characterized by ovarian fibrosis and changes in the oviduct and uterus which could conceivably have more prolonged effects on reproduction. Further study of this area is needed.

Sheep

- Decrease in ovulation rate and lambing percentage.
- *Fusarium* spp. growing on pasture is a recognized cause of exposure to estrogenic mycotoxins.

Diagnosis

- Zearalenone and zearalenol can be quantified by high performance liquid chromatography in feedstuffs at most veterinary diagnostic laboratories.
- Second choice screening tests include Neogen's Veratox, Agriscreen ®
  - ELISA test (used to screen feeds) for zearalenone

Differential Diagnosis

- Pseudorabies
- Leptospirosis
- Enterovirus
- Parvovirus

Management

- Recent research has suggested that permanent reproductive damage rarely occurs. Once animals are on clean feed and have excreted the zearalenone, normal reproductive function should occur.
- Recovery should occur in 7 - 10 days, although more time may be required for sows to start cycling. However, culling sows **may** be more economical than waiting for a return to a normal reproductive cycle.
- Recent studies indicate that zearalenone is extensively recycled through the enterohepatic system. Therefore, intestinal binding agents (activated charcoal, bentonite clays) or agents that decrease GI transit time (e.g., alfalfa fiber) may enhance elimination and decrease the time needed for animals to regain normal function.
- Other mycotoxins have been associated with reproductive abnormalities (experimental evidence). Also, interactions of mycotoxins must be considered in field conditions.

Ergot Alkaloids

Sources

The Term Ergot is Used in 2 Ways

- as the common name for the fungus *Claviceps* which invades the ovary of grasses and cereals
- used to refer to the sclerotium, the hard purple mass of mycelium hyphae that replaces the heads of grasses
  - In the midwest, *C. purpurea* is the most common fungus invading grasses. The host plant range includes: rye, triticale, barley, oats, brome grass, timothy and quack grasses.
  - In commercial grain trade, wheat or rye are classified as "ergoty" if more than 0.3% by weight are comprised of ergot sclerotia and oats, triticale or barley are so graded when they contain more than 0.1%.
  - In some parts of the world, *Claviceps* fungi have been isolated from sorghum grain that contained ergot alkaloids.
  - Ergot poisoning, sometimes of epidemic proportions has occurred in persons due to the ingestion of smutted rye. Toxic amounts were associated with abortifacient effects and this effect led to its use to hasten labor. Unfortunately, this use led to excessive uterine contraction frequently and often caused ischemic damage to the child. In the present use of ergot alkaloids, the only rational objective is to prevent postpartum bleeding.

Toxicity

- Animal responses vary with the total and individual alkaloid content, quantity of ergot in the feed, frequency of ingestion, climatic conditions (cool, wet weather) and animal species. All domestic animals, birds and man are susceptible. In human medicine, the gangrenous reaction sometimes occurs at therapeutic doses, although it occurs more often with excessive doses.

Toxic Principle

- The toxic action of ergot is due to the numerous alkaloids (ergotamine, ergocristine, ergonovine, etc.) present in the sclerotia and other components-choline, Ach, histamine, sterols. Over 40 alkaloids have been identified which are derivatives of lysergic acid, some of which are inactive.
- The important naturally occurring alkaloids are ergotamine and ergonovine. Of these, ergonovine is more readily absorbed. Both compounds are potent smooth muscle activators. LSD is also derived from ergot, and the smooth muscle contracting activity, although sometimes present, is not always seen. LSD causes depersonalization or hallucinations and may produce toxic psychosis.

Toxicokinetics

- Metabolism (detoxification) of the ergot alkaloids is assumed to take place in the liver, since toxic effects are more likely in animals with liver dysfunction.
- Meat and milk residues have not been detected in any field outbreaks.

Toxicodynamics

- The wide spectrum of pharmacological activity is attributed in part to the alkaloids' agonist/antagonist activity at alpha adrenoreceptors, 5-HT receptors and dopamine receptors. The primary effects are central/neurohormonal and peripheral. The peripheral effects include an oxytocic-like effect on the uterus and vasoconstriction from smooth muscle contraction.
- The central neurohormonal effect mimics the effects of dopamine. Dopaminergic action may result in a reduction in prolactin which can adversely affect (reduce) milk production.

- All smooth muscles, vascular and nonvascular, are contracted, and there is no dependence on innervation or any other chemical mediators.
- Only at term is uterine muscle more sensitive to ergot than is other smooth muscle. Therefore in early pregnancy, ergot cannot be used as an abortifacient. Furthermore in early pregnancy, these alkaloids are more stimulatory to the cervix, than to the uterus. Ergot is not recommended in any context as an abortifacient. For the induction of labor, oxytocin is very much preferred.
- The blood vessels in all vascular beds are constricted by the ergot alkaloids, but the larger arteries are most sensitive. Occlusion may occur, as shown by arteriograms. The result is ischemia of the tissues perfused by the artery. It is possible for blood flow to be reestablished without permanent damage, or the tissue may become gangrenous before the process reverses. The limbs, toes, ears and tail are often affected, but usually not all in the same animal.

Clinical Signs

- Ergot poisoning is commonly seen in cattle. Clinical signs include: reduced feed intake, unthriftiness, **lameness**, swelling and sloughing of feet below the fetlocks (generally the hind feet). Usually a line of demarcation separates the proximal viable tissue and the distal dry cold epidermis. Less commonly the ears and tail are sloughed.
- Affected extremities may become inflamed and then cold, with numbness and dry gangrene developing. Eventually, there is a painless loss of tissue. The gangrenous form results when animals ingest ergot alkaloids over periods of days or weeks.
- Other clinical signs may include poor milk production, nervous signs, and reduced conception.
- The primary signs in swine with ergotism are **agalactia**, early parturition, weak or dead pigs, infertility and **reduced rate of gain**.
- In sheep, necrosis of the tongue, gastroenteritis, abortions, gangrene and central nervous system involvement are reported.

Diagnosis

- Ingestion of ergoty small grains (ergot does **not** occur in corn).
- Ergot alkaloids in grains may be identified in toxicology laboratories by gas chromatography-mass spectrometry or less sophisticated methods including thin-layer and high pressure liquid chromatography.

Treatment

- Isolate from source.
- Control secondary bacterial infections.
- Move animals to a dry, warm environment.
- Keeping the animals warm is indicated to avoid the added insult of lower environmental temperature to the vascular insult. In warm weather, fly control is essential.
- Of several xenobiotics and maneuvers tried to alleviate the vasoconstriction, only nitroprusside infusions showed any promise.

Prevention

- Control of ergot - Climatic conditions are involved in yearly incidence.
- Mow grasses prior to flowering.

Festuca Arundinacea
(Tall Fescue)
Description

- Coarse perennial grass, deeply rooted, in vigorous clumps, reaching 3 - 4 feet in height when mature.
- Leaves broad, dark-green, ribbed, and rough on the upper surfaces.
- Inflorescence paniculate, nodding, to 1 foot in length
- Spikelets many-flowered.

Habitat

Tall fescue is a major forage grass,grown on an estimated 35 million acres and will tolerate being closely grazed. The grass is sometimes allowed to "accumulate or stockpile" for winter grazing. Fescue is sometimes cultivated as hay.

Toxic Principle

- The toxic principles are apparently produced by the endophytic (inside the grass) fungus, *Neotyphodium coenophialum*, previously known as *Acremonium coenophianum*; and before that, *Epichloe typhina*. This fungus is a *Clavicipitaceae fungus* which is transmitted in the seed (and not via spores) and can, produce ergot alkaloids. Ergovaline is the ergot alkaloid of greatest significance in endophyte-infected fescue. It is estimated that over 90% of tall fescue fields in the world are infected with the endophyte to some extent, with an average of 62% of the plants infected within each field.

- Pyrrolizidine alkaloids including N-acetylloline, N-formylloline, and dimethyl-N-acetylloline have been isolated from fescue. Also, the alkaloid perloline has been identified in endophyte-infected fescue. However, the significance of these types of alkaloids remains to be demonstrated.

Toxicodynamics

Ergovaline is believed to account for the decrease in prolactin, and other effects of endophyte-infected fescue, most of which are compatible with the effect of ergot alkaloids (gangrene and low milk production, for example).

Clinical Signs

The Syndromes Associated with Tall Fescue Include

- Summer syndrome in cattle.
- Fescue foot in cattle.
- Fat necrosis in cattle.
- Reproductive and lactation problems in cattle, horses and sheep

Cattle

- **Summer syndrome**:
- Poor weight gain, reduced feed intake
- Reduced conception rates
- Intolerance to heat
- Failure to shed the winter hair coat (rough hair)
- Elevated body temperature
- Nervousness, excessive salivation
- More prevalent where fescue is present as a monoculture and where high nitrogen fertilization is used.

Fescue Foot

- Some fescue fields have a history of repeated fescue foot outbreaks, but in general, the outbreaks are non-recurring. Conditions which favor the fescue foot syndrome include the feeding of the fall regrowth or the total yearly accumulated fescue (longer stockpiling increases incidence).

- Lameness most often occurs with the onset of cooler or cold weather (below 60 °F and especially with snow or ice).
- Cattle on low-quality rations, and underweight are predisposed, animals in good flesh are not immune.
- Onset is 5 - 15 days, up to weeks after on pasture, occasionally where continuously pastured.
- Slight arching of the back.
- Rough hair coat.
- Soreness in 1 or both rear limbs, weight shifting, holding 1 foot up.
- Knuckling.
- Loose stools.
- Reddening of the coronary band, then swelling.
- Redness, swelling and then purple-black discoloration of the tail.
- Sloughing of the ear tips.
- Sloughing of the feet, usually at or just above the coronary band, sometimes, higher.

Fat Necrosis

- Lipomatosis or fat necrosis is defined as the presence of masses of hard or necrotic fat in the adipose tissue of the abdominal cavity.
- Affected fat has yellowish or chalky white irregular masses of very hard fat, especially in the mesenteries.
- These may be detected on rectal exam. Subcutaneous fat is not affected.
- Digestive disturbances, due to obstruction or intestinal constriction, scanty faeces, bloating and occassionally death occur.
- Dystocia due to hardening of fat around the birth canal may also occur.
- Similarly urine retention has been encountered secondary to these fat deposits with associated postrenal uremia.
- Other signs associated with fat necrosis include; weight loss, poor appetite, listlessness and rough hair coat.
- Predisposing factors include the presence of fescue in monoculture and heavy nitrogen fertilization.

Horse, Sheep, Cattle

- Predisposition to laminitis in horses has also been associated with exposure to endophyte-infected fescue.

- **Reproductive and lactation problems** in cattle, horses and sheep: The primary problems are abortion, weak to stillborn young and moderate to severe agalactia. The effects result in the death of many neonates.
- Cattle
  - Typically a farmer with cows on a problem pasture will have a 70 - 80% calf crop, which is made worse by fertilization, but improves with the addition of clover to the pasture. Dairy cows may have a marked decrease in milk production. Prolactin concentrations are depressed in cows ingesting affected fescue.
- Horses
  - Horses may abort or more often have dystocia after a prolonged gestation, and may have a thick placenta that increases the need for human assistance during parturition. Serum cortisol concentrations did not increase normally near parturition in mares grazing a problem fescue pasture, and serum prolactin levels were extremely low. The low milk production may be attributable to the low prolactin levels. Prolactin is responsible for the initiation and maintenance of lactation and possibly for the initiation and maintenance of the corpus luteum as well. The decrease in prolactin may therefore also be responsible for the early abortion and fetal resorption in affected species, but this remains to be verified.
  - Predisposition to laminitis in horses has also been associated with exposure to endophyte-infected fescue.
- Ewes
  - Serum prolactin levels are depressed by ingestion of affected fescue.
  - Increased rate of return to estrus.

Treatment of Fescue Foot

- Remove from fescue pasture, when 1st signs occur.
- Rule out foot rot, frost bite, mechanical injuries such as stone bruising.

Management

- Mix legumes and other grasses with the fescue stand or supplement the diet with other feeds. This appears to work well with cattle but apparently dystocia in pregnant mares may occur with as little as 5 - 10% of the ground cover in a pasture as infected fescue.
- Rotational grazing.

- Do not fertilize with over 90 kg of nitrogen per acre per year.
- Feeding hay may lessen problems; field cured fescue hay, processed in the early dough to boot stage, when quality is at a maximum is considered safe for feeding to cattle. However, toxic fescue cut for hay remains toxic.
- Observe cattle daily for lameness or stiffness, especially during the first month on pasture and in cold weather. Observe in early AM before cattle warm out of the lameness. Move affected animals to another field or put them on another feed.
- Adequate protein and mineral supplementation should be assured.
- Avoid stress especially in cold weather.
- Addition of a legume to the pasture sharply increases gains. Ladino clover also improves conception rates.
- If new plantings of fescue are to be done, the use of old seed is recommended, since the fungus dies after 1 year under normal storage conditions. New cultivars of fescue are relatively free of the endophyte. Strains should be chosen with 0-5% infection rate.

Chapter 8

ZOOTOXICOLOGY

Introduction

A *toxin* (Greek: ôïîéêüí, *toxikon*, lit. (poison) for use on arrows) is a poisonous substance produced by living cells or organisms that is active at very low concentrations. Toxins can be small molecules, peptides, or proteins and are capable of causing disease on contact or absorption with body tissues by interacting with biological macromolecules such as enzymes or cellular receptors. Toxins vary greatly in their severity, ranging from usually minor and acute (as in a bee sting) to almost immediately deadly (as in botulinum toxin)

A toxin is simply a poison that can affect the body by internal or external means. A toxin can be a chemical which occurs naturally or in synthetic form. More than 120,000 human-made chemicals have been introduced into the environment, in one form or another, and this number continues to grow each year at a phenomenal rate. At the same time, microbial toxins, being influenced by the vast numbers of chemicals, are mutating beyond belief.

Each category of microbes produces species that generates toxins in host cells. Evidence is proving a definitive link between the accumulation of toxins in body tissues and the development of chronic diseases.

External toxins, either chemical or microbial, enter the body through food, water, air, or physical contact with the skin or mucous membranes. Internal toxins, as the free radicals, are produced inside the body through normal metabolic processes or through the decomposition of foods in the small and large intestines. Bacterial toxins and yeast overgrowth can also form in cases of chronic constipation.

Under normal circumstances, the body is able to eliminate toxins from the body via urine, feces, exhalation, and persperation. Thus, the major organs involved in elimination are the kidneys, liver, colon, lungs, and skin. In addition, WBCs (white blood cells) of the immune system are designed to neutralize microbial toxins. The liver is the organ primarily responsible for breaking toxins into harmless byproducts, which are eliminated into the stool or through the kidneys into the urine.

The process of elimination can be hampered for one reason or another. When a particular toxin overwhelms the normal excretion mechanisms, the body produces inflammation in the area of the toxin trying to rid itself of the problem. These inflammatory areas signal the start of a disease. They are actually signals the body is sending, stating that it cannot rid itself of accumulating toxins. If the toxins remain, the body then moves into the next stage, where they are deposited in areas where they will do the least harm. These areas are usually fat cells, cysts, polyps or tumors. After years of storage, the toxins move into body cells and tissues. They ultimately produce such degenerative diseases as cancer, diabetes, arthritis, and heart disease.

A *toxoid* is a treated toxin, often used in vaccines, that retains its immunological structure, but which no longer causes damage to tissues. For example, the diphtheria toxoid is a sterile preparation of formaldehyde-treated products produced from the growth of *Corynebacterium diphtheriae*. It is generally mixed with the tetanus toxoid and pertussis in the DPT vaccine, but it can be used alone (DT). The same holds true for the tetanus toxoid produced from the growth of *Clostridium tetani* and used either by itself or in mixtures with diphteria toxoid and pertussis vaccine.

There are two general categories of toxins which differ in potency and function:

1. Endotoxins, which are part of the cell wall of Gram-negative bacteria. Only small amounts may escape into surrounding fluids from living

bacteria. Greater amounts are released when the bacteria die and their cell walls disintegrate. Endotoxins are less potent, and larger amounts are needed to induce disease symptoms. Also, they are heat resistant and cannot be converted into toxoids.

2. Exotoxins are mainly proteins that are secreted by a bacterial cell into surrounding fluids, and are produced by both Gram-negative and Gram-positive bacteria. Most are readily destroyed by heat, but they can be converted into toxoids that are used as vaccines. Exotoxins are extremely powerful biological poisons as in the case of tetanus, where it has been estimated that 1 mg of purified tetanus toxin could kill millions of mice.

An *exotoxin* is a soluble protein excreted by a microrganism, including bacteria, fungi, algae, and protozoa. An exotoxin can cause damage to the host by destroying cells or disrupting normal cellular metabolism. Both gram negative and gram positive bacteria produce exotoxins. They are highly potent and can cause major damage to the host. Exotoxins may be secreted, or, similar to endotoxins, may be released during lysis of the cell.

Most exotoxins can be destroyed by heating. They may exert their effect locally or produce systemic effects. Well known exotoxins include the botulinum toxin produced by *Clostridium botulinum*, the *Corynebacterium diphtheriae* exotoxin which is produced during life threatening symptoms of diphtheria.

Exotoxins are susceptible to antibodies produced by the immune system, but many exotoxins are so toxic that they may be fatal to the host before the immune system has a chance to mount defenses against it.

Biotoxins

Biotoxins in nature have two primary functions:

- Predation (spider, snake, scorpion, jellyfish, wasp)
- Defense (bee, poison dart frog, honeybee, wasp)

Some of the more well known types of biotoxins include:

- Cyanotoxins, produced by cyanobacteria
- Hemotoxins target and destroy red blood cells, and are transmitted through the bloodstream. Organisms that produce hemotoxins include:
  - Pit vipers, such as rattlesnakes

- Necrotoxins cause necrosis (i.e., death) in the cells they encounter and destroy all types of tissue. Necrotoxins spread through the bloodstream. In humans, skin and muscle tissues are most sensitive to necrotoxins. Organisms that possess necrotoxins include:
  - The brown recluse or "fiddle back" spider
  - The "Puff Adder" - *Bitis arietans*
  - Necrotizing fasciitis (the "flesh eating" bacteria)
- Neurotoxins primarily affect the nervous systems of animals. Organisms that possess neurotoxins include:
  - The Black Widow and other widow spiders
  - Most scorpions
  - The box jellyfish
  - Elapid snakes
  - The Cone Snail
- Cytotoxins are toxic at the level of individual cells, either in a non-specific fashion or only in certain types of living cells:
  - Ricin is a plant toxin found in the castor bean plant

Some examples of toxins include

1. Bacterial toxins are produced by bacteria that include exotoxins, endotoxins, interotoxins, neurotoxins, and toxic enzymes.
2. Botulinus toxin is one of several type-specific exotoxins produced by *Clostridium botulinum*.
3. Cholera toxin is an exotoxin produced by *Vibrio cholerae*, in which a protein enterotoxin stimulates cells in such a way as to cause severe diarrhea characteristic of the disease.
4. Chlostridial toxin is one produced by species of *Clostridium*, which include those causing botulism, gas gangrene, and tetanus. In addition, *C.difficile* produces an exotoxin which causes severe intestinal necrosis. *C.perfringens* produces a number of potentially fatal exotoxins.
5. Diptheria toxin is a protein exotoxin produced by *Corynebacterium diphtheriae*.
6. Dysentry toxin is one produced by organisms of various species of *Shigella*.
7. Erythrogenic toxin is a bacterial toxin from certain strains of *Streptococcus pyogenes*. Extracellular toxin is an exotoxin.

8. Gas gangrene toxin is one of at least ten types of exotoxin produced by *Clostridium perfringens*. Intracellular toxin is endotoxin.
9. Streptococcal toxin is a mixture of exotoxins formed by *Streptococcus pyogenes*.
10. Tetanus toxin is a potent exotoxin produced by *Clostridium tetani*, consisting of two components, one a neurotoxin (tetanospasmin) and the other a hemolysin (tetanolysin).

Microbial Toxins and their Laboratory Diagnostic Methods

The term toxin was originally used for filterable (subcellur) substances inducing illness. Today hundreds of toxins are known,which are exerting some deadly effect on the living cells. Toxins are proteins of quite complex structure with very specific targets. Toxins of microbial origin can be classified based on the sources as 1) Bacterial toxins 2) Viral toxins and 3) Mycotoxins

Bacterial toxins are protein in nature and can be again subclassified in to Exotoxins and Endotoxins

Endotoxins

- Possessed solely by Gram negative organisms.
- Lipopolysaccharide (LPS) which occur on the outer membrane of Gram negative bacteria and are not secreted but are released only when cells are disrupted or destroyed.
- Elicit an antigenic response resulting in fever and altered resistance to bacterial infections. Exposure may cause hemorrhagic shock and severe diarrhea
- Examples: *Salmonella typhimurium, E. coli.*

Exotoxins

- Secreted by viable pathogenic cells and are soluble, heat labile, protein toxins that are usually released into other surrounding as they are produced by either Gram negative or Gram positive bacteria
- Their chemical nature is protein, loose their toxicity when heated at 60-80° C or acids, inactived by chemicals like formaldehyde and converted into toxoids and produce antitoxin upon injection into host.

Exotoxins can be categorized on the basis of site of affect as; 1) Neurotoxin- act on nervous tissue Ex. *Clostridium botulinum, Cl. Tetanii.* 2) Enterotoxin- act on GIT Ex. *Vibrio cholerae, E. coli.;* 3) Cytotoxin- act on general tissue. Ex. *Shigella spp., Cl. Perfringens*

According to mode action the bacterial toxins can be categorized as damaging the cell membrane, inhibiting the protein synthesis, activating the second messenger pathway, inhibiting the release of neurotransmitters.

Activities of extra cellular bacterial protein toxins

Name of toxin	Bacteria involved	Activity
Anthrax toxin (EF)	*Bacillus anthracis*	- Adenylatecyclase causes increased levels in cAMP in phagocytes and formation of ion permeable pores in membranes (hemolysis)
Cholera enterotoxin (CTX)	*Vibrio cholera*	- Stimulates adenylate cyclase and increases cAMP in GI tract causing secretion of water and electrolytes
E. coli LT toxin	*E.coli*	- Similar to cholera toxin
E. coli ST toxin	*E. coli*	stimulates guanylate cyclase and promotes secretion of water and electrolytes from intestinal epithelium
Perfringens enterotoxin	*Cl. Perfringens*	- Stimulates adenylate cyclase leading to increased CAMP in epithelial cells
Botulinum toxin	*Cl. Botulinum*	- Zn $^{++}$ dependent protease that inhibits neurotransmission at neuromuscular synapses resulting in flaccid paralysis
Tetanus toxin	*Cl. Tetani.*	-Do- spastic paralysis
Exotoxin A	*Pseudomonas aeruginosa*	- Inhibits protein synthesis, similar to diphtheria toxin
Anthrax toxin (LF)	*Bacillus anthracis*	- Cytotoxic to cells by an unknown mechanism
Staphylococcus enterotoxin	*Staph. aureus*	- Massive activation of the immune system including lymphocyte and macrophages leads to emesis
Exfoliatin toxin	*Staph. Aureus*	- Cleavage of epidermal cells

Laboratory Detection of Toxins

It requires demonstration of toxin in plasma or tissue before death or from fresh carcass.

Isolation of the organism: especially from intestinal contents or post-mortem demonstration of toxin is not definitive. Demonstration of toxin in feed stuffs, fresh stomach contents or vomitus supports diagnosis of toxins induced toxicity condition.

Toxin is extracted from suspected material (unless fluids) overnight with saline. The mixture is centrifuged and the clear portion filter, sterilized and trypnised (1% at 37^{0}C for 45 minutes). Guinea pig or mice are injected intraperitonially with the extract, mixture of extract and antitoxins and extract heated to 100^0 C for 10 minutes. Death due to toxin occurs within 10hrs to 3 weeks (average is 4 days) preceded by muscular weakness, limb paralysis and respiratory difficulties. Toxin must be neutralized by specific antitoxin.

Isolation of *Cl.botulinum* from suspected feeds to tissues begins with heating suspected material for 30 minutes at 65° C to 80° C to induce germination. Type E spores require in addition treatment with lysozyme (5mg/ ml of medium). Culture anaerobically on blood agar plates. Identification by biochemical reaction and toxin production. Immunoflurescence is used to identify some cultural grays. Primers designed to amplify the genes encoding the various toxins (by the polymerase chain reaction) can be used to support the demonstration that *Cl.botulinum* has been been isolated

The detection of microbial toxins can also be done in the laboratory by using a variety of serological tests mentioned below.

1) Agar Gel Diffusion Test

Since each antigen combines with its own specific antibody, and antigenic mixture will give rise to multiple bands,the immunological relationship between two antigens is assessed by setting up the reaction in adjacent wells. (a) when the lines confluent it indicates immunological identity in terms of antiserum used (b) the line crossing indicating unrelated antigens.

2) Radial Immunodiffusion

The basis of a single radial immunodiffusion test (SRID) used in the quantitative determination of antigens. Antigens from a well diffuse into antiserum incorporated agar. Initially since the concentration is high soluble complexes may be formed and with further diffusion of optimal proportions are reached resulting in a circular zone of precipitation. The diameter of the zone gives the amount of antigen and by running 4 or 5 different dilution of the antigen a standard curve is obtained which can used in the assay of unknowns. It is current method in use for the quantitative determination of immunoglobulin content.

3) Agglutination Test

Because antibodies are bivalent they can crosslink particulate antigens such as bacteria or foreign red cell, resulting in their clumping or agglutination. When a particular antigen is mixed with its antibody in the presence of electrolytes at a suitable temperature and pH the particles are clump or agglutinated.

Slide or Plate Agglutination test : is employed to screen sera within short period for preliminary testing.

Standard Tube Agglutination test: is used for diseases like brucellosis, salmonellosis are screened by these techniques.

4) Complement Fixation Test

Guinea pig complement gets fixed to antigen-antibody complexes and lyses them, but the antibodies or antigens are not capable of fixing the complement. This property of complement is made use of in detecting the reaction between soluble antigens and their antibodies. The presence or absence of complement in a system is detected by an indicator system of Ag-Ag complex, namely sheep erythrocytes and anti-sheep erythrocyte antibodies.

When a specific antigen is added to a serum sample containing its antibodies they form a complex and when complement is added to this system, gets fixed to this complex. Since no more free complement is available in this system, when the sheep erythrocytes complex us added to this, they are unaffected and the cells settle down to form a compact button. If a serum sample does not contain specific antibodies, the antigen is free and hence does not fix the complement. The free complement get fixed to sheep the erythrocytes is a visible reaction these results are read accordingly.

5) Neutralization Test

Neutralization tests estimate the ability of antibody to neutralize the biological activity of antigen when they are mixed in vitro. These tests may be used to identify *bacterial toxin such as Clostridium perfringens Alpha-toxin or the Staphylococcal* alpha-toxin.

Viruses may be prevented from infecting cells after specific antibody has combined with and blocked their critical attachment sites. This reaction is the basis of the neutralization tests that are employed either for the identification of unknown viruses or for the measurement of specific antiviral antibody.

6) Electrophoresis

Electrophoresis is the term which describes the movement of charged ions in solution in an electrical field. Counter-immuno electrophoresis is one of the quickest diagnostic technique for the diagnosis of the viral and bacterial diseases. In this technique the principle is based on the fact that if the antigen migrates in an electric field through a medium of diffusion towards the anode and the antibody migrates towards the cathode there will be precipitation at optimum levels. Under certain electrophoretic conditions in a suitable gel both immuno- reactants, meet in optimal proportions and give rise to precipitation lines. This method is quick when compared to get diffusion tests that are used for diagnosis of most of infections diseases.

7) Immuno Fluorescence Technique

This technique has proved a valuable tool in rapid detection of viral antigen and has been applied, in the detection of Foot and mouth disease virus, rabies virus etc., The technique would be highly advantageous in the conditions like (a) for quick diagnosis of the disease on the face of an outbreak so as to take suitable control measures immediately. (b) in those case where virus cannot be isolated from the sample because of inactivation or ,low titre of virus (c) for screening of large number of animal for carrier status etc.

8) Enzyme-Linked Immuno Sorbent Assay (ELISA)

ELISA's may be used to detect and quantitative either antibody or antigen. The technique is highly sensitive, specific, reliable and rapid.A soluble antigen is immobilized by coating a solid base such as plastic tube or plate. The test serum thought to contain antibody to the antigen is incubated in the coated tube. Any specific antibody present will react with the antigen. The tube then washed to remove all free immunoglobulin. A solution of conjugate consisting of antispecies globulin labeled with enzyme is then incubated in the tube. This reacts with the antibody fixed to the antigen. Further washing removes excess conjugate. The enzyme substrate is then added and its change in colour indicates the amount of enzyme in the tube. This amount is proportional to the concentration of antibody in the test serum. The different methods of ELISA employed are

a) Direct ELISA
b) Indirect ELISA
c) Double sandwich ELISA
d) Competitive ELISA
e) Dot-ELISA and many more alternatives of these methods in ELISA

9) Radio-Immunoassay

One primary binding test that is used to measure levels of specific IgE in allergic animal is the radio allergosorbent test (RAST).Competitive immunoassays are based on the principle that unlabeled antigen will displace radio labelled antigen from immune complexes. They are extremely sensitive and are commonly used to detect trace amounts of drugs.The technique has got many disadvantages like non availability, cost effective, non-feasibility by any person or laboratory, time consuming and requirement of license to do the work, difficulty in disposing of the waste etc. and hence ELISA's are taking over these techniques.

10) Cytotoxic Assays

The assay involves treatment of cell culture monolayers (usually in 96-well trays) with sterile extracts or filtrates of test materials and examination of cells for cytopathic effects after 48-72 h of incubation. The specificity of cell- culture cytotoxicity can be tested.

11) DNA-Based Assays

The DNA-based assays are colony hybridization and Polymerase chain reaction (PCR) assays can be used for detection bacterial which are toxin producing

The advantages and disadvantages of each immunodiagnostic test vary according to specific requirements of the investigator , the nature of antigen employed, the complexity, sensitivity and specificity of each method.

Tetanus

Sources

- Tetanus toxin is produced by *Clostridium tetani* a gram-positive, spore-forming bacillus under anaerobic conditions.
- *C. tetani* spores are also commonly present in the feces of domestic animals, especially those of horses, and in soil contaminated by the feces.
- *C. tetani* spores may persist in soil for many years and are resistant to many standard disinfection processes, including steam heat (100° C for 15 minutes).
- Poisoning is known to result from clostridial growth in contaminated wounds in which anaerobic conditions predominate. The usual incubation period is 1 - 3 weeks. It is possible for the original point of entry to heal without any evidence of infection and for subsequent trauma, even months later to set up the necessary environment for clostridial growth and toxin production.
- Animals given appropriate preventative measures (toxoid and antitoxin) are at low risk of developing tetanus.

Horse: The usual portal of entry in s deep puncture wounds. Clinical toxicosis is most likely when there is sufficient accompanying tissue damage to result in an anaerobic environment favorable to clostridial growth. Umbilical infections also occur in foals that receive no maternal immunity.

Cattle: The usual portal of entry in is via the reproductive tract at parturition. Outbreaks of tetanus in cattle have suggested that the toxin may have been produced in the gut or ingested preformed in the feed. Grazing of rough, fibrous feeds before such outbreaks is a common factor and it is possible that infection may have begun via wounds in the oral cavity. Castrating and dehorning with elastic bands can also result in clostridial infection.

Pigs: castration wounds are the most common point of infection.

Sheep : In lambs and adult sheep, infection is most often associated with castration, docking, or shearing. Docking with elastic bands is one of the most common causes of tetanus in lambs.

Susceptibility Order

Horses> Pigs>Cattle>Sheep>Dogs>Cats>Poultry.

Toxicodynamics

- Three exotoxins are produced by the vegetative form of *C. tetani*: tetanospasmin (causes clinical signs); tetanolysin (increases local tissue necrosis); and nonspasmogenic toxin (activates sympathetic nervous system).
- Tetanus toxin (tetanospasmin) is a protein (2 polypeptide fragments; total MW approximately 150,000). Transport to the CNS occurs retrograde within nerves and via the bloodstream.. The toxin binds to gangliosides in the brain stem or spinal cord, blocking inhibitory synaptic input, especially at glycine mediated sites, by binding to the presynaptic membrane and blocking the release of glycine, resulting in spastic paralysis. It may also inhibit release of GABA and other amino acid neurotransmitters.
- Tetanus toxin may also cause paralysis by inhibiting the release of acetylcholine at neuromuscular junctions (probably less important than inhibitory effect on release of glycine).
- Constant muscular spasticity may be produced and normally innocuous stimuli cause exaggerated responses.
- Death occurs as a result of rigidity of the muscles of respiration and associated asphyxia.

- Tetanus toxin may also cause cardiovascular symptoms in patients whose spastic paralysis was controlled.
- Nonspasmogenic toxin is poorly understood and is thought to cause paralysis of the peripheral nervous system.
- Tetanolysin is antiphagocytic and enhances local tissue necrosis.

Clinical Signs

- Hyperesthesia, tetany and convulsions with eventual rigidity of the muscles of respiration, asphyxia, and death. Tetany, the predominant clinical sign of tetanus, is characterized by sustained tonic contractions of muscle without twitching
- A sawhorse stance, protrusion of the third eyelid, rigidity of the generalized musculature, "sardonic grin", and secondary postural effects which diminish defecation and urination. Rigidity with extension of the tail has been described for cats "pump-handle tail".
- Opisthotonus and persistent rigid extension of all four limbs with stiff gait.
- In horses, spasms of the masseter muscles occur early in the disease, resulting in "lockjaw"
- Aspiration pneumonia may develop due to paralysis of laryngeal and pharyngeal musculature
- Excitation or loud noises may elicit convulsions in hyperesthetic animals.
- Excess stimulation of sympathetic nervous system with sweating, tachycardia, arrhythmias, vasoconstriction, colic. Being exhibited
- Complications due to recumbency occur, e.g., pressure induced neuropathy, decubital ulcers and as the dose of toxin is increased, paralysis can result.
- Localized tetanus involving only the muscle groups closest to the site of injury is relatively uncommon.

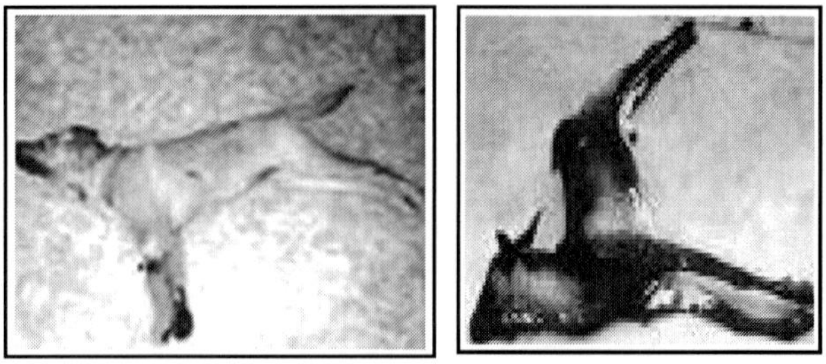

Picture showing sawhorse appearance of dog and a lamb effected with tetanus

Lesions : The only lesions which assist in the diagnosis of tetanus are the finding of appropriate wounds. Culture of the organism may be attempted.

Diagnosis

Based on

- Case history
- Symptoms
- Lesions
- Laboratory examination.

Differential Diagnosis

- Hypomagnesemia
- Encephalitis
- Eclampsia
- Strychnine toxicosis.

Treatment

- Keep the effected animal in dark quiet room
- Offending wound should be located and asepitcally cleaned
- Antibiotics (e.g., penicillin) are used to decrease bacterial numbers.
- Muscle relaxants most often used include guaifenesin guiacolate (5% to effect, keep standing), methocarbamol (10 - 20 mg/kg, q8h), and diazepam (0.05 - 0.4 mg/kg).
- Tranquilizers may be required. Promazine (0.5 - 1.0 mg/kg, IM) may provide 4 - 8 hours of relaxation.
- Administration of tetanus antitoxin will not reverse the clinical signs, once being exhibited
- Suggested dosages of antitoxin range from 10 - 220 IU/kg. Probably 5,000 - 10,000 IU given IV or IM in an adult horse is adequate.
- Tetanus toxoid is administered concurrently.
- Local infiltration of wounds with antitoxin has been recommended.

Prognosis

- Many animals become dysphagic which necessitates intensive support measures.

- If the animal is recumbent, generally the prognosis is poor . Mortality rate may be 50% for horses displaying neurologic signs at presentation.

Botulism

Introduction

- Botulism is the disease caused by any one of 7 serotypically different, but functionally similar toxins produced by strains of *Clostridium botulinum*. They are among the most potent toxins known. Of these 7 serotypes (A-G), types C and D have historically been the most commonly implicated in domestic mammals and poultry. These proteinaceous toxins are only slightly cross-reactive and can generally be regarded as immunologically specific.
- Serotypes of *C. botulinum* toxins:
  - A, B serotypes: primarily isolated from soil. B serotype has been a problem especially in horses, and also is implicated in toxicoses of cattle. Most often implicated with human infant botulism.
  - C serotype: is the most commonly implicated serotype in dogs, waterfowl, and poultry. Reports now also implicate this toxin in horses.
  - D serotype: birds are somewhat resistant to type D, but cattle are quite sensitive.
  - E serotype: isolated from mud and water of estuaries and sea food. Dogs are reportedly extremely sensitive to type E toxin.

Sources

- The most common source of botulinus toxin causing poisoning in most if not all species of domestic animals is carrion. Carcasses of decaying animals form an anaerobic environment and the toxin may be present in maggots feeding on the contaminated tissus.
  - Waterfowl: Decaying vegetation and invertebrates in flooded areas or other stagnant water, such as ponds, may serve as the primary source of botulinus toxin causing death in the first affected birds. Subsequently, birds which are simultaneously poisoned and inoculated with *C. botulinum*, become the anaerobic carcasses for additional toxin production and the source for additional animals to become poisoned. This often results in a mass die off due to botulism. Maggots often serve as the vector of botulinus toxin.

- Treatment: Drain areas, remove dead birds, frighten off incoming birds temporarily.
- Carnivores: Carrion.
- Cattle: Carrion incorporated into feed is one source (dead rodents or other animals in feed bins). "Osteophagia", the eating of the bones of dead animals associated with hypophosphatemia, is another source that occasionally results in botulism (sometimes referred to as "loin disease"). Adding pond water, from a stagnant pond, to corn silage resulted in a massive, highly lethal episode of botulism in dairy cattle.
- Feeding poultry litter is a strongly suspected cause of botulism in ruminants in Australia.
- Horses: Horses are extremely sensitive to the effects of botulinus toxin and suffer from toxicosis as a result of incorporation of carrion into their feed, as well as "toxicoinfectious botulism". The latter is a result of colonization of necrotic tissue in the animal by *C. botulinum* organisms and apparent production of toxin *in situ*. Sites may include the navel, wounds, gastric ulcers and possibly other necrotic areas, such as foci of necrosis in the liver and the gut in association with such problems as sand ingestions. Botulism has not been reproduced by the feeding of *C. botulinum* to healthy horses. "Toxico infectious botulism" (Shaker foal syndrome) of horses has been associated primarily with *C. botulinum* type B toxin. Signs suggestive of botulism have been reported in horses fed haylage. Proof of botulinus toxin involvement remains to be demonstrated in these cases.
- Affected foals are typically less than 8 months of age and are commonly less than 2 months of age.
- Humans: Three forms of the disease occur as a result of: 1) Ingestion of preformed botulinus toxin in improperly canned foods, especially in high protein foods such as meats and beans; 2) Wound botulism; and 3) Infantile (gastrointestinal) botulism. An association has been made with the latter and the feeding of honey.

❒ General

- Affected animals may shed *C. botulinum* spores in their feces which may result in further environmental contamination.

Toxicity

❒ One of most toxic compounds known, particularly on a mole/kg basis. Because of its high molecular weight, botulinus toxin is 36 times as toxic as parathion on a mg/body weight basis, but over 100,000 as toxic on a molecule/body weight dosage basis.

- LD50 mouse 0.3 mg/kg bw; minimal LD mouse 0.12 mg/kg.
- A single maggot from a dead pheasant was sufficient to kill a 3 week old chicken.

Toxicodynamics

- Botulinus toxin enters presynaptic membranes of cholinergic nerve endings via receptor mediated endocytosis. The toxin acts intracellularly via a metalloendoprotease action to cleave 3 proteins essential for neurotransmitter release (synaptobrevin, syntaxin, and SNAP-25). Thus, the toxin inhibits degranulation or exocytosis of acetylcholine granules. A small number of molecules of this toxin binds irreversibly to the sites of action, producing an essentially irreversible cessation of all cholinergic transmission. Death results from respiratory failure.

  Schematic drawing of the blockage of acetylcholine release by botulinal toxin at the neuromuscular junction. The toxin prevents exocytosis of acetylcholine. From: Greene CE. Clinical Microbiology and Infectious Diseases of the Dog and Cat. WB Saunders, 1984.
- Lower motor neuron effects include paresis to paralysis, hypotonia and hyporeflexia.
- Some pharmacologic actions of various botulinus toxins and specific binding difference between toxins indicate the possibility of different mechanisms of action.

Clinical Signs

- Myasthenia.
- Inability to swallow
- Progressive muscle paralysis with muscle weakness first in the hindquarters and then progressing to the forequarters, then the head and neck become involved. Humans are atypical in that in some aspects the effects are descending in sequence.

Dogs

- General weakness is followed by an ascending paresis and paralysis with cranial nerve involvement (facial paralysis may be present). Remain alert and responsive, wag tail and move head even when paralyzed.

- Mydriasis with slow pupillary reflexes, decreased palpebral reflexes.
- Poor jaw tone, dysphagia. Vomiting, pain in cranial abdomen.
- May have secondary dehydration and/or urinary tract infections as well as secondary respiratory infections.
- Occasionally may have slow heart rate, rarely see megaesophagus and associated regurgitation. Decreased gag reflex.

Cattle

- Inability or decreased ability to stand. Sternal and sometimes subsequent lateral recumbency. Often down with head down or turned to the side, like a cow with milk fever, may die in sternal recumbency.
- Rumen motility decreased or absent.
- Hypersalivation. Paralysis of muscles of mastication and cannot resist forced opening of the mouth.
- Tongue may have normal tone, but often exhibits varying degrees of flaccid paralysis. This is most apparent after pulling the tongue out of the mouth repeatedly.
- Urinary bladder distended: with severe toxicosis become less likely to urinate when "feathered" or may not urinate at all until stimulated by attempts to introduce a urinary catheter.
- Proteinuria in some cows exhibiting paresis or paralysis.
- Concentrated urine and reduced rumen fill indicate decreased ability to drink water and resultant dehydration. Dry feces with large amount of mucus.
- Slow pupillary response to light.
- Animals sense pain stimuli but withdrawal reflexes from pin pricks or other pain are weak or absent.
- Rectal temperature, heart rate and respiratory rate remain normal until late in the syndrome.
- Death occurs without agonal respiratory gasps.
- Deaths in a herd may occur in one to several cows per day every day or every few days.
- Hyperglycemia may be noted.

Foals and Horses

- Progressive symmetrical muscle paralysis, with stilted gait.

- Muscle tremors, inability to remain standing for longer than 4 - 5 minutes, drop to sternum. If helped to feet after a rest, signs reoccur and duration of standing decreases as time progresses.
- *Dysphagia*: In foals, milk runs out of their mouths as they attempt to suckle. Difficulty swallowing water, tongue and pharyngeal paralysis. Loss of tongue tone is often an early clinical sign in adult horses.
- Reduced intestinal peristalsis. Constipation. Frequent attempts to urinate with voiding of only a few ml of urine.
- Mydriasis.
- Later see dyspnea with extension of the head and neck. Tachycardia.
- Respiratory arrest, generally after a period of lateral recumbency, with the neck extended.
- Generally, the body temperature and hemograms remain normal throughout the syndrome.
- Creatine kinase may be elevated due to prolonged recumbency.
- Mortality is high in all ages, and is greater than 90% in foals. Foals less than 3 weeks old usually die within 24 hours and those 4 weeks or older live up to 72 hours.

Birds: All (waterfowl) are susceptible (other species vary).

- Signs start with the progressive paralysis of the neck (limberneck), legs and wings.
- Gasping for air and sometimes greenish diarrhea.
- Usually die in coma within 24 - 48 hours due to respiratory and circulatory failure.
- May drown from inability to hold head and body in normal positon.

Lesions

- In all species, lesions are generally nonspecific.
- Cattle:
  - Abomasal hyperemia.
  - Fluid-filled large intestine.
  - Aspiration pneumonia may be present.
- Horses
  - Abscesses may occur in the navel, the lungs or in wounds of the skin or muscle. These may be sites of toxin production.

- Foci of necrosis may occur in the liver.
- Gastric ulcers may be present at the margo plicatus or less often at the pyloris.
- Congestion and edema of the lungs.
- Excessive pericardial fluid with free floating strands of fibrin.
- Often there is generalized fatty change of the liver.
- The urinary bladder is often distended with urine.
- Aspiration pneumonia is sometimes present.
- The rectum is often filled with hard, mucus-coated feces.
- Occasionally the mare and foal are both affected and in such cases, the mare often has adrenocortical hyperplasia.

Diagnosis

- Most species
  - Diagnosis is difficult to confirm.
  - Tests for botulinus toxin can be used in cases where the animal is still alive or has just died. After a longer postmortem interval, the carcass may no longer represent the antemortem state.
  - Mouse inoculation test:Positive test is manifested by a "wasp-wasted" appearance with respiratory distress and progressive paralysis and death within 24 hours in most cases.
  - Specimens to test include: food,spoiled bone meal, silage, bones, decaying vegetation; serum, gastrointestinal tract contents, feces, etc.
  - These specimens may be tested to determine if the toxin is present by the mouse inoculation test and may also serve as materials for the culture and identification of *C. botulinum*.
  - Mouse inoculation/protection test procedure: Mice are inoculated with a suspect specimen with and without a specific or polyvalent antiserum. The production of typical botulism, and concurrent protection of the appropriate antitoxin treated mice allow delineation of the specific toxin type.
- An immunodiffusion test using agar impregnated with antitoxins may sometimes be recommended as an alternative to the mouse protection test. Poultry labs are generally set up to run tests to identify the Type C toxin, commonly implicated in small animals.

Differential Diagnosis

- Cattle
  - Mineral imbalances (Ca or Mg deficiencies), including parturient paresis.
  - Other paralytic toxicoses (cholinesterase inhibitors and many others).
- Horse
  - Dysphagia-esophageal or pharyngeal obstruction, leukoencephalomalacia, yellow star thistle, rabies.
  - Tick paralysis, hypocalcemia, white snakeroot poisoning.

Treatment

- In cases of recent ingestion of preformed botulinus toxin, measures to remove the contents of the gastrointestinal tract as well as activated charcoal and a cathartic are indicated.
- Antitoxins are the product (serum) of an animal (horse), which has received injections of a toxoid (inactivated toxin). Use of polyvalent antitoxin early in the course of the syndrome greatly enhances survival rates. The following dosage schedules have been recommended.
- Horse
  - 200 ml for foal and 500 ml for adult (> 400 kg bw).
  - Restrain and treat any deep wounds.
  - Sodium/potassium penicillin 22,000 - 44,000 IU/kg QID IV to eliminate proliferating *C. botulinum* organisms.
  - Oral penicillin therapy as well as aminoglycosides and tetracyclines are contraindicated in the horse.
- Dog
  - 5 ml of a polyvalent antitoxin was administered IV and IM
- Antibiotic therapy with 20,000 IU/kg penicillin IM BID and ampicillin 16 mg/kg PO or 8 mg/kg IM QID has been recommended.
- Supportive care including padding, provision of a warm, dry environment and turning the animal with assistance in eating, drinking, urination and defecation are indicated.
- In cattle, carbamylcholine to stimulate gastrointestinal motility and enhance removal of the toxin seemed to enhance the probability of survival in a small number of animals.

- The use of guanidine HCl at 15 - 30 mg/kg/day orally in divided doses to increase the release of acetylcholine has been debated. Is not advocated for therapy.
- Recently a therapeutic regimen of cholinesterase inhibitors, such as physostigmine and neostigmine, have been recommended along with atropine sulfate to block the muscarinic effects of the cholinesterase inhibition. Such measures should be used only in life-threatening toxicoses and with the utmost caution
- Recovery Recovery in dogs may occur within 14 days or longer. Recovery of function occurs in the reverse order of the loss of function during the development of the syndrome.

Blue-Green Algae

Description

Blue-green algae cells in water are green, blue-green or blue depending on their degree of deterioration. Fresh blooms are green, and the colonies of cells are approximately the size of grains of sand and often float at or near the surface of the water. Microscopically, colonies of *Microcystis* cells contain hundreds or thousands of marble-like cells grouped in a common mucilaginous matrix. Colony shape may be round or irregular. The individual cells are approximately the size of erythrocytes.

Habitat

- Potentially toxic blooms of *Microcystis aeruginosa, Anabaena flos-aquae, Nostoc* spp., and *Oscillatoria aghardii* occur during sunny weather in stagnant bodies of freshwater with high nutrient (especially phosphate) concentrations, such as in eutrophic ponds, lakes, and reservoirs.
- Commonly animals are exposed to potentially toxic amounts when pastures or holding pens uphill have fertilized the pond with animal wastes and wind has concentrated the bloom near the side of the pond where the animals drink.
- Nutrient enrichment associated with fish food and excreta may encourage algal growth.Shrimp are relatively tolerant of microcystins and may bioaccumulate potentially toxic amounts.

Toxic Principle

- Microcystins and nodularin; microcystins were termed as "fast-death factor".

- Blue-green algae also have lipopolysaccharide endotoxins in their cell walls.

Toxicodynamics

- Hepatocytes are the primary target cell in liver.; Specificity for hepatocytes is related to cell uptake of the toxins via bile acid carriers.
- The biochemical mechanism(s) of action of microcystins and nodularin is inhibition of protein phosphatases 1 and 2A; which results in excessive phosphorylation of specific intracellular proteins including cytokeratins 8 and 18 which are the major proteins in cytoskeletal intermediate filaments of hepatocytes.
- The hepatocytes round-up apparently due to a loss of the normal arrangement of intermediate filaments, microtubules, and actin microfilaments, the three major components of the hepatocyte cytoskeleton. The hepatic sinusoids are severely disrupted. The resultant intrahepatic hemorrhage and necrosis, as well as acute hepatic insufficiency, possibly accompanied by hypoglycemia, may result in severe circulatory shock and death.

Clinical Signs

- Acute lethal syndrome often lasting less than 24 hours from the onset , characterized by gastrointestinal disturbances (vomiting depending on species, abdominal pain and often diarrhea which may be bloody), followed by weakness, pallor of the mucous membranes, severe reduction in both activity and responsiveness, and death.
- Sublethal toxicoses with substantial liver damage , not lethally exposed often seem to make a successful recovery.
- Secondary (hepatogenous) photosensitization sometimes develops in surviving herbivores.

Lesions

- The liver tends to be swollen and to contain abnormal amounts of blood.
- Often the lobular pattern may be exaggerated (depending on species) due to hemorrhage into the liver lobules. There may be significant edema in and around the wall of the gallbladder.
- Marked edema of the gall bladder

Microscopically, the picture is one of acute separation of hepatocytes from one another, toxic centrilobular apoptosis followed in some cells by necrosis which may extend nearly to the entire liver lobule with replacement by hemorrhage.

Diagnosis

- History, and clinical signs
- Gross and microscopic lesions, and identification of the algae in the water.
- The gastrointestinal tract contents of lethally poisoned animals may also contain the readily identifiable colonies of *Microcystis* cells.
- A 1 ml specimen of cells should be shipped chilled (not frozen) to a laboratory capable of culturing the cells as rapidly as possible. A smaller specimen (5 ml) should be combined with an equal amount of buffered, neutral 10% formalin in order to fix the algae and prevent its physical deterioration.

Treatment

- No specific treatment
- Avoid further exposure by fencing off contaminated ponds and lakes, as well as streams emanating from them. It has been theorized that, immediately after treatment with copper sulfate, an algal bloom may be of increased toxicity due to cell breakdown and a greater access to the toxin(s) present. This now seems unlikely in the case of the hepatotoxin but may be true for the neurotoxins.
- Animals recently exposed should have measures taken to thoroughly evacuate their gastrointestinal tracts at the earliest possible time, and should be given activated charcoal and saline cathartic. In small animals, cholestyramine would be preferred over activated charcoal.
- To maintain respiration , artificial respiration may be needed, which without additional therapy may not do anything more than prolong the onset of death
- Steps to combat hemorrhagic shock are indicated, such as intravenous fluids and possibly blood transfusions, corticosteroids, and, if marked metabolic acidosis is present, sodium bicarbonate should be given slowly IV

- For hepatotoxin poisoning, prognoses are poor in severely affected animals. Combatting shock and hemorrhage with fluids and blood are clearly indicated as is dextrose if hypoglycemic and measure to counteract hyperkalemia (if present), but severe liver damage may often preclude an uneventful recovery. Regeneration of hepatocytes in sublethal toxicosis has, however, been documented in mice.

Chapter 9

ENVIRONMENTAL TOXICOLOGY

Pollution is the introduction of contaminants into an environment that causes instability, disorder, harm or discomfort to the physical systems or living organisms they are in.

Pollution can take the form of chemical substances, or energy, such as noise, heat, or light energy.

Pollutants, the elements of pollution, can be foreign substances or energies, or naturally occurring; when naturally occurring, they are considered contaminants when they exceed natural levels. Sometimes the term **pollution is extended to include any substance when it occurs at such unnaturally high concentration within a system that it endangers the stability of that system**. For example, water is innocuous and essential for life, and yet at very high concentration, it could be considered a pollutant.

Major Forms of Pollution

- *Air pollution* : the release of chemicals and particulates into the atmosphere. Common gaseous air pollutants include carbon monoxide, sulfur dioxide, chlorofluorocarbons (CFCs) and nitrogen oxides produced by industry and motor vehicles. Photochemical ozone and smog are created as nitrogen oxides and hydrocarbons react to sunlight.

- *Water pollution* : the release of waste products and contaminants into surface runoff, river drainage systems, leaching into groundwater, liquid spills, wastewater discharges, eutrophication and littering.
- *Soil contamination* : occurs when chemicals are released by spill or underground leakage. Among the most significant soil contaminants are hydrocarbons, heavy metals herbicides, pesticides and chlorinated hydrocarbons.
- *Radioactive contamination* : resulting from activities in atomic physics, such as nuclear power generation and nuclear weapons research, manufacture and deployment
- *Noise pollution* : which encompasses roadway noise, aircraft noise, industrial noise as well as high-intensity sonar.
- *Light pollution* : includes light trespass, over-illumination and astronomical interference
- *Thermal pollution* : is a temperature change in natural water bodies caused by human influence, such as use of water as coolant in a power plant.

Air Pollution

Air pollutants are substances which, when present in the atmosphere, may become injurious to life or property or interfere with their enjoyment or use. The definition also emphasizes the importance of receptors: that is, the effects that substances have on living things or property. There are three important stages in the lifetime of a pollutant:

1) Emissions
2) Atmospheric transport and transformation
3) Sinks: receptor response

Emissions vary according to the rate and type of emission, and the configuration of the source. Sources can be points (e.g. a factory or power station), lines (e.g. roads) or areas (e.g. a city), and may be mobile or stationary.

Atmospheric transport and transformation is very important in understanding pollutants. The state of the atmosphere determines whether pollutants are concentrated or dispersed, and whether they are likely to remain in areas and concentrations that put life or health at risk. Atmospheric processes may also transform primary pollutants into secondary pollutants (e.g. the formation of photochemical smogs), or allow the settling and removal of pollutants.

Receptor response covers a wide range of effects, including health effects, vegetation damage, soiling of surfaces, or corrosion of metals or other materials.

Sources and Types of Air Pollutants

1. Aerosols (Particulates)

Aerosols are solid or liquid particles dispersed in air, kept aloft by upward air currents. Aerosols may cover a wide range of sizes: from less than 0.1 microns to greater than 100 microns (fine sand). They may act as pollutants in several ways: as poisons ;by contributing to synthesis of poisons in atmosphere; by soiling surfaces or by absorbing, scattering or blocking solar radiation

The behaviour and effects of aerosols mainly dependent on size:

- Large aerosol particles settle out quickly, where as smaller particles can be transported to greater distances.
- Large particles cause greatest nuisance close to source: e.g. quarry dust or soot from diesel exhausts soiling laundry, cars, houses, vegetation.
- *Small particles pose the greatest health hazard*: larger particles (>0.5 μm otherwise known as microns or micrometres) are trapped in the nose and throat, while smaller particles (< 10 μm) can travel into the windpipe and lungs, where they lodge and cause damage (e.g. asbestos, fine coal dust). These smaller particles are termed *respirable* or *thoracic particles*. This is a particularly serious form of aerosol pollution: cumulative doses can give rise to serious and fatal illnesses such as silicosis and lung cancers.

Composition

Solids : Carbon (soot: smoky fires, biomass burning, diesel engines), silica (sand or silt particles: windblown material, volcanic ejecta, mining waste), lead, asbestos, salts, and many more.

Liquids : Cloud droplets are a natural liquid aerosol. Most important pollutant aerosols are acidic droplets (sulphur and nitrogen compounds).

Sulphur Compounds

Naturalsources: bacteria, sea-spray, volcanoes.

Human sources: burning of sulphur-bearing materials, such as coal and oil. oil refineries and ore smelters.

Anthropogenic sulphur compounds are mainly in the form of Sulphur dioxide (SO_2), but other compounds, such as Hydrogen sulphide (H_2S) may also be important. Sulphur dioxide is transformed on contact with atmospheric water into acidic solutions.

Transformed in atmosphere to sulphurous and sulphuric acids (H_2SO_3 and H_2SO_4). Component of certain types of smogs and acid rain.

Nitrogen

Oxides of nitrogen (particularly NO) produced by combustion, transformed in atmosphere into Nitric acid (H+ and NO_3).

2. Gaseous Air Pollutants

Certain kinds of atoms or molecules exist in the atmosphere as gases. These may act as pollutants in the following ways: by contributing to the synthesis of poisons in atmosphere, as greenhouse gases, by contributing to destruction of other atmospheric components (e.g. ozone) or accelerating weathering.

Nitrogen Compounds

These may be produced naturally as the result of organic decomposition in soil or oceans. Human sources include the combustion of fuels under pressure at high temperatures: e.g. in internal combustion engines. They are also produced during the manufacture of explosives and fertilizers.

The most common gaseous nitrogen compound produced by combustion is NO (nitric oxide): a relatively harmless gas. But it tranforms readily into NO_2 (Nitrogen dioxide), a yellow-brown, irritant gas, which is a major component of urban smogs. NO also transforms into nitric acid and nitrous oxide (N_2O, a greenhouse gas). Oxides of nitrogen include NO, NO_2, NO_3, N_2O_5.

Hydrocarbons

Hydrocarbons are compounds of hydrogen and carbon, naturally produced by decomposition of vegetation. Anthropogenic hydrocarbons are produced by incomplete combustion or evaporation of fuels (e.g. petrol, lighter fuels, and solvents). One of the most important hydrocarbons is Methane (CH_4) produced in biomass burning and agricultural activities. This is a major greenhouse gas, with 21 times more effect on atmospheric energy budgets, per molecule, than CO_2. Methane is created by decomposition in rice paddies, and in the guts of grazing animals.

Ozone

Ozone is the triatomic form of oxygen (O_3) [Most oxygen in atmosphere is in form of O_2] Ozone in upper atmosphere is essential to life on earth, but in the lower atmosphere it is a serious pollutant, formed by the transformation of hydrocarbons and nitrogen compounds in presence of sunlight, and is a major component of urban smogs. Ozone causes irritation of the lungs, and can lead to asthma attacks.

Chlorofluorocarbons

(CFCs) are entirely man-made compounds, created by modifying hydrocarbon molecules. They were produced in quantity as refrigerants, propellants, solvents and fillers. They were initially thought to be inert and harmless, but are now identified as major greenhouse gases and play a part in crucial reactions in the stratosphere leading to destruction of stratospheric ozone.

Carbonmonoxide (CO)

This is an odourless, colourless gas, lethal in high concentrations. Carbon monoxide, though thought of as a pollutant today, has always been present in the atmosphere, chiefly as a product of volcanic activity. It occurs dissolved in molten volcanic rock at high pressures in the earth's mantle. Carbon monoxide has an indirect radiative forcing effect by elevating concentrations of methane and tropospheric ozone through chemical reactions with other atmospheric constituents (e.g., the hydroxyl radical, $OH^{\cdot}$) that would otherwise destroy them. Through natural processes in the atmosphere, it is eventually oxidized to carbon dioxide. Carbon monoxide concentrations are both short-lived in the atmosphere and spatially variable.

Anthropogenic CO from automobile and industrial emissions may contribute to the greenhouse effect and global warming. In urban areas carbon monoxide, along with aldehydes, reacts photochemically to produce peroxy radicals. Peroxy radicals react with nitrogen oxide to increase the ratio of NO_2 to NO, which reduces the quantity of NO that is available to react with ozone. Carbon monoxide is also a constituent of tobacco smoke. Carbon monoxide, nitrogen oxides, hydrogen cyanide and ammonia are all present in cigarette smoke.

Sources: incomplete combustion of carbon compounds, and as a product of engines, metal processing, oil refineries, and cigarettes.

Cigarettes are single most important source of CO to which humans are exposed. When inhaled, CO fixes onto blood haemoglobin, reducing its ability to fix oxygen and reducing efficiency of respiration.

Carbon monoxide is a significantly toxic gas and has no odor or color. It is the most common type of fatal poisoning in many countries. Exposures can lead to significant toxicity of the central nervous system and heart. Following poisoning, long-term sequelae often occurs. Carbon monoxide can also have severe effects on the fetus of pregnant animals. Symptoms of mild poisoning include dizziness at concentrations less than 100 ppm. Concentrations as low as 667 ppm can cause up to 50% of the body's haemoglobin to be converted to carboxy-haemoglobin (HbCO). Carboxy-haemoglobin is quite stable but this change is reversible. Carboxy-haemoglobin is ineffective for delivering oxygen, resulting in failure in oxygen delivery to certain tissues. As a result, exposures of this level can be life-threatening. The mechanisms by which carbon monoxide produces toxic effects are not yet fully understood, but haemoglobin, myoglobin, and mitochondrial cytochrome oxidase are thought to be compromised. Treatment largely consists of administering 100% oxygen or hyperbaric oxygen therapy, although the optimum treatment remains controversial.

CO_2 (Carbondioxide)

Carbon dioxide is not poisonous, but it can have harmful effects. It is best known as a greenhouse gas, and is produced naturally as by-product of metabolism and by volcanoes.

Deforestation of rainforests is currently of major concern, but deforestation in temperate regions was important in the past, providing a larger source of atmospheric CO_2 than fossil fuels. In high concentrations CO_2 can displace oxygen, causing asphyxiation

Smog is a recent compound word from "smoke" and "fog" refers to locally high concentrations of acids, dry acid-forming compounds, particulates, or other pollutants in stagnant, stable air. Smog form when emissions are prevented from dispersing by stable or sinking air masses.

Sulphurous Smog

These are produced by high outputs of SO_2, which are converted to acids on contact with atmospheric moisture. Usually, sulphurous smog also contain elevated concentrations of suspended soot.

Photochemical Smog

With the increase in vehicle use in cities, there has been a major change in the character of air pollution. Combustion of fossil fuels contributes to photochemical smog, so-called due to the role of sunlight in forming a cocktail of harmful chemicals from other gases. They form when Nitrogen compounds (NOx) and hydrocarbons react in the atmosphere, fuelled by solar energy in the form of ultraviolet radiation. The smog form in a complex series of reactions, forming nitric acid and other secondary oxidizing pollutants such as ozone (O_3). The main source of NOx is vehicle exhausts, and therefore occurs in cities where vehicle density is very high. As such, they are a major problem in many cities. Other vehicle pollutants include particulates and lead, adding to the noxious character of urban smog.

Toxic Gases

General Considerations

The air livestock breathe is frequently contaminated with potential toxicants. Usually these gases are dissipated and diluted by the normal environmental air movement. However, in today's modern confinement-rearing buildings, adequate ventilation of the animals surroundings is often dependent upon proper mechanical function of systems intended to move air and proper management including that of ventilation systems by the producer. When one or both of these components is faulty, problems can arise.the various important toxic gases that are effecting the health of livestock are as follows

Nitrogen Dioxide (NO_2)

- Yellowish brown; bleach-like smell.
- Heavier than air.
- Primary source is fermentation of ensiled forages; "silo-filler's disease".
- Formed during first 2 weeks after silage is cut and stored.
- Highest concentrations in first 48 hours.
- Human nose can detect very low concentrations.
- 5 ppm has caused lesions in lab animals - concentrations in silo gas may exceed 100 ppm.

Clinical Signs

- Forms nitric acid when combines with H_2O on respiratory mucosa - permanent lung damage.

- May die instantly or hours, days, or months later.
- Dyspnoea, salivation, coughing, methemoglobinemia.

Lesions

- Severe pulmonary edema, "dark red" kidneys, hemorrhage, and bronchiolitis may be seen. Emphysema may occur in chronic cases.

Treatment

- No specific treatment; even fresh air has no direct beneficial effect other than removing the source of the problem.

Hydrogen Sulfide (H_2S)

- Rotten egg smell.
- Heavier than air.
- Produced by bacterial action on sulfur-containing amino acids and other sources of sulfur.
- Rapidly paralyzes olfactory nerves at high concentrations.
- Death from respiratory paralysis.

Methane (CH_4)

- Colorless, odorless.
- Lighter than air.
- Produced by bacterial decomposition of carbonaceous materials such as excreta.
- Not notably toxic; biologically inert.
- Would need 90% methane to deprive of O_2.
- Principle danger lies in its flammability and explosiveness.

Carbon Dioxide (CO_2)

- Odorless.
- Heavier than air, therefore collects in lower areas of buildings.
- Present in normal atmospheric air at 300 ppm.
- Can cause "suffocation" in overcrowded, inadequately ventilated enclosures.

Sources

- Normal respiration of animals.
- Decomposing excreta.
- Rarely approaches dangerous levels.

Toxicity and Signs

When concentrations exceed 400,000 ppm, may see anxiety, staggering, coma, cyanosis, and death.

Lesions

Dark tissues and blood.

Treatment

Provide fresh air, artificial respiration if needed.

Prevention

Maintenance of proper humidity in winter and proper temperature in summer helps to keep CO_2 in confinement buildings within acceptable levels.

Note

It has been suggested that if all ventilation were stopped in an air-tight building, animals would generally die from hyperthermia before CO_2 toxicosis.

Carbon Monoxide (CO)

- Odorless, colorless, slightly lighter than air.

Sources

- Background concentrations in air range from 0.02 ppm (fresh air) to 40 ppm (high traffic area).
- Incomplete combustion of hydrocarbon fuels (inadequate oxygen to form CO_2).
- Exhaust fumes of internal combustion engines.
  - Dogs in trunks of cars with faulty exhaust system, or in enclosed garages have been affected.
  - Metabolite of methylene chloride (dichloromethane).

Toxicodynamics

- Competes with O_2 for binding sites on several proteins including hemoglobin (Hb).
  - Affinity of Hb for CO = 250X that for O_2.
- When CO is bound to Hb, its affinity for O_2 molecules already bound increases (oxygen-dissociation curve shifted to the left). This prevents release of that O_2 to tissues. Net result is tissue hypoxia.
- Fetal Hb has a greater affinity for CO and O_2 than does adult Hb. In cats, dogs, and pigs, the fetal hemoglobin is the same as maternal, but the fetal blood cells have lower amounts of 2,3-diphosphoglycerate (2,3-DPG) which enables the fetus to take up O_2 from the dam. Amount of blood COHb depends on:
  - The rate of formation of COHb - is proportional to the atmospheric carbon monoxide concentration.
  - The disappearance half-life of COHb - approximately 2 hours.

Toxicity and Clinical Signs

- High exposures may produce rapid deaths.
- Lower exposures produce drowsiness, incoordination, dyspnoea, and coma.
- Relationship of blood carboxyhemoglobin to clinical manifestations:

% Blood COHb	Effects
1 - 3	None
6 - 8	Decreased ability to maintain attention
20	Definite psychomotor disturbance
20 - 40	Lethargy, disturbance in gait, EEG changes
60 - 70	Death

- Possible permanent deafness in small animals (rare).

Lesions

- Characteristic cherry-red blood.
- Pink or red coloration of tissues and nonpigmented skin.
- Bronchial dilation and distension of major blood vessels (occasionally)

Histopathology

- Necrosis of cortex and focal leukoencephalomalacia in the white matter of the cerebral hemispheres, the globus pallidus, and brain stem
- There may also be glial-vascular proliferation, edema, and hemorrhage in the brain.
- Demyelination.
- Brain lesions may coincide with permanent deafness in dogs and cats.

Diagnosis

Based on

- History
- Measurement of CO in air
- Measure COHb in blood. COHb is stable for several days if the blood is refrigerated.
- COHb greater than 2% in fetal thoracic fluid.
- Fetal heart blood may range from 20 - 60% COHb; sow's blood may be greater than 10% COHb.

Treatment

- Fresh air.
- Best treatment is 90 - 95% O_2 with 5 - 10% CO_2.

Nitrogen Oxides (Silo Filler's Disease)
Sources

- Nitrogen dioxide is formed when nitric oxide in fresh silage comes in contact with oxygen in the air.
- Toxicosis is primarily seen when animals are near silos shortly after they are filled. The risk is highest when feedstuffs are high in nitrates (drought years), since in the ensiling process these form nitric acid as the silage reacts with oxygen in the air.
- Gas production is greatest in alfalfa silage, reaching a peak in 24 hours and apparently ending in 2 or 3 days. Concentrations as great as 1500 ppm can be reached during the first 48 hours after filling a silo.
- Nitrogen dioxide usually is seen as a yellowish-brown haze if any amount of it has been formed. Other toxic by-products such as NO or N_2O_4 are colorless and odorless.

- This gas has an irritating odour. It is heavier than air and therefore remains in the silo below the upper edge of the last door or settles down through the chute to the silo room and into the barn.
- Oxides of nitrogen play a very important role in air pollution because in urban areas, large quantities of these oxides are constantly being generated from such sources as automobiles, diesel engines, thermal power plants, boilers, industrial gaseous wastes, etc.
- Combustion of x-ray films results in the production of nitrogen dioxide.
- Plastic plants also have the potential of giving off this gas.

Toxicodynamics

- Nitrogen dioxide dissolves in water to form a mixture of nitric and nitrous acids, both of which are very irritating and corrosive to the mucous membranes. Due to its relatively low solubility in water, however, the transient passage of nitrogen dioxide through the upper respiratory tract may not cause significant signs but may result in considerable damage to the lower respiratory tract, where the duration of contact and the amount of moisture are greater.
- The acid is only slowly absorbed and removed from the lung. The ultimate effect is local irritation which results in pulmonary edema. Because of a short residency time, the upper airways are generally less affected. Prior exposure can produce a degree of tolerance to subsequent inhalation of comparatively high concentrations of nitrogen oxides.
- NO_2 also acts by causing lipid peroxidation, which is maximal at 24 hours after exposure and lasts at least 24 hours thereafter. Vitamin E deficiency increases susceptibility to nitrogen dioxide. Nitrogen dioxides, in turn, increase the susceptibility to infection by decreasing the ability of the lung to remove pathogenic microorganisms.

Toxicity

- "Silo-filler's disease", or silage gas poisoning, also called bronchiolitis fibrosa obliterans due to inhalation of nitrogen dioxide, is especially hazardous for agricultural workers and animals.
- Inhalation of low concentrations of the oxides of nitrogen may cause little or no discomfort of the upper respiratory tract but may result in death hours later due to pulmonary edema. A brief exposure to 200 ppm can be fatal.

- Though it is an invisible gas in smaller concentrations, it is still dangerous. Humans are able to detect NO_2 at levels as low as 0.1 - 0.2 ppm in the air.

Clinical Signs

- Clinical manifestations vary according to the intensity of exposure and the period of inhalation.
- Inhalation of nitrogen dioxide can produce serious respiratory symptoms with feeling of suffocation in the chest, dyspnea, cyanosis, syncope, pulmonary edema and death.
- An increase in respiratory rate, a decrease in compliance and an increase in airway resistance occurs.

Lesions

- Extent of pathological changes in the lungs corresponds to the degree of exposure.
- Cyanosis.
- Pulmonary mast cells are ruptured, degranulated and the alveoli become markedly expanded.
- Pulmonary congestion, edema.
- Emphysema.

Diagnosis

KI starch papers are available commercially—turn dark when exposed to NO_2 gas.

Treatment

- Treatment consists of immediate administration of oxygen and artificial respiration if necessary.
- Corticosteroids are very effective in relieving the pulmonary edema and other clinical signs.
- Additional supportive care includes controlling pulmonary edema and administering broad-spectrum antibiotics for bronchopneumonia.
- Recovery may require 1 - 6 months. Some emphysematous changes may persist indefinitely.

Prevention

- Education of the farmer to the dangers of toxic silo gas, as well as the safety measures that should be carried out to prevent undue exposure and inhalation by both humans and animals, is paramount in the elimination of this serious type of poisoning.
- This hazard of farming can be avoided simply by not entering a silo during filling and for a week or 10 days after completion thereof. Animals should not be allowed to gather in a barn near the base of a silo shortly after filling.

Ozone Layer Depletion

The atmosphere modifies solar energy as it passes through by acting as a filter, reducing certain types of incoming radiation by absorption. One of the most important filtering effects for life on earth is the reduction of ultraviolet radiation (UV).This is radiation of shorter wavelength than the visible spectrum. Low levels of UV are useful to life, it is used in Vitamin D synthesis. However, high levels of UV are harmful, causing skin cancers, genetic damage and climate change.

UV radiation can be subdivided into three bands:

- UVA: 0.32-0.40 microns,
- UVB: 0.28-0.32 microns,
- UVC: 0.20-0.28 microns.

UVC is entirely filtered out by the atmosphere, and of the UV that reaches sea-level, organisms are most sensitive to UVB.

The most important component of the atmosphere for filtering UV is ozone (O_3). Ozone is bluish in colour, and has strong, pungent smell (its name comes from the Greek word ozein: to smell). Atmospheric ozone occurs in the stratosphere between 10-50 km, with maximum concentrations at 20-25 km. - it is this part of the atmosphere that is referred to as the Ozone layer. Stratospheric ozone is very important, as it removes almost all incoming UVC, and 70% of the incoming UVB at equator, 90% at poles. It is processes of UV absorption by ozone that gives the stratosphere its characteristic thermal structure.

Atmospheric ozone is measured in Dobson Units (DU). 100 DU is equivalent to a 1mm thick layer of pure ozone at surface pressure (1000 mbar). The average amount of ozone in the atmosphere is about 300 DU.

Ozone levels fluctuate on a daily basis (30%) and multi-annually (10%). In general though, a natural dynamic equilibrium exists between processes of creation and destruction. In recent years, this equilibrium has been disrupted by human activities, resulting in widespread destruction of ozone.

Natural Processes in the Ozone Layer

Ozone is formed by the impact of UV on the common form of oxygen (diatomic oxygen: O_2). The energy of the radiation causes O_2 to split into single O atoms. These free oxygen atoms then combine with O_2 to form O_3. This reaction is reversible:

$$O_3 + O = 2 \times O_2; \text{ or } O_3 + UV = O + O_2,$$

Each reaction being associated with the absorption of UV radiation of a specific wavelength. The ozone levels in the stratosphere reflect the relative rates of creation and destruction. In nature, the two rates are linked, high rates of O_3 production also encourage high rates of destruction. The turnover is highest in equatorial areas, where the received solar radiation flux is at its maximum. Reactions involving ozone are accelerated by the presence of catalysts, substances that aid a reaction, but are themselves left unchanged. The same catalyst can cause very many reactions before being removed from the system by other processes. The main natural catalysts for ozone destruction are:

OH (known as the hydroxyl radical), derived from H_2O (water), CH_4 (methane) and H_2 in the stratosphere. OH has an important effect, especially at altitudes greater than 40km, and accounts for 11% of natural ozone destruction.

NO (nitric oxide) which accounts for 50-70% of natural ozone destruction. Some nitrogen oxides are formed by the action of cosmic rays. Supernovas (exploding stars) may have caused brief spikes of NO, reducing O_3 by 90% for decades. Nitrogen dioxide (NO_2) in lower stratosphere can encourage survival of ozone, by combining with chlorine monoxide (ClO), but higher in the stratosphere it is a precursor of nitric oxide, and contributes to ozone destruction.

Chlorine is a very efficient catalyst. Each free Chlorine atom can destroy up to 100,000 ozone molecules before it is removed.

Br Bromine is about 10 times more effective that chrorine in depleting ozone. Fortunately it is also less common. Natural sources are mainly in the form of methyl bromide (CH_3Br), a by-product of biologic productivity in the oceans. Methyl bromide is also widely used as a fumigating agent for soil pests.

The single most important point about catalysts is that minute amounts of trace gases can vastly accelerate ozone destruction. In nature, catalysts are in long-term balance with ozone cycle. Human modification has severely disrupted this balance by the input of anthropogenic catalysts, especially chlorine compounds.

Anthropogenic Ozone Destruction

Three potential sources of manmade ozone destroying compounds:

- nuclear explosions
- Supersonic aircraft
- Halocarbons.

Nuclear Explosions

The rapid release of energy in a nuclear explosion forms NOx from O_2 and Nitrogen. The gases are carried into the stratosphere by the intense convection associated with the explosion. NOx destroys ozone, so atmospheric bomb tests should have had an effect.

Supersonic Transport

All aircraft produce water, CO_2, CO, NOx in exhaust gases. Most commercial flights are confined to the troposphere, but high-level supersonic aircraft inject pollutants into the stratosphere (20km altitude). Of these nitrogen oxides are believed to be especially harmful. Theoretical fears about ozone destruction were used to argue against widespread adoption of plans to build fleets of supersonic passenger aircraft, and were partly responsible for such plans being adopted in the USA. Europe (Concorde) and USSR (Concordski) went ahead anyway, but the fleet remained small for commercial reasons. The Space Shuttle is also believed to harm stratospheric ozone, but is not used heavily enough to pose an important threat.

Halocarbons

These are artificial molecules made up of chlorine, fluorine, bromine and carbon, made by alteration of hydrocarbons by replacement of some atoms. They are called halocarbons because Chlorine, Fluorine and Bromine are all halogens, occupying the same column in the Periodic Table of elements. Examples of halocarbons are: CFC-11: C F Cl 3; CFC-12: C F2 Cl 2. These particular compounds are also known as CFCs, or Chlorofluorocarbons, composed of chlorine, fluorine, and carbon. CFCs were invented in the1920s by Thomas Midgely. At sea-level, they are non-poisonous and non-flammable, and were thus an ideal replacement for toxic compounds then in common use (SO_2 was used as a refrigerant). Production rose as result of lifestyle changes in late 20th Century, with CFCs used in refrigeration and air conditioning; propellants for spray cans (paint to hair spray); Foaming agents for polystyrene foam (fast food containers, furniture, and insulation).

The gases were released into the atmosphere during the manufacturing processes (foam), during use (spray cans), or at end of life of the product (e.g. fridge). Whereas CFCs are Non-toxic and Inert at sea-level temperatures and pressures, they remain in the atmosphere, and gradually rise into the stratosphere, where conditions of higher energy exist. Under heavy UV bombardment, the gases are no longer inert. CFCs are very susceptible to breakdown under UV radiation, releasing chlorine and bromine, which is a powerful catalyst in ozone destruction. Chlorine molecules are only neutralized when bonded with hydrogen (from hydrogen oxides or CH_4).

The Effects of Ozone Loss

Biological : High intensities of UVB are harmful to all life. Small fluctuations can be coped with, but large and long-term increases are potentially very dangerous. High UVB causes cell damage (altering proteins) and genetic damage (DNA). Humans and animals (especially pale skinned varieties) can suffer immediate effects (sunburn and eye damage); and long term effects (skin cancer). Most cancers are non-malignant and curable, but melanomas are malignant and usually fatal. The link between UVB and skin cancer is well established. Eye damage and Cataracts are also potential problems. About 200 plant species have been studied for UVB sensitivity, and half show significant adverse effects, including decreased photosynthesis, reduced leaf area, and restricted growth.

Marine ecosystems : Increased UVB may reduce photosynthesis in phytoplankton, with knock-on effects for food chains. Studies are underway in Antarctic waters.

Climatological : absorption of UVB by ozone reduces incoming shortwave (tending to reduce surface temps), but it also has an effect on the outgoing long wave (tending to increase surface temps). In balance, ozone depletion is thought to result in slight cooling, but is probably insignificant. CFCs, however, are significant greenhouse gases, as are their replacements.

Remedial Measures

Montreal Protocol : this was major legislation introduced in1987 under the UN Environmental Program. 31 countries signed an agreement to protect the stratospheric ozone layer. The US EPA proposed a 95% reduction by 2000 AD, but participants agreed to 50%. Also, 3rd World countries were allowed to increase CFC use to allow increased use of refridgerators, etc. Overall, the protocol amounted to only a 35% reduction by 2000. This was a historic agreement, but scientific evidence indicated that it was not enough.

Helsinki (1989) : 80 signatories agreed to complete CFC elimination by 2000. Production bans were brought forward in 1992 (Copenhagen) to 1996 (CFCs) and 1994 (Halons). Manufacturers responded positively, reducing production and searching for alternatives. The substitutes were designed to break down rapidly in the troposphere. They still have a negative effect, but much less so than CFCs. The rapidity of agreements related to new, powerful scientific data, but also to new economic conditions created by consumer awareness and government funding. Funding from US, Europe and Japan (the main CFC users) was provided to pay for 3rd World uptake of alternative technologies, guaranteeing the participation of India and China.

On September 17, 1997, at the 9th Meeting of Montreal Protocol participants agreed to an accelerated phase out of **methyl bromide** and proposed further amendments to the Montreal Protocol. Industrialized countries will now be subject to a phase out of methyl bromide by the year 2005, with exemptions for "critical uses," and interim deductions of 25% by the year 1999, 50% by the year 2001, and 70% by the year 2003. Developing countries that are covered by Article 5 of the treaty, have agreed to a 20% reduction in consumption by the year 2005 and phase out by the year 2015.

Acid Rain

One of the most important long-range air pollution issues is the problem of acid rain. Acids can be precipitated as snow or dew, as well as rain. Also, acid-forming compounds can be precipitated as dry gases or adhering to the surfaces of solid particles, such as soot (dry deposition). So, strictly speaking, we should refer to acid precipitation, although often the term *acid rain* is used to cover all kinds of wet and dry deposition. Acid rain is due to the widespread dispersion of acidic aerosols (Nitrogen and Sulphur compounds) in unstable or windy conditions. Acid rain is the regional equivalent of acidic air pollution (sulphurous or photochemical smog) from cities or industrial complexes. Acid rain is much more dilute than local acidic air quality crisis levels, and its effects are more complex.

Acids; A Definition

Acids are molecules that release hydrogen ions into solution.

Hydrogen ions consist of a single free proton without an electron: they therefore have positive charge and are written H^+. Hydrogen ions are very reactive: they are able to combine with a wide range of substances, altering their chemistry. Acids release hydrogen ions, increasing the hydrogen ion concentration in a solution, and increasing its tendency to react with other substances.

Acidity is measured by the concentration of hydrogen ions in a solution on the pH scale (potential hydrogen). The scale is *negative*: lower numbers relate to higher acidity, and *logarithmic*: a change of one point on the pH scale means a tenfold change in Hydrogen ion concentration. Thus an acid with a pH of 4 has a hydrogen ion concentration ten times that of an acid with pH 5.

Distilled water has a pH of 7, and is neutral. Substances with pH> 7 are alkaline, and those with pH < 7 are acidic. All rainwater is slightly acidic (pH ~5.5) due to the presence of naturally-occurring acids produced by biological and volcanic processes, thunderstorms, and the absorption of CO_2 by atmospheric water (weak carbonic acid). This weakly acidic rain participates in natural processes, the return of nitrogen and sulphur to soil helps in maintaining nutrient levels, and causes the weathering of limestone.

Human activities increase acidity, mainly by the input of SO_2 and NOx into the atmosphere. These compounds form Nitric acid (HNO_3 or H^+ and NO_3^-), and sulphurous and sulphuric acids (H_2SO_3 or H^+ and HSO_3^- and H_2SO_4 or H^+ and HSO_4^-) when they dissolve in water. The main polluters are the industrialized nations of N. America and W.Europe, but E. Europe, Japan and China are also major contributors. SO_2 output in N. America and Europe peaked in 1970s/ early 1980s and has declined since, but NOx continues to rise (vehicles). SO_2 outputs remaining high or increasing in E. Europe and China (China's economic growth is largely fuelled by sulphurous coal).

Acid Rain increased partly due to the response to earlier acid smog problems. One of the responses to urban smog was to introduce a Tall Stacks policy, higher stacks were built in power stations and factories to prevent pollutants from accumulating locally. These undoubtedly reduced local smog problems, but caused pollutants to remain in the atmosphere longer, increasing the areas affected and increasing the acidity of cloud droplets (though they tended to be more dispersed) because of the longer time available for reactions to be completed before deposition. There was consequently a significant increase in the geographical extent of problems of acid deposition.

The effects of acid precipitation depend on water chemistry in the areas where it falls. In turn, this reflects geology and land use.

Geology : some rocks can buffer acidity, by weathering and neutralizing acid (e.g. chalk, limestone). Other rocks yield naturally acid soils (e.g. granite, quartz-rich rocks), and acid levels Can seriously rise.

Land Use : conifer plantations tend to elevate local acidity because they have a high ability to capture acidic aerosols from passing air.

Pollutants cross national boundaries, and there is thus a need for international cooperation in pollution control. The rapid industrialization is fuelled by sulphur-rich coal, and clean technologies are slow to be introduced due to cost. Downwind pollution is severely affecting Japan, and it is feared that the effects on forests will be as bad as in Europe.

Effects of Acid Rain

Vegetation damage : Effects on vegetation may be *direct* due to acid particles coming into contact with leaves, or *indirect,* via soils and groundwater. Vegetation can concentrate acids: dry deposition occurs on leaves, and acids are then washed off into the soil. This acidity affects soil processes: disturbing nutrient cycles, interfering with bacterial activity; leaching nutrients, and mobilizing toxic metals (especially aluminium (Al), copper (Cu), iron (Fe), lead (Pb), zinc (Zn), mercury (Hg). The released metals then enter groundwater and lakes. In combination, the effects of acidity cause leaf dieback, beginning with the crown and spreading to the whole tree, giving it a skeletal appearance. Forest damage is known in Germany as *Waldsterben* ('Forest Death').

Role of acid rain in damage has been questioned, as natural factors can also cause damage (e.g. water-table changes, insects, fungi). However, man-made and natural factors are not mutually exclusive. The multiple stress hypothesis conveys the idea that acid rain can make trees more susceptible to other stressors, and thus more likely to die or suffer due to a dry season or fungal attack.

Lakes

Acidification of lake water, and associated increase of toxic metals, is a major problem in most parts of the world. Acid lakes have low nutrient levels, and high concentrations of Al, Mg, Mn, Zn and Pb. Al is especially problematic. In lakes with pH below 5.6, Al is usually sufficiently concentrated to kill fish. Acidification also causes changes to ecosystem structure: acid-tolerant species thrive (Sphagnum, green algae, water boatmen) and others perish.

Built Environment

Limestone is a common building material, which is attacked by acidic water. Calcium and Magnesium carbonates react with sulphuric acid, and form soluble sulphates. The sulphates are washed out, weakening the stone and destroying fine decoration. Water in such solutions also evaporates, precipitating calcium and magnesium sulphate crystals, which cause disintegration of the surrounding stone. The buildings of ancient Greece & Rome have suffered more damage in the last 50 yr than in previous 2000. Damage has also been done to the great Medieval cathedrals. Even the Taj Mahal has suffered (minor) damage from local sulphur pollution.

Solutions

Previous solutions to acid smog (tall stacks) merely passed on the problem. Two other types of solution can be employed:

- Alleviating effects on affected area
- Controlling emissions.

Alleviating Effects

Acidified lakes can be neutralized by the addition of powdered lime (CaCO3). This buffers acidity, increasing pH, and allowing ecosystem re-establishment. In such practices acidity returned to normal and nutrient levels increased, although Cu and Ni remained at toxic levels at lakes closest to treated lakes.The lower organisms recover first (plankton) followed by invertebrates, amphibians and fish. This is, however, a temporary measure (similar to taking antacid tablets for indigestion). The problem will return in 3-5 yr if acid loading continues. Liming only tackles consequences, not causes.

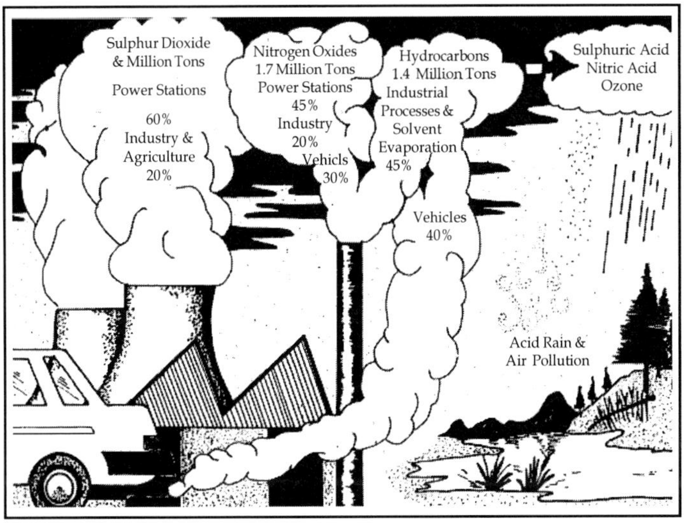
Sulphur Dioxide
& Million Tons
Power Stations
60%
Industry &
Agriculture
20%
Nitrogen Oxides
1.7 Million Tons
Power Stations
45%
Industry
20%
Vehicls
30%
Hydrocarbons
1.4 Million Tons
Industrial
Processes &
Solvent
Evaporation
45%
Vehicles
40%
Sulphuric Acid
Nitric Acid
Ozone
Acid Rain &
Air Pollution

A graphic illustration of problems of air pollution & acid rain that occur in industrialized countries

Water Pollution

Water pollution is the contamination of water bodies such as lakes, rivers, oceans, and groundwater caused by human activities, which can be harmful to organisms and plants which live in these water bodies.

Although natural phenomena such as volcanoes, algal blooms, storms, and earthquakes also cause major changes in water quality and the ecological status of water, water is typically referred to as polluted when it is impaired by anthropogenic contaminants and either does not support a animals use (like serving as drinking water) or undergoes a marked shift in its ability to support its constituent biotic communities. Water pollution has many causes and characteristics.

The primary sources of water pollution are generally grouped into two categories based on their point of origin.

1. Point-source pollution refers to contaminants that enter a waterway through a discrete "point source". Examples of this category include discharges from a wastewater treatment plant, outfalls from a factory, leaking underground tanks, etc.
2. Nnon-point source pollution, refers to contamination that does not originate from a single discrete source. Non-point source pollution is often a cumulative effect of small amounts of contaminants gathered from a large area. Nutrient runoff in storm water from sheet flow over an agricultural field, or metals and hydrocarbons from an area with high impervious surfaces and vehicular traffic are examples of non-point source pollution.

The primary focus of legislation and efforts to curb water pollution for the past several decades was first aimed at point sources. As point sources have been effectively regulated, greater attention has come to be placed on non-point source contributions, especially in rapidly urbanizing/ suburbanizing or developing areas.

The specific contaminants leading to pollution in water include a wide spectrum of chemicals, pathogens, and physical or sensory changes. While many of the chemicals and substances that are regulated may be naturally occurring (iron, manganese, etc) the concentration is often the key in determining what is a natural component of water, and what is a contaminant. Many of the chemical substances are toxic. Pathogens can produce waterborne diseases in either human or animal hosts. Alteration of water's physical chemistry include acidity, electrical conductivity, temperature, and eutrophication. Eutrophication is the fertilization of surface water by nutrients that were previously scarce. Water pollution is a major problem in the global context. It has been suggested that it is the leading worldwide cause of deaths and diseases accounting for thousands of deaths daily.

Contaminants may include organic and inorganic substances.

Organic water pollutants

- Insecticides and herbicides, a huge range of chemicals
- Bacteria, often is from sewage or livestock operations
- Food processing waste, including pathogens
- Tree and brush debris from logging operations
- Volatile organic compounds such as industrial solvents, from improper storage
- Dense non-aqueous phase liquids such as chlorinated solvents, which may fall at the bottom of reservoirs, since they don't mix well with water
- Petroleum Hydrocarbons including fuels (petrol, diesel, jet fuels, and fuel oils) and lubricants (motor oil) from oil field operations, refineries, pipelines, retail service station's underground storage tanks, and transfer operations.
- Detergents
- Various chemical compounds found in personal hygiene and cosmetic products

Inorganic Water Pollutants

- Spill of oil over the seas.
- Heavy metals including acid mine drainage
- Acidity caused by industrial discharges (especially sulfur dioxide from power plants)
- Pre-production industrial raw resin pellets, an industrial pollutant
- Chemical waste as industrial by products
- Fertilizers, in runoff from agriculture including nitrates and phosphates
- Silt in surface runoff from construction sites, logging, slash and burn practices or land clearing sites

Transport and Chemical Reactions of Water Pollutants

Most water pollutants are eventually carried by the rivers into the oceans. In some areas of the world the influence can be traced hundred miles from the mouth by studies using hydrology transport models. Each successive step up the food chain causes a stepwise concentration of pollutants such as heavy metals (e.g. mercury) and persistent organic pollutants such as DDT. This is known as biomagnifications which is occasionally used interchangeably with bioaccumulation.

Many chemicals undergo reactive decay or chemically change especially over long periods of time in groundwater reservoirs. A noteworthy class of such chemicals is the chlorinated hydrocarbons such as trichloroethylene (used in industrial metal degreasing and electronics manufacturing) and tetrachloroethylene used in the dry-cleaning industry. Both of these chemicals, which are carcinogens themselves, undergo partial decomposition reactions, leading to new hazardous chemicals (including dichloroethylene and vinyl chloride).

Groundwater pollution is much more difficult to abate than surface pollution because groundwater can move great distances through unseen aquifers. Non-porous aquifers such as clays partially purify water of bacteria by simple filtration (adsorption and absorption), dilution, and, in some cases, chemical reactions and biological activity. However, in some cases, the pollutants merely transform to soil contaminants. There are a variety of secondary effects stemming not from the original pollutant, but a derivative condition. Some of these secondary impacts are:

- Silt bearing surface runoff can inhibit the penetration of sunlight through the water column, hampering photosynthesis in aquatic plants.
- Thermal pollution can induce fish kills and invasion by new thermophilic species. This can cause further problems to existing wildlife

Chapter 10

RADIATION HAZARDS

Definition

Radiation poisoning, also called "radiation sickness" or a "creeping dose" is a form of damage to organ tissue due to excessive exposure to radiation. The term is generally used to refer to acute problems caused by a large dosage of radiation in a short period, though this also has occurred with long term exposure to low level radiation. Many of the symptoms of radiation poisoning occur as ionizing radiation interferes with cell division.

The clinical name for "radiation sickness" is acute radiation syndrome . A short exposure can result in acute radiation syndrome; chronic radiation syndrome requires a prolonged high level of exposure. A chronic radiation syndrome does exist but is very uncommon;

History

What may be the earliest confirmed cases of acute radiation poisoning occurred in 1879 in Barry County, Missouri, where three men were fatally poisoned and a fourth permanently injured under mysterious circumstances. After chasing an animal they were hunting to the mouth of a cave, they discovered what the cave appeared to be several large veins of silver. They returned the next day to begin prospecting, but fled when they began to fall ill; by the time they had left, one of them was so ill that he was paralyzed and had to be carried to aid. In 1912, after the discovery of radium was announced, a local entrepreneur who had recalled the story investigated the cave to find that the metal was in fact radium, the first isolated veins of the metal ever found (previously, radium was only known from samples extracted from uranium-bearing pitchblende ore). The mine would be the first in the world to be excavated specifically for radium.

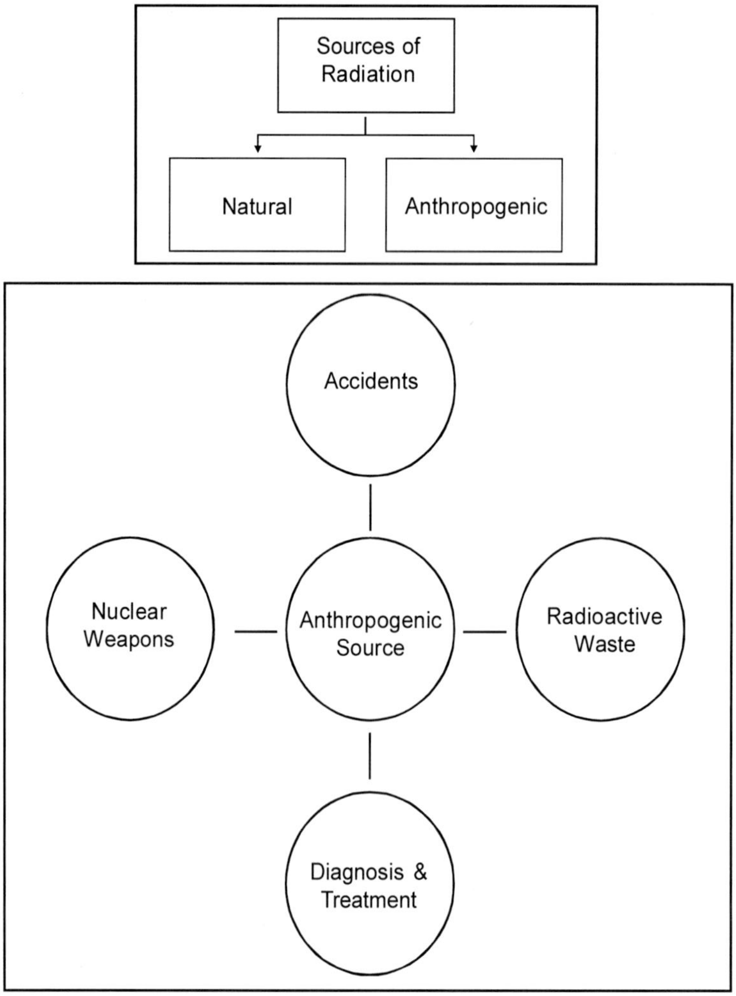

Although radiation was discovered in late 19th century, the dangers of radioactivity and of radiation were not immediately recognized. Acute effects of radiation were first observed in the use of X-rays when the Serbo-Croatian-American electric engineer Nikola Tesla intentionally subjected his fingers to X-rays in 1896. He published his observations concerning the burns that developed, though he attributed them to ozone rather than to X-rays. His injuries healed later.

By the 1930s, after a number of cases of bone necrosis and death in enthusiasts, radium-containing medical products had nearly vanished from the market. Atomic bombings of Hiroshima and Nagasaki resulted in a large number of incidents of radiation poisoning, allowing for greater insight into its symptoms and dangers.

Nuclear Reactor Accidents

Radiation poisoning was a major concern after the Chernobyl reactor accident. It is important to note that in humans the acute effects were largely confined to the accident site. Thirty-one people died as an immediate result.

Of the 100 million curies (4 exabecquerels) of radioactive material, the short lived radioactive isotopes such as I^{131} Chernobyl released were initially the most dangerous. Due to their short half-lives of 5 and 8 days they have now decayed, leaving the more long-lived Cs^{137} (with a half-life of 30.07 years) and Sr^{90} (with a half-life of 28.78 years) as main dangers.

Other Accidents

Improper handling of radioactive and nuclear materials lead to radiation release and radiation poisoning. The most serious of these, due to improper disposal of a medical device containing a radioactive source (teletherapy), occurred in Goiania, Brazil in 1987.

Ingestion and Inhalation

When radioactive compounds enter the animal body, the effects are different from those resulting from exposure to an external radiation source. Especially in the case of alpha radiation, which normally does not penetrate the skin, the exposure can be much more damaging after ingestion or inhalation. The radiation exposure is normally expressed as a committed effective dose equivalent (CEDE)

Measuring of Radiation Dosage

The rad is a unit of absorbed radiation dose defined in terms of the energy actually deposited in the tissue. One rad is an absorbed dose of 0.01 joules of energy per kilogram of tissue. The more recent SI unit is the gray (Gy), which is defined as 1 joule of deposited energy per kilogram of tissue. Thus one gray is equal to 100 rad.

To accurately assess the risk of radiation, the absorbed dose energy in rad is multiplied by the relative biological effectiveness (RBE) of the radiation to get the biological dose equivalent in rems. Rem stands for "Röntgen equivalent in man." In SI units, the absorbed dose energy in grays is multiplied by the same RBE to get a biological dose equivalent in sieverts (Sv). The sievert is equal to 100 rem.

The RBE is a "quality factor," often denoted by the letter Q, which assesses the damage to tissue caused by a particular type and energy of radiation. For alpha particles Q may be as high as 20, so that one rad of alpha radiation is equivalent to 20 rem. The Q of neutron radiation depends on their energy. However, for beta particles, x-rays, and gamma rays, Q is taken as one, so that the rad and rem are equivalent for those radiation sources, as are the gray and sievert.

Units of Radioactivity

- Curie = Ci = 3.7×10^{10} nuclear disintegrations per second.
- Roentgen = R = a measurement of the quantity of ionizations induced in air.
  - 1R = 2.58×10^{-4} coulomb/kg of air.
  - 1R = 0.0096 joules/kg of tissue for gamma radiation.
- Rad = A unit used to express doses of radiation absorbed by living matter.
  - 1 Rad = 100 ergs/g tissue or
  - 1 Rad = 0.01 J/kg of any medium.
- Gray (of gamma radiation) = 1J/kg = 100 rads or 100 rems.
- Rem = Amount of any radiation that produces a biological effect equivalent to that resulting from 1 rad or 0.01 gray of gamma radiation.
- Seivert = Amount of any radiation that is equivalent in biological effect to 1 gray of gamma radiation.
  - 1 Seivert = 100 rems or 100 rads.

- For a given dose of differing types of radiation as measured in roentgens, rads, or grays, there is wide variation in effects. Usually particulate radiation is more injurious than electromagnetic.
- Quality of radiation is sometimes described in terms of linear energy transfer = LET.
  - LET = rate of energy transfer = a function of energy and velocity.
  - Higher LET = means greater injury for a given absorbed dose.

Ionizing Radiation

- Ionization - removal or addition of electrons.
- Direct ionization - ionization due to the mass and motion of a charged particle which imparts an electrical force to electrons in orbit.
- Indirect ionization - ionization attributable to collision of an atom with a particle bearing no charge but which thereby liberates ionized (charged) particles.

Types of electromagnetic radiation.

- Gamma rays and x-rays - short wavelength; high frequency, good penetration.
  - Gamma (γ) rays originate from unstable atomic nuclei which release energy to gain stability. Ionization occurs primarily via indirect ionization.
  - X-rays originate outside of the nucleus of atoms, and ionization occurs primarily via indirect ionization.

Types of particulate radiation (subatomic particles of varying masses and charges).

- Alpha (a) particle: Two neutrons and 2 protons; arise from decay of heavy metals such as U, Pl, Ra, Th. Have high mass and 2 positive charges which results in large direct ionization potential but very little penetration.
- Beta (b) particle = b-: An electron which arises from conversion of a neutron to a proton in the nucleus. Have high penetration but low ionizing power as compared to an alpha particle.
- Positron particle = b+: Like a beta particle but positively charged. Same mass; arises when a proton is converted to a neutron.

- Neutron: An electron combined with a proton which therefore has no charge and can only cause indirect ionization. Readily penetrates; free neutrons undergo β decay.
- Proton: A hydrogen ion; potent ionizer, produced by neutron interactions.

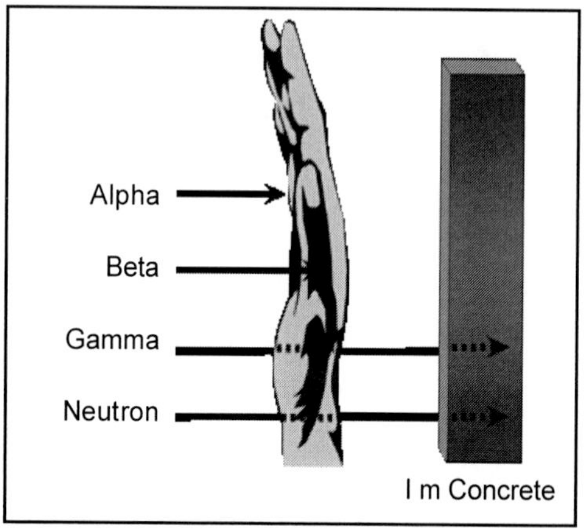

Figure showing the penetrating power of different ionizing rays

Radioactive Decay

- Radioactive decay is decay of unstable isotopes by the emission of subatomic particles and gamma or x-rays.
- Heavy elements generally decay by emission of á particles , Lighter elements by b .

$$T\,½ = \frac{0.693}{\text{lambda}}$$

where lambda = the radioactive decay constant.

Sources of Ionizing Radiation

- Natural Background Radiation
  - Cosmic rays.
  - Disintegration of radioactive elements in earth's crust.
  - Emission from naturally occurring isotopes in the body.

- Average background exposure - human - is: 80 millirems/year = 0.8 milliseiverts/year at sea level.
  - In mountains exposure is 2 times as high due to cosmic rays which are 3 times as intense.
  - In areas where radium or other isotopes are in abundance exposure increases.
- Man-made Exposure
  - Medical diagnostic - average = 70 millirems/year
  - Nuclear power - average = 0.003 millirems/year
  - Global fallout - average = 4.0 millirems/year
  - Radiopharmaceuticals - average = 1.0 millirems/year
  - **Subtotal 75 millirems/year**
  - Occupational and miscellaneous = 2 - 8 millirems/year
  - e.g.: Industrial, television, air travel.
  - **Total average exposure = 150 - 180 millirems/year**

Toxicodynamics

- **Ionization**, e.g. orbital electron is ejected which results in the formation of an ion pair.
- Example: ionization of water.

$HOH \rightarrow HOH^+ + e-$

$HOH^+ \rightarrow H^+ + OH$

ion pair

Excitation

- An electron is raised to a higher energy state.
- Molecule may be excited with energy exceeding that required for ionization and may lose energy by dissociation into free radicals (i.e., H. and OH.) without passing through the stage of ionization.
- In biological systems, the free radicals H. or OH. exist for only a fraction of a second and react to form H2O, H2, or hydrogen peroxide or may react with macromolecules such as DNA. The most fundamental effect of ionizing radiation on biological systems is the ionization of water with the formation of free radicals, H· and OH·.

Note: There are 5 classes of cells with regard to radiosensitivity.

In decreasing order of sensitivity these are:

- Vegetative intermitotic cells (most sensitive).
  - Hematopoietic stem cells.
  - Intestinal gland cells.
  - Spermatogonia type A cells.
  - Ovarian granulosa cells.
  - Large and intermediate lymphocytes.
  - Germinal cells of the epidermis.
  - Gastric and holocrine glands.
- Differentiating intermitotic cells.
  - Hematopoietic cells in differentiation.
  - Differentiated spermatogonia, spermatocytes, oocytes.
- Multipotential connective tissue cells.
  - Endothelial cells.
  - Fibroblasts.
  - Mesenchymal cells.
- Reverting post mitotic cells.
  - Epithelial parenchymal cells.
  - Salivary gland duct cells.
  - Liver.
  - Kidney.
  - Pancreas.
- Fixed post mitotic cells.
  - Neurons.
  - Muscle.
  - Neutrophils.
  - Erythrocytes.
  - Spermatids.

Extrinsic and intrinsic factors influence the response of a living organism to a given dose of radiation.

1. Extrinsic factors: Dose, quality of radiation and part of body exposed.
2. Intrinsic factors: Species, sex and age

Effects of Radiation Toxicosis

Early to Intermediate Effects

- At greater than 50 rads radiation sickness occurs as does pulmonary fibrosis.
- A sensitive indicator of irradiation is the frequency of chromosomal aberrations in lymphocytes. This measurement is useful when the whole body or a major part is exposed to 25 rads or more.
- Cell death causes most early effects of radiation toxicosis.
- The rate of mitosis is generally related to radiosensitivity.

Acute Whole Body Exposure to Radiation

Whole Body Exposure - Acute LD_{50} for Irradiation of Various Species

Animal	Rads
Mouse	638
Rabbit	751
Dog	244
Pig	247
Sheep	205
Goat	237
Monkey	546
Burro	246

Clinical manifestations most commonly involve 4 forms.

- Hematopoietic and immune.
- GI.
- Skin
- Reproductive

Manifestation of early effects occur only after doses of greater than 50 rads, and this must be at a relatively high rate of dosing such as several rads per hour.

- At 50 - 1000 rads
- Bone marrow is damaged.

- The first decrease seen is in lymphocytes and this occurs in 1 - 2 days.
  - There is an early increase in PMNs which may be followed by a leveling off; this is termed an "abortive rise". Failure to see the abortive rise is a bad sign and results in a poorer prognosis.
  - PMNs may decrease in numbers for 4 - 6 weeks then increase slowly to normal within a few months.
  - Platelet sensitivity is similar to that of PMNs. Hemorrhage occurs if platelet counts fall too low.
  - Anorexia, Nausea, Vomiting, and Diarrhea may be seen at different doses
- At very high doses of greater than or equal to 1000 rads, the prodromal response merges with a fatal gastrointestinal syndrome.
- One-thousand to 5000 rads results in a 5 - 10 day survival, death attributable to uncontrollable bloody diarrhea.
  - At over 5000 rads death due to neurologic and cardiovascular degeneration occurs in minutes to 48 hours.

Partial Body Exposure to Radiation

- Usually results in atrophy and fibrosis of some organs and late focal necrosis in others.
  - With partial body exposure to irradiation at doses of:
  - 10 - 100 rads: there may be a decrease in sperm count.
  - 500 rads: redness of skin; permanent sterility.
  - Less than 500 - 1000 rads: serious effects are usually not immediately evident except in skin, eyes, and gonads.

Late Effects of Low Level Exposure to Radiation

- Carcinogenesis
  - Increase in leukemia occurred in areas of Japan hit by atomic bombs.
- Mutagenesis and chromosomal aberrations.
  - Somatic and germinal cells.
  - Point or gene mutations.
  - Deletions.
  - Duplication.
  - Inversion.
  - Translocation.

Diagnosis

When a animal has exposed to known or probable exposure to high-energy radiation from an accident or attack, veterinarian will take a number of steps to determine the absorbed radiation dose. This information is essential for determining how severe the illness is likely to be, which treatments to use and whether a animal is likely to survive. Information important for determining an absorbed dose includes:

Known exposure : Details about distance from the source of radiation and duration of exposure can provide a rough estimate of the severity of radiation sickness.

Vomiting and other symptoms : The time between radiation exposure and the onset of vomiting is a fairly accurate screening tool to estimate absorbed radiation dose. The shorter the time before the onset of this sign, the higher the dose is. The severity and timing of other signs and symptoms may also help veterinarian to determine the absorbed dose.

Blood tests : Frequent blood tests over several days enable to look for drops in disease-fighting white blood cells and abnormal changes in the DNA of blood cells. These factors indicate the degree of bone marrow damage, which is determined by the level of an absorbed dose.

Dosimeter : A device called a dosimeter can measure the absorbed dose of radiation but only if it was exposed to radiation at the same time as the animal was exposed.

Survey meter : A device such as a Geiger counter can be used to survey animal to determine the body location of radioactive particles.

Type of radiation : A part of the larger emergency response to a radioactive accident or attack would include identifying the type of radiation animals have been exposed to. This information would guide some decisions for treating animals with radiation sickness.

Prevention and Treatment

First Aid

1. Only provide medical care if you have appropriate protective gear to prevent possible contamination:
2. Check for adequate breathing and circulation.
3. Start **CPR** if necessary.

4. Vigorously wash body with soap and water.
5. Dry body and wrap with soft, clean blanket.
6. Report exposure to emergency officials.

If Symptoms Occur During or After Medical Radiation Treatments

7. Notify veterinarian or seek medical treatment.
8. Handle affected areas gently.

Do Not

9. Do not remain in area where exposure occurred.
10. Do not apply ointments to burned areas.
11. Do not remain in contaminated clothing.
12. Do not minimize the potential danger - radiation exposure is dangerous.
13. Do not hesitate to seek emergency medical treatment.
14. The best prevention for radiation sickness is to minimize exposure to high levels of ionizing radiation. The use of radionuclides in science and industry is strictly regulated in most countries. In the event of an accidental or deliberate release of radioactive material, evacuation or sheltering in place are the recommended measures. Potassium iodide (KI), administered orally immediately after exposure, may be used to protect the thyroid from ingested radioactive iodine in the event of an accident or terrorist attack at a nuclear power plant, or the detonation of a nuclear explosive. KI would not be effective against a dirty bomb unless the bomb happened to contain radioactive iodine, and even then it would only help to prevent thyroid cancer.
15. Neumune, a drug designed to combat the most deadly effects of radiation, is currently under development by Hollis-Eden Pharmaceuticals.

❑❑❑

Chapter 11

DEFENSE TOXICOLOGY

Dr. U. SUNIL CHANDRA
Assistant Professor, Department of Pharmacology and Toxicology
Veterinary College, KVAFSU, Bidar, Karnataka

Chemical warfare involves using the toxic properties of chemical substances to kill, injure or incapacitate an enemy.

Chemical warfare is different from the use of conventional weapons or nuclear weapons because the destructive effects of chemical weapons are not primarily due to any explosive force. The offensive use of living organisms (such as anthrax) is considered to be biological warfare rather than chemical warfare; the use of nonliving toxic products produced by living organisms (e.g., toxins such as botulinum toxin, ricin, or saxitoxin) *is* considered chemical warfare under the provisions of the Chemical Weapons Convention. Under this Convention, any toxic chemical, regardless of its origin, is considered as a chemical weapon unless it is used for purposes that are not prohibited (an important legal definition, known as the General Purpose Criterion)

About 70 different chemicals have been used or stockpiled as Chemical Warfare (CW) agents during the 20th century. Chemical weapons are classified as weapons of mass destruction by the United Nations, and their production and stockpiling was outlawed by the Chemical Weapons Convention of 1993. Under the Convention, chemicals that are toxic enough to be used as chemical weapons, or may be used to manufacture such chemicals, are divided into three groups according to their purpose and treatment:

- **Schedule 1** – Have few, if any, legitimate uses. These may only be produced or used for research, medical, pharmaceutical or protective purposes (i.e. testing of chemical weapons sensors and protective clothing). Examples include nerve agents, ricin, lewisite and mustard gas. Any production over 100 g must be notified to the OPCW and a country can have a stockpile of not more than one ton of these chemicals.
- **Schedule 2** – Have no large-scale industrial uses, but may have legitimate small-scale uses. Examples include dimethyl methylphosphonate, a precursor to sarin but which is also used as a flame retardant and Thiodiglycol which is a precursor chemical used in the manufacture of mustard gas, also widely used as a solvent in inks.
- **Schedule 3** – Have legitimate large-scale industrial uses. Examples include phosgene and chloropicrin. Both have been used as chemical weapons but phosgene is an important precursor in the manufacture of plastics and chloropicrin is used as a fumigant. Any plant producing more than 30 tonnes per year must be notified to, and can be inspected by, the OPCW.

Chemical Warfare Agents

A chemical used in warfare is called a *chemical warfare agent* (CWA). About 70 different chemicals have been used or stockpiled as chemical warfare agents during the 20th century and the 21st century. These agents may be in liquid, gas or solid form. Liquid agents are generally designed to evaporate quickly; such liquids are said to be *volatile* or have a *high vapor pressure*. Many chemical agents are made volatile so they can be dispersed over a large region quickly.

The earliest target of chemical warfare agent research was not toxicity, but development of agents that can affect a target through the skin and clothing, rendering protective gas masks useless. In July 1917, the Germans employed mustard gas, the first agent that circumvented gas masks. Mustard gas easily penetrates leather and fabric to inflict painful burns on the skin.

Chemical warfare agents are divided into *lethal* and *incapacitating* categories. A substance is classified as incapacitating if less than 1/100 of the lethal dose causes incapacitation, e.g., through nausea or visual problems. The distinction between lethal and incapacitating substances is not fixed, but relies on a statistical average called the LD_{50}.

An Update in Chemical Warfare Substances

Year	Agents	Dissemination	Protection	Detection
1900s	Chlorine Chloropicrin Phosgene Mustard gas	Wind dispersal		Smell
1910s	Lewisite	Chemical shells	Gas mask Rosin oil clothing	
1920s		Projectiles w/ central bursters	CC-2 clothing	
1930s	G-series nerve agents	Aircraft bombs		Blister agent detectors Color change paper
1940s		Missile warheads Spray tanks	Protective ointment (mustard) Collective protection Gas mask w/ Whetlerite	
1950s				
1960s	V-series nerve agents	Aerodynamic	Gas mask w/ water supply	Nerve gas alarm
1970s				
1980s		Binary munitions	Improved gas masks (protection, fit, comfort)	Laser detection
1990s	Novichok nerve agents			

Persistency

One way to classify chemical warfare agents is according to their *persistency*, a measure of the length of time that a chemical agent remains effective after dissemination. Chemical agents are classified as *persistent* or *nonpersistent*.

Agents classified as *nonpersistent* lose effectiveness after only a few minutes or hours. Purely gaseous agents such as chlorine are nonpersistent, as are highly volatile agents such as sarin and most other nerve agents. Tactically, nonpersistent agents are very useful against targets that are to be taken over and controlled very quickly. Generally speaking, nonpersistent agents present only an inhalation hazard.

By contrast, *persistent* agents tend to remain in the environment for as long as a week, complicating decontamination. Defense against persistent agents requires shielding for extended periods of time. Non-volatile liquid agents, such as blister agents and the oily VX nerve agent, do not easily evaporate into a gas, and therefore present primarily a contact hazard.

Classes

Chemical warfare agents are organized into several categories according to the manner in which they affect the living organism. The names and number of categories varies slightly from source to source, but in general, types of chemical warfare agents are as follows:

Classes of Chemical Weapon Agents

Class of agent	Agent Names	Mode of Action	Signs and Symptoms	Rate of action	Persistency
Nerve	Cyclosarin (GF) Sarin (GB) Soman (GD) Tabun (GA) VX VR Some insecticides Novichok agents	Inactivates enzyme acetylcholine sterase, preventing the breakdown of the neurotransmi the acetylcholine in the victim's synapses and causing both muscarinic and nicotinic effects	Miosis (pinpoint pupils) Blurred/dim vision Headache Nausea, vomiting, diarrhea Copious secretions/swe ating Muscle twitching/fasci culation Dyspnoea Seizures Loss of consciousness	Vapors: seconds to minutes; Skin: 2 to 18 hours	VX is persistent and a contact hazard; other agents are non-persistent and present mostly inhalation hazards.
Asphyxiant/ Blood	MostArsines Cyanogen chloride Hydrogen cyanide	**Arsine**: Causes intravascular hemolysis that may lead to renal failure.	Possible cherry-red skin Possible cyanosis Confusion	Immediate onset	Non-persistent and an inhalation hazard.

Contd...

		Cyanogen chloride/hydrogen cyanide: Cyanide directly prevents cells from utilizing oxygen. The cells then uses anaerobic respiration, creating excess lactic acid and metabolic acidosis.	Nausea Patients may gasp for air Seizures prior to death Metabolic acidosis		
Vesicant/Blister	Sulfur mustard (HD, H) Nitrogen mustard (HN-1, HN-2, HN-3) Lewisite (L) Phosgene oxime (CX)	Agents are acid-forming compounds that damages skin and respiratory system, resulting burns and respiratory problems.	Severe skin, eye and mucosal pain and irritation Skin erythema with large fluid blisters that heal slowly and may become infected Tearing, conjunctivitis, corneal damage Mild respiratory distress to marked airway damage	**Mustards**: Vapors: 4 to 6 hours, eyes and lungs affected more rapidly; Skin: 2 to 48 hours **Lewisite**: Immediate	Persistent and a contact hazard.
Choking/Pulmonary	Chlorine Hydrogen chloride Nitrogen oxides Phosgene	Similar mechanism to *blister agents* in that the compounds are acids or acid-forming, but action is more pronounced in respiratory system, flooding it and resulting in suffocation; survivors often suffer chronic breathing problems.	Airway irritation Eye and skin irritation Dyspnoea, cough Sore throat Chest tightness Wheezing Bronchospasm	Immediate to 3 hours	Non-persistent and an inhalation hazard.

Contd...

Lachrymatory agent	Tear gas Pepper spray	Causes severe stinging of the eyes and temporary blindness.	Powerful eye irritation	Immediate	Non-persistent and an inhalation hazard.
Incapacitating	Agent 15 (BZ)	Causes atropine-like inhibition of acetylcholine in subject. Causes peripheral nervous system effects that are the opposite of those seen in nerve agent poisoning.	May appear as mass drug intoxication with erratic behaviors, shared realistic and distinct hallucinations, disrobing and confusion Hyperthermia Ataxia (lack of coordination) Mydriasis (dilated pupils) Dry mouth and skin	Inhaled: 30 minutes to 20 hours; Skin: Up to 36 hours after skin exposure to BZ. Duration is typically 72 to 96 hours.	Extremely persistent in soil and water and on most surfaces; contact hazard.
Cytotoxic proteins	Non-living biological proteins, such as: Ricin Abrin	Inhibit protein synthesis	Latent period of 4-8 hours, followed by flu-like signs and symptoms Progress within 18-24 hours to: Inhalation: nausea, cough, dyspnoea, pulmonary edema Ingestion: Gastrointestinal hemorrhage with emesis and bloody diarrhea; eventual liver and kidney failure.	4-24 hours; see *symptoms*. Exposure by inhalation or injection causes more pronounced signs and symptoms than exposure by ingestion	Slight; agents degrade quickly in environment

There are other chemicals used militarily that are not scheduled by the Chemical Weapons Convention, and thus are not controlled under the CWC treaties. These include:

- Defoliants that destroy vegetation, but are not immediately toxic to human beings and animals . Dioxins, rather than Agent Orange itself, have long-term cancer effects and for causing genetic damage leading to serious birth deformities.
- Incendiary or explosive chemicals (such as napalm) because their destructive effects are primarily due to fire or explosive force, and not direct chemical action.
- Viruses, bacteria, or other organisms. Their use is classified as biological warfare. Toxins produced by living organisms are considered chemical weapons, although the boundary is blurry. Toxins are covered by the Biological Weapons Convention.

Delivery

The most important factor in the effectiveness of chemical weapons is the efficiency of its delivery, or *dissemination*, to a target. The most common techniques include *munitions* (such as bombs, projectiles, warheads) that allow dissemination at a distance and *spray tanks* which disseminate from low-flying aircraft. Developments in the techniques of filling and storage of munitions have also been important.

Although there have been many advances in chemical weapon delivery since World War I, it is still difficult to achieve effective dispersion. The dissemination is highly dependent on atmospheric conditions because many chemical agents act in gaseous form. Thus, weather observations and forecasting are essential to optimize weapon delivery and reduce the risk of injuring friendly forces. Dispersion is the simplest technique of delivering an agent to its target. It consists of placing the chemical agent upon or adjacent to a target immediately before dissemination, so that the material is most efficiently used.

Thermal Dissemination

Thermal dissemination is the use of explosives or pyrotechnics to deliver chemical agents. This technique, developed in the 1920s, was a major improvement over earlier dispersal techniques, in that it allowed significant quantities of an agent to be disseminated over a considerable distance. Thermal dissemination remains the principal method of disseminating chemical agents today.

Most thermal dissemination devices consist of a bomb or projectile shell that contains a chemical agent and a central "burster" charge; when the burster detonates, the agent is expelled laterally.

The efficacy of thermal detonation is greatly limited by the flammability of some agents. For flammable aerosols, the cloud is sometimes totally or partially ignited by the disseminating explosion in a phenomenon called *flashing*. Explosively disseminated VX will ignite roughly one third of the time. Despite a great deal of study, flashing is still not fully understood, and a solution to the problem would be a major technological advance.

Despite the limitations of central bursters, most nations use this method in the early stages of chemical weapon development, in part because standard munitions can be adapted to carry the agents.

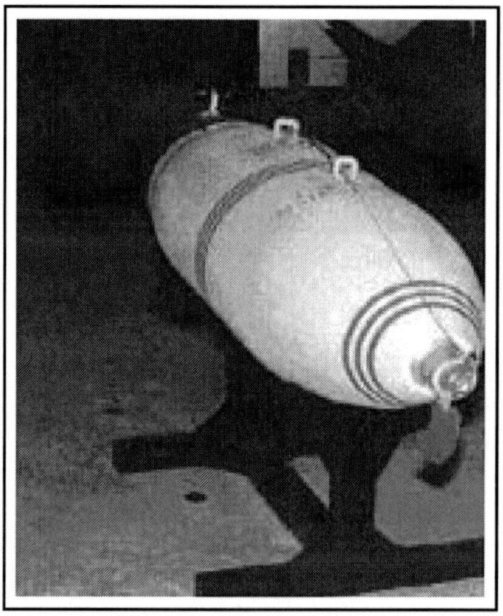

An American-made MC-1 gas bomb used for thermal dissemination

Aerodynamic Dissemination

Aerodynamic dissemination is the non-explosive delivery of a chemical agent from an aircraft, allowing aerodynamic stress to disseminate the agent. This technique is the most recent major development in chemical agent dissemination, originating in the mid-1960s.

This technique eliminates many of the limitations of thermal dissemination by eliminating the flashing effect and theoretically allowing precise control of particle size. In actuality, the altitude of dissemination, wind direction and velocity, and the direction and velocity of the aircraft greatly influence particle size.

Drawback : ideal deployment requires precise knowledge of aerodynamics and fluid dynamics, and because the agent must usually be dispersed within the boundary layer (less than 200–300 ft above the ground), it puts pilots at risk.

Protection Against Chemical Warfare

Ideal protection begins with nonproliferation treaties such as the Chemical Weapons Convention, and detecting, very early, the *signatures* of someone building chemical weapons capability. These include a wide range of intelligence disciplines, such as economic analysis of exports of dual-use chemicals and equipment, human intelligence (HUMINT) such as diplomatic, refugee, and agent reports; photography from satellites, aircraft and drones (IMINT); examination of captured equipment (TECHINT); communications intercepts (COMINT); and detection of chemical manufacturing and chemical agents themselves (MASINT).

If all the preventive measures fail and there is a clear and present danger, then there is a need for detection of chemical attacks, collective protection, and decontamination. Since industrial accidents can cause dangerous chemical releases (e.g., the Bhopal disaster), these activities are things that civilian, as well as military, organizations must be prepared to carry out. In civilian situations in developed countries, these are duties of HAZMAT organizations, which most commonly are part of fire departments.

Detection has been referred to above, as a technical MASINT discipline; specific military procedures, which are usually the model for civilian procedures, depend on the equipment, expertise, and personnel available. When chemical agents are detected, an alarm needs to sound, with specific warnings over emergency broadcasts and the like. There may be a warning to expect an attack. Civilian authorities dealing with an attack or a toxic chemical accident will invoke the Incident Command System, or local equivalent, to coordinate defensive measures. Individual protection starts with a gas mask and, depending on the nature of the threat, through various levels of protective clothing up to a complete chemical-resistant suit with a self-contained air supply.

Collective protection allows continued functioning of groups of people in buildings or shelters, the latter may be fixed, mobile, or improvised. With ordinary buildings, this may be as basic as plastic sheeting and tape, although if the protection needs to be continued for any appreciable length of time, there will need to be an air supply, typically a scaled-up version of a gas mask. Decontamination varies with the particular chemical agent used. Some *nonpersistent* agents, such as most pulmonary agents such as chlorine and phosgene, blood gases, and nonpersistent nerve gases (e.g., GB) will dissipate from open areas, although powerful exhaust fans may be needed to clear out building where they have accumulated. In some cases, it might be necessary to neutralize them chemically, as with ammonia as a neutralizer for hydrogen cyanide or chlorine. Riot control agents such as CS will dissipate in an open area, but things contaminated with CS powder need to be aired out, washed by people wearing protective gear, or safely discarded.

Mass decontamination is a less common requirement for living organisms than equipment. It is a requirement when human beings and animals have been contaminated with persistent agents. Treatment and decontamination may need to be simultaneous, with the medical personnel protecting themselves so they can function.

There may be a need for immediate intervention to prevent death, such as injection of atropine for nerve agents. For decontaminating equipment and buildings exposed to persistent agents, such as blister agents, VX or other agents made persistent by mixing with a thickener, special equipment and materials might be needed,e.g. in the form of a spraying device with neutralizing agents such as Chlorine, Fichlor, strong alkaline solutions or enzymes. In other cases, a specific chemical decontaminant will be required.

Chapter 12

APPENDIX

Appendix - 1

Differential Diagnosis of Poisons based on Clinical Signs

Clinical sign	Possible causes
Abdominal pain	Acids, alkalis, ammonium salts, arsenic, carbamates, chlorate, chlorophenoxy herbicides, copper (sheep), fluoroacetate, lead, mercury (inorganic), nicotine, nitrate/ nitrite, organophosphorus insecticides, paraquat, phenol, phenothiazines, phosphorus, selenium, thallium, urea, zinc, zinc phosphide
Anaemia	Cadmium, copper (sheep), lead, molybdenum, phenothiazines
Blindness	Arsanilic acid, benzoic acid (cat), carbon monoxide, lead, mercury (inorganic and organic), molybdenum (lambs), phenothiazines (poultry), selenium, sodium chloride (pigs and cattle)
Coma	Alphachloralose, arsenic, barbiturates, carbamates, carbon monoxide, chloral hydrate, chlorophenoxy herbicides, chlorpromazine, cyanide, ethylene glycol, hydrogen sulphide, metaldehyde, narcotics, nicotine, organochlorine and organophosphorus insecticides, phenol, phosphorus, zinc phosphide

Contd...

Appendix 1. Contd...

Constipation	Calciferol, lead, phenothiazine (horse), sodium chloride (pig)
Convulsions	Alphachloralose, benzoic acid (cat), caffeine, carbamates, carbon tetrachloride, chlorophenoxy herbicides, copper (sheep), crimidine, cyanide, DNOC, ethylene glycol, fluoroacetate, garbage (staphylococcal enterotoxin; dog), hydrogen sulphide, lead, metaldehyde, narcotics, nitrate/nitrite, organochlorine insecticides, organophosphorus insecticides, phenol, phosphorus, red squill, sodium chloride (pig), strychnine, thallium
Cyanosis	Acrolein, ANTU, carbamates, chlorate, DNOC, hydrogen sulphide, metaldehyde, organochlorine insecticides, organophosphorus insecticides, paraquat
Depression and weakness	Alphachloralose, anticoagulant rodenticides, arsenic, barbiturates, benzalkonium chloride, cannabis, carbon monoxide, carbon tetrachloride, chloral hydrate, chlorophenoxy herbicides, chlorpromazine, copper (sheep), DNOC, ethylene glycol, fluoride, fluoroacetate, garbage (staphylococcal enterotoxin; dog) Heavy metals like lead and mercury (organic). Narcotics, nicotine, nitrate/nitrite, organochlorine insecticides, kerosene (paraffin), paraquat, pentachlorophenol phenol, phenothiazine (horse), phosphorus, red squill, reserpine, rotenone, salicylates (cat), thallium, triazine herbicides, urea herbicides, zinc phosphide
Diarrhoea	Acids, alkalis, ammonium salts, anticoagulant rodenticides, ANTU, arsenic, cadmium, calciferol, carbamates, carbon tetrachloride, chlorate, chlorophenoxy herbicides, chromate, detergents, garbage (staphylococcal enterotoxin; dog), lead, mercury (inorganic), molybdenum, nicotine, nitrate/nitrite, organophosphorus insecticides, phenothiazine (horse), red squill, reserpine, thallium, TOCP, urea, urea herbicides, zinc
Dilated pupils	Barbiturates, cyanide, metaldehyde, strychnine,snake venom.
Dyspnoea	Acrolein, ammonium salts, anticoagulant rodenticides, ANTU, carbamates, carbon monoxide, chlorate, chromate, cyanide, DNOC, hydrogen sulphate, lead (horse), nitrate/nitrite, organophosphorus insecticides, kerosene (paraffin), paraquat, phenothiazine, selenium, sulphur, thallium, TOCP, triazine herbicides, urea
Excitement	Alphachloralose, benzoic acid (cat), caffeine, cannabis, cyanide, ethylene glycol, fluoroacetate, lead, metaldehyde, narcotics (cat, horse), nicotine, organochlorine insecticides, strychnine
Haematuria	Anticoagulant rodenticides, chlorate, mercury (inorganic and organic)
Haemoglobinuria	Chlorate, copper (sheep), phenothiazines

Contd...

Appendix 1. Contd...

In appetence	Anticoagulant rodenticides, arsenic, benzoic acid (cat), calciferol, carbon tetrachloride, chlorate, chlorophenoxy herbicides, chromate, copper, DNOC, fluoride, hydrogen sulphide, lead, mercury (inorganic and organic), organophosphorus insecticides, kerosene (paraffin), paraquat, pentachlorophenol, phenol, phenothiazines, phosphorus, salicylates (cat), sodium chloride (pig), thallium, TOCP, triazine herbicides, urea, urea herbicides, zinc phosphide
Incoordination	Alphachloralose, ammonium salts, ANTU, arsenic, barbiturates, benzoic acid (cat), caffeine, cannabis, carbamates, carbon monoxide, carbon tetrachloride, chloral hydrate, chlorate, chlorophenoxy herbicides, chlorpromazine, ethylene glycol, garbage (staplyococcal enterotoxin; dog), mercury (inorganic and organic), metaldehyde, molybdenum, nicotine, nitrate/nitrite, organochlorine insecticides, organophosphorus insecticides, paraquat, phenol, phenothiazines (pig), red squill, salicylates (cat), selenium, sodium chloride (pig), TOCP, triazine herbicides, urea, urea herbicides
Jaundice	Arsenic, carbon tetrachloride, copper (sheep), paraquat, phenol, phenothiazines, phosphorus
Lameness	Anticoagulant rodenticides, fluoride, molybdenum, selenium
Muscle tremors	Carbamates, cyanide, lead, mercury (inorganic), metaldehyde, organochlorine insecticides, organophosphorus insecticides, phenol, sodium chloride (pig), strychnine, triazine herbicides. *(Note: kerosene (paraffin) and reserpine cause shivering)*
Paralysis	Carbon monoxide (pig), copper (sheep), cyanide, nicotine, organophosphorus insecticides, phenothiazines, phosphorus, selenium, sodium chloride (pig), TOCP
Salivation	Alphachloralose, ANTU, arsenic, benzalkonjum chloride, benzoic acid (cat), cannabis, carbamates, copper, cyanide, detergents, lead, mercury (inorganic), metaldehyde, nicotine, organochlorine insecticides, organophosphorus insecticides, phosphorus, sodium chloride (pig), strychnine, thallium, triazine herbicides
Thirst	Arsenic, calciferol, chlorate, chromate, DNOC, sodium chloride
Vomiting	Acids, alkalis, anticoagulant rodenticides, ANTU, arsenic, benzalkonium chloride, carbamates, chlorophenoxy herbicides, copper, ethylene glycol, fluoroacetate, garbage (staphylococcal enterotoxin; dog), lead, narcotics (dog), nicotine, organochlorine insecticides, organophosphorus insecticides, kerosene (paraffin), paraquat, phosphorus, red squill, reserpine, rotenone, salicylates (cat), thallium, zinc

Appendix - 2

Diagnosis of Poisons based on Biochemical Values

Poison	Species	Lab. tests	Results
Dicumarol	All species	OSPT, APTT, ACT, Platelet Count	Increased OSPT, APTT, ACT Platelets normal in number.
Organophos-phate	All species	Cholinesterase	Cholinesterase activity < 25% normal activity.
Oxalate	All species	Chemistry profile	Azotemia, hypocalcemia in ruminants.
Mercury	All species	BUN, Creatinine	Azotemia
Ethylene glycol	Dogs, Cats	BUN, Creatinine, Urinalysis	Azotemia, Oxalate crystals in urine.
Thallium	Dogs, Cats	CBC, Chemistry Profile, UA	Stress Leukogram, Azotemia, Glycosuria.
Sodium Flouroacetate	Dogs, Cats	Chemistry Profile	Hyperglycemia
Salt	Pigs	Serum Electrolyte	Sodium > 160 MEq
Iron	Pigs	Serum iron, liver enzymes	Hyperferremia, increase in enzyme activity.
Lead	Dog	CBC	Many NRBC with little or no anemia. Basophilic stippling of RBC.
Urea	Ruminants	Rumen pH.. Blood ammonia	Rumen pH > 7.5.Increased blood ammonia.
Nitrate	Ruminants	Methemoglobin	Increased
Selenium (chronic)	Ruminants	CBC, liver enzymes	Anemia, Increased enzyme activity.
Bracken fern	Herbivores	CBC, OSPT, APTT	Non-regenerative anemia, leukopenia thrombocytopenia, normal OSPT,APTT.
Molybdenum (Cu deficiency)	Ruminants	CBC	Microcytic hypochromic anemia.
Copper (acute)	Ruminants	CBC	Hemolytic anemia
Polybrominated biphenyls	Ruminants	Chemistry profile	Increased liver enzymes, azotemia, hypocalcemia, hypoalbuminemia.

Note:

CBC = Complete blood count UA = Urine analysis OSPT = One step prothrombin time

APTT = Activated partial thrombo-plastin time ACT = Activated clotting time

Appendix - 3

Classification of Poisons based on Systems Affected

Neurological Toxicants	Gastrointestinal Toxicants	Nephrotoxicants
Excitation (or stimulation) of nervous system	***Stomatitis, pharyngitis***	Arsenic
		Bismuth
Amphetamine	Acids and alkalis	Cadmium
Aminopyridine	Aldehydes	Cresols
Caffeine	Chromium salts	Dichromate
Cyanide	Fertilizer	Ethylene glycol
Ergot	Mercuric salts	Halogenated hydrocarbons
Fluoroacetate	Detergents	Mercury
Lead	Petroleum distillates	Ochratoxin
Metaldehyde	Phenol	Oxalates
Mycotoxins		Petroleum distillates
Nicotine	***Salivation***	Phenols
Organochlorine insecticides	Cyanogenatic glycosides	Thallium
Organophosphate insecticides	Amanita muscaria	Turpentine
Phenols and chlorophenols	Ammonia	Volatile oils
Strychnine	Cresol	
Theobromine	Metaldehyde	***Nephrotoxic xenobiotics***
Theophylline	Nicotine	Acetaminophen
Water hemlock	Organophosphates	Amphotercin B
Depression, coma	Thallium	Bacitracin
Alcohols	***Dry mouth***	Cephalosporins
Antihistamines	Amphetamine	Gentamicin
Barbiturates	Antihistamine	Kanamycin
Carbon monoxide	Atropine	Neomycin
Hydrocarbons-aliphatic	Belladonna	Polymyxin-B
Hydrocarbons-aromatic	Opiates	Sulfonamides
Hydrocarbons-halogenatd		Vancomycin
Lead	***Gastroenteritis***	
Mercury	Amanita spp.	**Blood Toxicants**
Morphine derivatives	Antimony	
Salicylates	Arsenic	***Methemoglobin***
Snake venoms	Barium	Acetaminophen
Loss of motor control	Bismuth	Aniline derivatives
Botulinum	Cantharidin	Chlorate
Carbon disulfide	Copper salts	Copper
Curare	Croton oil	Methylene blue
Ergot	Detergents, soaps, sanitizers	Nitrite
Ethylene glycol	Digitalis toxins	Nitrobenzene
Hexachlorophene	Iron	
Lead	Lead	***Hemolysis***
Nicotine	Mercury	Acetaminophen
Organophosphates	Mushrooms	Aniline

Contd...

Appendix 3. Contd...

Triaryl phosphates	Phenoxy herbicides	Arsenic
Autonomic stimulation	Phosphorus	Chlorates
Atropine	Plants (many)	Copper
Carbamate insecticides	Staphylococcus toxin	Methylene blue
Fly mushroom (Amanita muscaria)	Thallium	Nitrobenzene
Organophosphate insecticides	Zinc phosphide	Onions
Behavioural changes		Snake venoms
Belladonna alkaloids	Hepatotoxins	Turpentine
Ergot	Acetaminophen	
Lead	Aflatoxin	***Aplastic anemia, leukopenia***
Lysergic acid diethylamide (LSD)	Amanita phalloides	Arsenicals
Marijuana	Blue-green algae	Aspirin
Nutmeg	Coal tar derivatives	Benzene
Opium derivatives	Copper	Chloramphenicol
Organochlorine insecticides	Halogenated hydrocarbons	Cytostatic agents
Periwinkle (Vinka rosea)	Iron	Estrogens
Phosphorus	Petroleum distillates	Phenylbutazone
Sulfonamides	Phosphorus	Toluene
		Trichlorethylene
Cardiovascular Toxicants	**Respiratory Toxicants**	
Tachycardia & arrhythmias	Air pollutants (nitrogen dioxide,	***Coagulopathy***
Adrenaline	sulfur dioxide)	Aflatoxin
Aminophylline	Allergens	Aspirin
Amphetamine	Ammonia	Coumarin rodenticides
Aminoglycoside antibiotics	ANTU rodenticide	
Atropine	Gasoline, kerosene	***Hypothermia***
Caffeine	Organophosphate insecticides	Alcohol
Cyanide	Ozone	Arsenic
Dinitrophenol	Paraquat herbicide	Barbiturates
Fluorocarbons	Thallium	Heroin
Nicotine		Morphine
Thallium	**Ocular Toxicants**	Oxalates
Bradycardia	***Mydriasis***	Phenols
Barium	Amanita mushrooms	***Cyanosis***
Cardiac glycosides	Atropine	Carbon dioxide
Digitalis	Barbiturates	Hydrogen sulfide
Morphine	Belladonna	Nitrite
Opiates	Methanol	Paraquat
Oleander	Snake venom	
Red squill	***Miosis***	***Pink skin color***
Myocardial damage	Heroin	Arsenic
Amanita phalloides	Morphine	Carbon monoxide
Barium	Nicotine	Cyanide
Carbon monoxide	Organophosphates	Mercury
Oleander	***Optic neuropathy***	Thallium
Phosphorus	Arsenicals	—
Thallium	Lead	—
Vascular necrosis	Mercury	—
Ergot	Methanol	—
Lead	Thallium	—
Mercury	Vitamin A	—
Selenium	Phenothiazins(corneal ulcer)	—

Appendix - 4

Materials to be sent to the Laboratory in Various Poisoning Conditions

S.No.	Suspected Xenobiotic for Analysis	Specimen required	Amount required	Remarks
1.	Ammonia/Urea	Whole Blood or serum	5ml	Frozen or add 1-2
		Urine	5ml	drops of saturated
		Rumen contents	100 g	mercuric chloride.
2.	Arsenic	Liver, kidney	100g	
		Whole blood	15ml	
		Urine	50ml	--
		Ingesta	100 g	
		Feed	1-2 kg	
3.	Chlorinated hydrocarbons	Cerebrum	½	Use only glass
		Fat	100g	containers
		Liver, Kidney, Ingesta	100g	Avoid aluminum foil for wrapping specimens
4.	Copper	Kidney, Liver	100g	
		Serum	2-5ml	
		Whole blood	10ml	--
		Feed	1-2kg	
		Faces	100g	
5.	Cyanide/HCN	Forage /Ingesta	1-2kg	Rush sample to
		Whole blood	10ml	laboratory
		Liver	100g	Frozen in air tight bottle. Stomach contents in 1% mercuric chloride
6.	Fluoride	Bone	20g	Ideal sample will be
		Water	100ml	lesion seen in organal
		Forage	100g	bone
		Urine	50ml	
7.	Herbicides	Treated weedy	1-2kg	
		Urine	50ml	--
		Ingesta	500g	
		Liver, Kidney	100g	
8.	Lead, Mercury	Kidney	100g	Heparinized, do not
		Whole blood	10ml	use EDTA
		Liver	100g	
		Urine	15ml	
9.	Mycotoxins	Forages, Feed sample,	100g	Airtight containers or
		Liver, Kidney, Brain.	100g	plastic bags. Cloth bags for dry feeds
10.	Nitrate/Nitrite	Forage/Ingesta	1kg	Ingesta in chloroform
		Water	100ml	or formalin filled air
		Body fluids	10-20ml	tight container

Contd...

Appendix 4. Contd...

11.	Organophosphates and Organocarbametes	Feed	100g	
		Ingesta	100g	--
		Liver	100g	
		Urine	50ml	
12.	Oxalates	Fresh forage	100g	Fixed in formalin
		Kidneys	100g	
13.	Sodium (NaCl)	Brain	100g	
		Serum	5ml	--
		CSF	1ml	
		Feed	1-2kg	
14.	Znic phosphide	Liver, Kidney	100g	--
		Gastric contents	100g	

Appendix - 5

Industries and Principal Constituents of Effluents

Industries	Important Constituents of Effluent
Acetate rayon	Acetic acid
Aluminium anodising	Chromium
Atomic energy plants	Fluorides
Battery manufacture	Lead, mineral acids
Bleaching industries	Sulphite, free chlorine
Breweries	Sugars, mineral acids
Ceramic plants	Fluorides
Chemical manufacture	Mineral acids, phenols, ammonia, organic acids such as tartaric acid, nitro compounds
Chocolate and sweet making units	Sugars
Chrome tanning	Chromium
Copper pickling	Copper, mineral acids
Copper plating	Copper
Cotton mercerizing	Alkalis
Cotton and straw kiering	Alkalis
Cuprammonium rayon manufacture	Copper
Dairies	Sugars
DDT manufacture	Mineral acids
Distilleries	Organic acids
Dyeing industries	Tartaric acid
Dye manufacture	Phenolic compounds

Contd...

Appendix 5. Contd...

Engineering works	Fats, oil and grease
Explosive factories	Nitro compounds
Fertilizer plants	Phosphates, fluorides
Food processing	Starch
Galvanizing industries	Zinc
Gas and coke manufacture	Ammonia, cyanides, sulphides, phenols
Glass etching	Fluorides
Iron pickling	Iron, mineral acids
Laundries	Alkalis, free chlorine, fats, oils and grease
Leather manufacture	Tartaric acid
Metal cleaning	Cyanides
Metal refineries	Fluorides
Oil refineries	Mercaptans
Paint manufacture	Lead
Paper mills	Free chlorine
Penicillin manufacture	Formaldehyde
Peroxide bleaching of textiles	Hydrogen peroxide
Petrochemical industries	Hydrocarbons
Petroleum refineries	Hydrocarbons, phenols, fats, oils and grease
Photo-engraving	Mineral acids
Photography	Silver
Pickle manufacture	Acetic acid
Plating industries	Copper, chromium, nickel, cadmium, zinc and silver
Preserve manufacture	Sugars
Pulp mills	Mercaptans
Rocket motor testing	Hydrogen peroxide
Rubber processing	Zinc
Saw mills	Tannic acid
Scrubbing of flue gases	Fluorides
Sheep dipping	Arsenic, phenols
Soft drinks manufacture	Critic acid
Sugar factories	Sugar
Sweets manufacture	Sugars
Synthetic resin manufacture	Phenols, formaldehyde
Synthetic rubber factories	Hydrocarbons
Tanneries	Sulphides, chromium, phenols, tannic acid
Tar distilleries	Phenols

Contd...

Appendix 5. Contd...

Textile bleaching	Free chlorine, sulphites
Textile industries	Mineral acids, fats, oils and grease
Transistor factories	Fluorides
Viscose film manufacture	Sulphites
Viscose rayon manufacture	Sulphides, zinc
Wall-paper manufacture	Starch
Wood processing	Sugars
Wood pulp processing	Alkalis and sulphites
Wool scouring	Alkalis, fats, oil and greas

Appendix - 6

List of Teratogens and their Teratogenic Dosage

Chemical	Teratogenic dosage
Acetazolamide	0.6% (in diet)
ACTH	5 mg q 6 h/3 days
Actinomycin D	25 - 100 mcg/kg
Alcohol	1.0 - 210 gm/kg
Aldosterone	0.05 mg/day
Amantadine HCl	10 mg/kg
Aminophylline	100 - 200 mg/kg
Aminopterin	0.1 mg/kg
Anesthetics	-
Antibodies	-
Apomorphine	0.025 mg/embryo (chick)
Barbituric Acid	0.16% (mice) (in diet)
Busulfan	18 - 34 mg/kg
Caffeine	75 - 150 mg/kg
Chlorambucil	8 - 12 mg/kg
Chloramphenicol	100 - 200 mg/kg
Chlortetracycline	10 mg/kg
Colchicine	1 - 2 mg/kg (monkey)
Cortisone	-
Coumarin Derivatives	4 mg/kg (mice)
Dextroamphetamine Sulfate	1 mg/kg
Diazepam	200 mg/kg
Diethylstilbestrol	10 - 42 mg
Dimethyl Sulfoxide	4.0 ml/kg

Contd...

Appendix 6. Contd...

Diphenylhydantoin	75 - 150 mg/kg (mice)
Disulfiram	100 mg (in diet)
L-Dopa	10 mg/kg
Epinephrine	1 - 50 mcg
Fluorouracil	12 - 37 mg/kg
Griseofulvin	50 - 500 mg/kg
Hypervitaminosis A	35,000 I.U.
Imipramine	15 mg/kg
Isoniazid	-
Lithium	212 mg/kg hen 85 mg/kg
Marihuana	4.2 mg/kg
Meclizine	20 - 80 mg/kg
Methaqualone	0.8% (in diet)
Methotrexate	10 mg/kg (mice)
Nitrous oxide	50% (by inhalation)
Noradrenalin	25 mcg/embryo
Phenobarbital	0.16% (mice) (in diet)
Physostigmine	0.05 - 15.0 mg/embryo (chick)
Pilocarpine	3 - 12 mg/embryo (chick)
Prednisolone	2.5 mg/kg
Prochlorperazine	2.5 - 10 mg/day
Reserpine	1.5 mg/kg
Salicylate	300 mg/kg
Sulphonamides	50 mg/kg
Tetracycline	40 - 80 mg/kg
Tolbutamide	300 mg/day

Appendix - 7

Drugs and Toxicants Modifying Cholinergic Neurotransmission

Toxicant	Effect
Hemicholinium	Block choline uptake with consequent depletion of ACh
4-Aminopyridine	Increased release of ACh
Black Widow spider venom	Explosive release of ACh
Botulinum toxin	Blocks release of ACh
Acetylcholine Muscarine	Muscarinic receptor activation

Contd...

Appendix 7. Contd...

Methacholine	Stimulates muscarinic receptor especially in
Carbachol	exocrine glands
Bethanechol	"
Pilocarpine	"
Arecoline (from areca nut)	"
Slaframine	"
Muscarinic/histaminic mushrooms	"
Atropine	Muscarinic receptor blocker
Benztropine	"
Scopolamine	"
Belladonna (*Atropa belladonna*)	"
Henbane (*Hyoscyamus niger*)	"
Jimson weeds (*Datura stramonium*)	"
Tomato, etc.	"
Acetylcholine	Nicotinic-receptor activation
Nicotine sulfate	"
Tobacco (*Nicotiana*)	"
Indian tobacco (*Lobelia*)	"
Poison hemlock (*Conium maculatum*)	"
Kentucky coffee tree (*Gymnocladus dioica*)	"
Lupine (*Lupinus*)	"
Mescal bean (*Sophora* spp.)	"
Goldenchain (*Laburnum anagyroides*)	"
Blue green algae - Anatoxin-A	"
(+)-Tubocurarine	Nicotinic receptor blocker at neuromuscular
Hexamethonium	junction
Gallamine	"
Pancuronium	"
Larkspur (*Delphinium*)	"
Organophosphate insecticides	Anticholinesterases
Carbamate insecticides	"
Blue green algae - Anatoxin-A(s)	"
Solanum spp. (significance of this mechanism is	"
controversial in *solanum* and other Solanaceae)	"
Black nightshade (*S. nigrum*)	"
Potato (*S. tuberosum*)	"
Horse nettle (*S. tuberosum*)	"
European bittersweet (*S. dulcamara*)	"
Jerusalem cherry (*S. pseudocapsicum*)	"

Appendix - 8

Drugs and Toxicants Modifying Noradrenergic Neurotransmission

Mechanism	Drug	Effect
Synthesis	α-methyl-DOPA	Synthesis of false transmitter
	γ-methyl-p-tyrosine	Inhibits tyrosine hydroxylase
	Disulfiram (Antabuse®)	Inhibits dopamine-α-hydroxylase
Storage	Reserpine	Disrupt norepinephrine (NE) storage
	Tetrabenazine	
	MAO inhibitors	Enhance NE storage
Release	(+)-amphetamine	Indirectly acting sympathomimetic amines, cause release of NE
	Tyramine	
	Ephedrine	
	Guanethidine	Adrenergic neuron blockers, decrease NE release
	Debrisoquine	
	Bethanidine	"
	Bretylium	"
Receptors	NE	
	Phenylephrine (α1)	α -adrenoceptor activation
	α-methyl-NE	"
	Clonidine (α2)	"
	Phentolamine	α -adrenoceptor blockers
	Phentoxybenzamine	"
	NE	
	Adrenaline	"
	Isoproterenol (α1,2)	"
	Albuterol	α -adrenoceptor activation
	Terbutaline (α2)	"
	Dobutamine (α1)	"
	Propranolol (α1, α2)	α - adrenoceptor blockers[1]
	Metoprolol (α1)	"
	Esmolol (α1)	"
	Oxprenolol	"
	Sotalol	
	Alprenolol	

Contd...

Appendix 8. Contd...

Postreceptor	Methylxanthines:	
	Caff eine	Phosphodiesterase inhibitors (minor site of action)
	Theophylline	
	Aminophylline	"
Inactivation of uptake	Cocaine	Neuronal-uptake inhibitors
	Imipramine	"
	Amitriptyline	"
	Iproniazid	MAO inhibitors
of metabolism	Nialamide	"
	Phenelzine	"
	Tranylcypromine	"
	Pargyline	

Appendix - 9

Drugs and Toxicants Modifying Dopaminergic Neurotransmission

Mechanism	Drug	Effect
Synthesis	L-DOPA	Increased synthesis
	α-methyl-p-tyrosine	Inhibits tyrosine hydroxylase
	Carbidopa	Inhibit DOPA decarboxylase
	Benserazide	outside CNS
Storage	Reserpine	Disrupt dopamine storage
	Tetrabenazine	Enhance dopamine storage
	MAO inhibitors	
Release	(+)-amphetamine	Increase release of dopamine
	Phenmetrazine	
	Mazindol	
	Tyramine	
Receptors	Dopamine	Dopamine-receptor activation
	Apomorphine	
	Bromocriptine	
	ADTN	
	Piribedil	
	Chlorpromazine	Dopamine-receptor blockers
	Fluphenazine	
	Haloperidol	
	Pimozide	
	Metoclopramide	
Postreceptor	Methylxanthines:	Phosphodiesterase inhibitors
	Caffeine	
	Theophylline	
	Theobromine	
Inactivation of Uptake	Amphetamines	Neuronal dopamine uptake inhibitors
	Nomifensine	
	Benztropine	
	Benzhexol	
	Mazindol	
of metabolism	Iproniazid	MAO inhibitors
	Tranylcypromine	
	Phenelzine	

Appendix - 10

Drugs and Toxicants Modifying 5-Hydroxytryptaminergic Neurotransmission

Mechanism	Drug	Effect
Synthesis	L-tryptophan	Increases synthesis
	p-chlorophenylalanine	Inhibits tryptophan hydroxylase
Storage	Reserpine Tetrabenazine	Disrupt 5-HT storage
	MAO inhibitors	Enhance 5-HT storage
Release	Fenfluramine Chlorphentermine Amphetamines	Release 5-HT onto receptors
Receptors	5-HT LSD DMT Quipazine	Activate 5-HT-receptor
	Cyproheptadine Methysergide Mianserin	Block 5-HT-receptor
Inactivation of uptake	Tricyclic antidepressants Mianserin Fenfluramine	Inhibit neuronal 5-HT uptake
of metabolism	Phenelzine Iproniazid Tranylcypromine	Inhibit MAO

Appendix - 11

Drugs and Toxicants Modifying Histaminergic Mechanisms

Mechanism	Drug	Effect
Synthesis	-	-
Storage	-	-
Release	Injury (+)-tubocurarine Morphine Dextran	Release histamine onto receptors
	Cromolyn sodium	Inhibits histamine release
Receptors	Histamine 2-methyl histamine	Activate H1-histamine-receptor
	Mepyramine Promethazine Chlorpheniramine	Block H1-histamine-receptor
	Histamine Betazole	H2-histamine-receptor activation
	Cimetidine Burimamide Metiamide Ranitidine	H2-histamine-receptor blockers
Inactivation	-	-

Appendix - 12

Drugs and Toxicants Modifying GABA Neurotransmission

Mechanism	Drug	Effect
Synthesis	Allylglycine 3-mercaptopropionic acid	Inhibit glutamic acid decarboxylase
Storage	-	-
Release	Ivermectin	Increases release of GABA
Receptors	GABA Muscimol Ivermectin	Activates GABA receptors
	Benzodiazepines Barbiturates Ivermectin Piperazine	Enhance GABA-receptor activity
	Bicuculline Picrotoxin Benzylpenicillin α CN-pyrethroids Cyclodiene organochlorine insecticides	Block GABA receptors
Inactivation of uptake	α-alanine Nipecotic acid	Inhibit GABA uptake
of metabolism	Ethanolamine-O-sulphate Sodium valproate	Inhibit GABA transaminase (GABA-T)

Appendix - 13

Drugs and Toxicants Modifying Glycine Neurotransmission

Toxicant	Mechanism of Effect
Tetanus toxin	Inhibits release of glycine
Strychnine Brucine *Gelsemium* *Calycanthus*	Block glycine receptors
Penitrem A (tremorgenic mycotoxin)	Competitively inhibits glycine and GABA at receptors

Chapter 13

BIBLIOGRAPHY

Ahn.,J.H., Robertson, B.M., Elliot, R., Gutterridge, R.C. and Ford C.W. 1989. Quality Assessment of Tropical Browse Legumes: Tannin Content and Protein Degradation. Animal Feed Science and Technology 27: 147–156.

Air Pollution, Heart Disease and Stroke from the Website of The American Heart Organization January 5, 2008.

Aktories K. Rho Proteins: Targets for Bacterial Toxins. Trends Microbiol 1997;5:282-8.

Allison, M.J., Hammond, A.C. and Jones, R.J. 1990. Detection of Ruminal Bacteria That Degrade Toxic Dihydroxy Pyridine Compounds Produced From Mimosine. Applied and Environmental Microbiology 56: 590–594.

Andreu A, Stapleton AE, Fennell C, Lockman HA, Xercavins M, Fernandez F, Et Al. Urovirulence Determinants In *Escherichia Coli* Strains Causing Prostatitis. J Infect Dis 1997;176:464-9.

Anonymous(1993): Surveillance of Food Contaminants In India-Report of An ICMR Task Force Study (Part-I), New-Delhi, pp15-40.

Arnon SS. Human Tetanus and Human Botulism. In: Rood JI, Mcclane BA, Songer JG, Titball RW, *Editors*. The Clostridia: Molecular Biology and Pathogenesis. San Diego: Academic Press; 1997. p. 95-115.

Averbuch-Heller L, Leigh RJ. Medical Treatments for Abnormal Eye Movements: Pharmacological, Optical and Immunological Strategies. Aust. NZ. J. Ophthalmol 1997; 25:7-13.

B. F. Stone, K. C. Binnington, M. Gauci, J. H. Aylward (1989). "Tick/Host Interactions Forixodes Holocyclus: Role, Effects, Biosynthesis and Nature of Its Toxic and Allergenic Oral Secretions". Experimental and Applied Acarology 7 (1): 59–69.

Bamualin, A., Jones, R.J. and Murray, R.M. 1980. Nutritive Value of Tropical Browse Legumes in the Dry Season. Proceedings of The Australian Society of Animal Production 13: 229–232.

Barry, T.N. 1987. Secondary Compounds of Forages. In: Nutrition of Herbivores. Hacker, J.B. and Ternouth, J.H. (Eds.) A.P. Sydney pp. 91–120.

Behl, C.R., Pande, M.B., Pande, D.P. and Radadia, N.S. 1986. Nutritive Value of Wilted Castor (Ricinus Communis L.) Leaves for Crossbred Sheep. Indian Journal of Animal Science 56: 473–474.

Benoit Morel and Kyle Olson; Shadows and Substance: The Chemical Weapons Convention. Westview Press, 1993.

Betley MJ, Borst DW, Regassa LB. Staphylococcal Enterotoxins, Toxic Shock Syndrome Toxin and Streptococcal Pyrogenic Exotoxins: A Comparative Study of Their Molecular Biology. Chem Immunol 1992; 55:1-35.

Beychok, M.R. (2005). Fundamentals of Stack Gas Dispersion, 4th Edition, Author-Published.

Bhakdi S, Bayley H, Valeva A, Walev I, Walker B, Weller U, *et al.* Staphylococcal Alpha-Toxin, Streptolysin-O and *Escherichia Coli* Hemolysin: Prototypes of Pore-Forming Bacterial Cytolysins. Arch Microbiol 1996; 165:73-9.

Binaykumar Sinha, 1994. PM Techniques and Diagnostic Procedures with Interpretations. First Edition Pushpa Prakashan, Bihar, pp : 81-93.

Blum G, Falbo V, Caprioli A, Hacker J. Gene Clusters Encoding the Cytotoxic Necrotizing Factor Type 1, Prs-Fimbriae and -Hemolysin form The Pathogenicity Island II of the Uropathogenic *Escherichia Coli* Strain J96. FEMS Microbiol Lett 1995; 126: 189-96.

Bohach GA, Stauffacher CV, Ohlendorf DH, Chi YI, Vath GM, Schlievert PM. The Staphylococcal and Streptococcal Pyrogenic Toxin Family. In: Singh BR, Tu AT, Editors. Natural Toxins II. New York: Plenum Press; 1996. p. 131-54.

Bokoch GM, Katada T, Northup JK, Hewlett EL, Gilman AG. Identification of the Predominant Substrate for ADP-Ribosylation by Islet Activating Protein. J Biol Chem 1983; 258:2072-5.

Boyce TG, Swerdlow DL, Griffin PM. *Escherichia Coli* O157:H7 and the Hemolytic-Uremic Syndrome. N Engl J Med 1995; 333:364-8.

Buckley Na, Isbister Gk, Stokes B, Juurlink Dn. (2005). "Hyperbaric Oxygen For Carbon Monoxide Poisoning : A Systematic Review And Critical Analysis Of The Evidence" (Abstract). Toxicol Rev 24 (2): 75–92.

Carter SR, Seiff SR. Cosmetic Botulinum Toxin Injections. Int Ophthalmol Clin 1997; 37:69-79.

Centers for Disease Control and Prevention. Addressing Emerging Infectious Disease Threats: A Prevention Strategy for the United States. MMWR Morb Mortal Wkly Rep 1994; 43:1-18.

Centers for Disease Control. Isolation of *E. Coli* O157:H7 from Sporadic Cases of Hemorrhagic Colitis United States. MMWR Morb Mortal Wkly Rep 1982;31:580-5.

Chadha P.V. 1984. Handbook of Forensic Medicine and Toxicology. pp:212-223. Fifth Edition, Jaypee Brothers.

Chatani, N.; Murai, S. "Carbon Monoxide" In Encyclopedia of Reagents for Organic Synthesis (Ed: L. Paquette) 2004, J. Wiley & Sons, New York.

Chauhan, R.S. 1998. Alphamethrin Induced Immunosuppression In Calves and its Modulation Using Herbal Immunomodulator. The Immunologist- Supplement 1: 496.

Chauhan, R.S. and Chandra, R. 1998. Immunodeficiency in Animals. In : An Introduction To Immunopathology. pp. 52-63. (Ed: R.S. Chauhan) Pantnagar.

Chauhan. R.S. and Mahipal. S.K. 1994. Immunotoxicity of Pesticides in Poultry. In: Advances in Veterinary Research and their Impact on Animal Health and Production Pp. 101-107. (Eds. R. Verma and T. N. Jaiswal).

Chauhan. R.S.; Baharat Bhushan; Khurana, S. K. and Mahipal, S.K. 1994. Effect of Pesticides on Immunocopetence of Animals and their Public Health Significance. In: Impact of Modern Agriculture on Environment (Eds. S.K. Arora, R, K. Behl and P. Tauro) CCSHAU, Hisar & Max Muller Bhawan, New Delhi. pp 169-178.

Chauhan. R.S.; Khurana, S. K.; Sharma, R. and Mahipal, S.K. 1995. Pesticide Induced Glomerulonephritis - An Indication of Type 10 Hypersensitivity Reaction. In: International Conference on Sustainable Agriculture & Environment, Jan. 11-13, 1995. Hisar.

Cheeke, P.R. and Shull, L.R. 1985. Natural Toxicants in Feeds and Livestock. AVI Publishing Inc., West Port, Connecticut.

Cherry JD. Comparative Efficacy of Acellular Pertussis Vaccines: An Analysis of Recent Trials. Pediatr Infect Dis J 1997; 16:S90-6.

Choinière M, Melzack R (December 1987). "Acute and Chronic Pain in Hemophilia". Pain 31 (3): 317–31.

Christopher H. Goss, Stacey A. Newsom, Jonathan S. Schildcrout, Lianne Sheppard and Joel D. Kaufman (2004). "Effect of Ambient Air Pollution on Pulmonary Exacerbations and Lung Function in Cystic Fibrosis". American Journal of Respiratory and Critical Care Medicine. 169: 816-821.

Collier RJ. In: Moss J, Vaughan M, Editors. ADP-Ribosylating Toxins and G Proteins. Washington: American Society for Microbiology; 1990. p. 3-19.

Conn, E.E. 1979. Cyanide and Cyanogenic Glycosides. In: Herbivores: Their Interaction with Secondary Plant Metabolites. Rosenthal, G.A. Janzen, D.H. (Eds.) A.P., New York. pp. 387–412.

CSWRI 1987, 1988, 1989. Processing of Tannin Feeds for their Increased Utilization. Report. Central Sheep & Wool Research Institute, Avikanagar-304 501, Rajasthan.

D'mello, J.P.F. and Acamovic, T. 1989. Leucaena Leucocephala in Poultry Nutrition: A Review. Animal Feed Science and Technology 26: 1–28.

Damgaard In, Skakkebæk Ne, Toppari J, *et al.*, Persistent Pesticides in Human Breast Milk and Cryptorchidism, Environ. Health Perspect. 2006, 114:1133-1138.

Davis, Devra (2002). When Smoke Ran Like Water: Tales of Environmental Deception and the Battle Against Pollution. Basic Books.

Derycke J, Gonzalez EA, Blanco J, Oswald E, Blanco M, Boivin R. Evidence for Two Types of Cytotoxic Necrotizing Factor in Human and Animal Clinical Isolates of *Escherichia Coli*. Journal of Clinical Microbiology 1990;28:694-9.

Descostes, G. and Mazue, G. 1987. Immunotoxicology. Adv. Vet. Sci. Comp. Med. 31 :95-199.

Dworkin MS, Shoemaker PC, Anderson D (1999). "Tick Paralysis: 33 Human Cases in Washington State, 1946–1996".

Eaton Dl and Klaasen Cd. Principles of Toxicology. In: Klaasen Cd, Ed. Casarett and Doull's Toxicology: The Basic Science of Poisons. 6th Edition. New York: Mcgraw-Hill, 2001; 11-34.

Eilert Ej (2005). "New Packaging Technologies for The 21st Century". Journal of Meat Science 71 (1): 122–27.

Elschenbroich, C.; Salzer, A. "Organometallics : A Concise Introduction" (2nd Ed) Wiley-VCH.

Endo Y, Tsurugi K, Yutsudo T, Takeda Y, Ogasawara Y, Igarashi K. Site of Action of A Vero Toxin (VT2) From *Escherichia Coli* O157:H7 and of Shiga Toxin on Eucaryotic Ribosomes. Eur J Biochem 1988;171:45-50.

Falbo V, Pace T, Picci L, Pizzi E, Caprioli A. Isolation and Nucleotide Sequence of the Gene Encoding Cytotoxic Necrotizing factor 1 of *Escherichia Coli*. Infect Immun 1993;61:4909-14.

Flatau G, Lemichez E, Gauthier M, Chardin P, Paris S, Fiorentini C, *et al.* Toxin-Induced Activation of the G Protein P21 Rho by Deamidation of Glutamine. Nature 1997; 387: 729-33.

Frasier ME, Chernaia MM, Kozlov YV, James MNG. Crystal Structure of the Holotoxin from *Shigella Dysenteriae* At 2.5 Å Resolution. Nature Structural Biology 1994; 1:59-64.

G. H. Coleman, David Craig (1943). "P-Tolualdehyde". Org. Synth.; Coll. 2: 583.

Ghetie MA, Ghetie V, Vitetta ES. Immunotoxins for the Treatment of B-Cell Lymphomas. Mol Med 1997; 3: 420-7.

Giannella RA. *Escherichia Coli* Heat-Stable Enterotoxins, Guanylins, and their Receptors: what are they and what do they do? J Lab Clin Med 1995;125:173-81.

Golbert Me, Mack CM,Crofton KM.Pyrethroids and Enhanced Inhibition in the Hippocampus of the Rats.Brain Res 1989; 477: 314-21.

Gordon M. Burck and Charles C. Flowwer; International Handbook on Chemical Weapons Proliferation 1991.

Gothe R, Kunze K, Hoogstraal H (1979). "The Mechanisms of Pathogenicity in the Tick Paralyses".

Grunfeld Ht, Bonefeld-Jorgensen Ec, Effect of *in vitro* Estrogenic Pesticides on Human Oestrogen Receptor Alpha and Beta MRNA Levels, Toxicol. Lett., 2004, 151(3): 467-80.

Gupta.P.K. 1988. Veterinary Toxicology. pp: 344-365. Cosmo Publications.

Halpern JL, Neale EA. Neurospecific Binding, Internalization and Retrograde Axonal Transport. Curr Top Microbiol Immunol 1995; 195: 221-41.

Harborne, J.B. 1989. Biosynthesis and Function of Antinutritional Factors in Plants. Aspects of Applied Biology 19: 21–28. D.V.Reeddy (2007). A Text Book of Principles of Animal Nutrition and Feed Technology, Oxford and IBH Publishing Company Co. Pvt. Ltd. Reprint, 2007.

Harborne, J.B. 1989. Biosynthesis and Function of Antinutritional Factors in Plants. Aspects of Applied Biology 19: 21–28.

Harnett MM. Analysis of G-Proteins Regulating Signal Transduction Pathways. Methods Mol Biol 1994; 27: 199-211.

Harrington DJ. Bacterial Collagenases and Collagen-Degrading Enzymes and their Potential Role in Human Disease. Infect Immun 1996; 64: 1885-91.

Hegarty, M.P. 1978. Toxic Amino Acids of Plant Origin. In: Effect of Poisonous Plants on Livestock. Keeler, R.F., Van Kampen, K.R. and James, L.F. (Eds.) Academic Press New York. pp. 575–585.

Henderson I, Davis T, Elmore M, Minton NP. The Genetic Basis of Toxin Production in *Clostridium Botulinum* and *Clostridium Tetani*. In: Rood JI, Mcclane BA, Songer JG, Titball RW, Editors. The Clostridia: Molecular Biology and Pathogenesis. San Diego: Academic Press; 1997. p. 261-94.

Hiremath, N.B. 1981. Subabool (Leucaena Leucocephala) - A Wonder Plant. Indian Dairyman 33: 351–356.

Holland Ww, Reid Dd. The Urban Factor in Chronic Bronchitis. Lancet. 1965;I:445-448.

Holleman, A. F. and Wiberg, E. "Inorganic Chemistry" Academic Press: San Diego, 200.

Holmgren J, Lycke N, Czerkinsky C. Cholera Toxin and Cholera-B Subunit as Oral Mucosal Adjuvant and Antigen Vector Systems. Vaccine 1993;11:1179-84.

Horigome, T., Kumar, R. and Okamoto, K. 1988. Effects of Condensed Tannins Prepared from the Leaves of Fodder Plants on Digestive Enzyme *in vitro* and in the Intestine of Rats. British Journal of Nutrition 60: 275–285.

Horiguchi Y, Inoue N, Masuda M, Kashimoto T, Katahira J, Sugimoto N, *et al. Bordetella Bronchiseptica* Dermonecrotizing Toxin Induces Reorganization of Actin Stress Fibers Through Deamidation of GLN-63 of the GTP-Binding Protein Rho. Proceeding of National Academy of Science, USA. 1997; 94: 11623-6.

Hrelia *et al.* 1996 - The Genetic and Non-Genetic Toxicity of the Fungicide Vinclozolin. Mutagenesis. 11: 445-453.

Ibarluzea JMJ, Fernandez MF, Santa-Marina L, *et al.*, Breast Cancer Risk and the Combined Effect of Environmental Estrogens, Cancer Causes Control, 2004, 15(6):591-600.

J. Sunyer. 2001. "Urban Air Pollution and Chronic Obstructive Pulmonary Disease: A Review". European Respiratory Journal 17: 1024-1033.

Jahn R, Hanson PI, Otto H, Ahnert-Hilger G. Botulinum and Tetanus Neurotoxins: Emerging Tools for the Study of Membrane Fusion. Cold Spring Harb Symp Quant Biol 1995; 60: 329-35.

James W. Hammond Jr.; Poison Gas: The Myths Versus Reality Greenwood Press, 1999

Jaouen, G., Ed. 2006. Bioorganometallics: Biomolecules, Labeling, Medicine. Wiley-VCH.

Jonathan B. Tucker. Chemical Warfare From World War I To Al-Qaeda (2006).

Jones, R.M., Mclennan, M.W. and Dowsett,K.F. 1989. The Effect of Leucaena Leucocephala on the Reproduction of Beef Cattle Grazing Leucaena/Grass Pastures. Tropical Grasslands 23: 108–114.

Jones, R.J. and Hegarty, M.P. 1984. The Effect of Different Proportion of Leucaena Leucocephala in the Diet of Cattle on Growth, Feed Intake, Thyroid Function and Urinary Excretion of 3-Hydroxy-4 (Ih)-Pyridone. Australian Journal of Agriculture Research 35:317.

Jones, R.J., Blunt, C.G. and Nurnberg, B.I. 1978. Toxicity of Leucaena Leucocephala. The Effect of Iodine and Mineral Supplements on Penned Steers Fed A Sole Diet of Leucaena. Australian Veterinary Journal 54: 387–392.

Joshi, D.C. Katiyar, R.C., Khan, M.Y., Banerji, R., Misra, G. and Nigam, S.K. 1989. Studies on Mahua (*Bassia Latifolia*) Seed Cake Saponin (Mowrin) In Cattle. Indian Journal of Animal Nutrition 6: 13–17.

Kakkar, B.B.; Mahipal, S.K. and Chauhan, R.S. 1996. Effect of Carbaryl and Malathian on Cell Mediated Immune Response in Chickens. Int. J. Anim. Sci. 11: 231-233.

Keeler, R.W. 1984. Teratogenes in Plants. Journal of Animal Science 58: 1029–1039.

Kellogg Rl, Nehring R, Grube A, Goss DW, and Plotkin S (February 2000), Environmental Indicators of Pesticide Leaching and Runoff from Farm Fields. United States Department of Agriculture Natural Resources Conservation Service.

Kessler KR, Benecke R. Botulinum Toxin: From Poison to Remedy. Neurotoxicology 1997; 18: 761-70.

Khurana, R.; Chauhan, R.S. and Mahipal, S.K 1997. Immunotoxic Effect of Cypermethrin and Endosulfan on Macrophage Functions in Broiler Chicks. Ind. J. Anim. Sci. 68:105-106.

Khurana, R.; Mahipal, S.K. and Chauhan, R.S. 1997. Effect of Insecticides on Peritoneal Macrophages in Sheep . Ind. J. Vet. Res. 6: 32-36.

Khurana, R.; Mahipal, S.K. and Chauhan, R.S. 1997. Insecticide Induced Biochemical Alterations in Sheep. Ind. J. Vet. Res. 8: 31-38.

Khurana, R.; Mahipal, S.K. and Chauhan, R.S. 1998. Effect of Carbofuran on Cell Mediated Immunity in Sheep. Ind. J. Toxicol. 5 : 1-6.

Koch, H.; Haaf, W. (1973). "1-Adamantanecarboxylic Acid". Org. Synth.; Coll. 5:20.

Koller, L.D. 1979. Effects of Environmental Contaminants on the Immune System. Adv. Vet. Sci. Comp. 23:267-295.

Kraulis PJ. Molscript: A Program to Produce both Detailed and Schematic Plots of Protein Structures. Journal of Applied Crystallography 1991; 24: 946-50.

Kumar, R. 1983. Chemical and Biochemical Nature of Fodder Tree Leaf Tannins. Journal of Agriculture and Food Chemistry 31: 1364– 1367.

Kumar, R. and Horigome, T. 1986. Fractionation, Characterization, and Protein Precipitating Capacity of the Condensed Tannins from Robinia *Pseudoacacia L.* Leaves. Journal of Agriculture and Food Chemistry 34:487.489.

Kumar, R. and Sing, M. 1984. Tannins: Their Adverse Role in Ruminant Nutrition. Journal of Agriculture and Food Chemistry 32: 447–453.

Kumar, R. And Vaithiyanathan, S. 1990. Occurrence, Nutritional Significance and Effect on Animal Procuctivity if Tannins in Tree Leaves. Animal Feed Science and Technology 30: 21–38.

L.F. Haber. The Poisonous Cloud: Chemical Warfare in the First World War Oxford University Press.

Lacasse EC, Saleh MT, Patterson B, Minden MD, Gariepy J. Shiga-Like Toxin Purges Human Lymphoma from Bone Marrow of Severe Combined Immunodeficient Mice. Blood 1996; 88:1551-67.

Latijnhouwers M, De Wit Pj, Govers F. Oomycetes and Fungi: Similar Weaponry to Attack Plants. Trends In Microbiology. 11 462-469

Lee PK, Schlievert PM. Molecular Genetics of Pyrogenic Exotoxin "Superantigens" of Group A Streptococci and Staphylococcus. Curr Top Microbiol Immunol 1991;174:1-19.

Lemichez E, Flatau G, Bruzzone M, Boquet P, Gauthier M. Molecular Localization of the *Escherichia Coli* Cytotoxic Necrotizing Factor CNF1 Cell-Binding and Catalytic Domains. Mol Microbiol 1997; 24:1061-70.

Leo P. Brophy and George J.B. Fisher; The Chemical Warfare Service: Organizing for War Office of the Chief of Military History, 1959; L.P. Brophy, W.D. Miles and C.C. Cochrane, the Chemical Warfare Service: From Laboratory to Field (1959); and B.E. Kleber and D. Birdsell, The Chemical Warfare Service in Combat (1966). Official US History.

Lesieur C, Vecsey-Semjen B, Abrami L, Fivaz M, Gisou Van Der Goot F. Membrane Insertion: The Strategies of Toxins. Mol Membr Biol 1997;14:45-64.

Levine SR. Thrombolytic Therapy for Stroke: The New Paradigm. Hosp Pract. 1997; 32: 57-73.

Liener, I.E. 1985. Anti-Nutritional Factors. In: Legumes, Chemistry, Technology and Human Nutrition. pp. 339–382. Matthews, R.H. (Ed.) Marce Dekker Inc., New York.

Lock E.A,Berry P.N.Biochemical Changes in the Rat Cerebellum following Cypermethrin Administration.Toxicol Appl Pharmacol 1981; 59: 508-14.

López P, Sánchez C, Batlle R, Nerín C (August 2005). "Solid- and Vapor-Phase Antimicrobial Activities of Six Essential Oils: Susceptibility of Selected Foodborne Bacterial and Fungal Strains". J. Agric. Food Chem. 53 (17): 6939-46. US Patent 6174920.

Lorgue .G, Lechenet J and Riviere. A (1996). Clinical Veterinary Toxicology Blackwell Science Publishers, UK, pp:19-30.

Lottenberg R, Minning-Wenz D, Boyle MD. Capturing Host Plasmin (Ogen): A Common Mechanism for Invasive Pathogens? Trends Microbiol 1994; 2: 20-4.

Lowry, J.B. 1990. Toxic Factors and Problems: Methods of Alleviating Them in Animals. In: Shrubs and Tree Fodders for Farm Animals. C. Devendra (Ed.) IDRC, Canada pp.76–88.

Lu, C.D. and Jorgensen, N.A. 1987. Alfalfa Saponins Effect Site and Extent of Nutrient Digestion in Ruminants. Journal of Nutrition 117: 919–927.

Luster, M.I.; Germolec, D.R. and Rosenthal, G. J. 1990. Immunotoxicology : A Review of Current Status. Ann. Allergy. 64: 427-432.

M. I. Yousef, F. M. El-Demerdash, K. S. Al-Salhen Protective Role of Isoflavones Against the Toxic Effect of Cypermethrin on Semen Quality and Testosterone Levels of Rabbits, *http://www.informaworld.com/smpp/title~content=t713597269~db=all http://www.informaworld. com/smpp/title~content = t713597269~db=all~tab= issueslist~branches = 38 - v3838, 4 : 2003,* Pages 463 - 478.

Mahipal, S.K.; Khurana, S.K. and Chauhan. R.S. 1995. Endosulfan Induced Delayed Neurotoxicity in Chickens. Indian J. Toxicol. 2: 83.

Maseri A, Andreotti F. Targeting New Thrombolytic Regimens At Specific Patient Groups: Implications for Research and Cost-Containment. Eur Heart J 1997; 18: F28-35.

Masina S, Broady K.W. (1999). "Tick Paralysis: Development of A Vaccine". International Journal for Parasitology 29.

Mcsweeney, C.S., Kennedy, P.M. and John, A. 1988. Effect of Ingestion of Hydrolysable Tannins in Terminalia Oblongata on Digestion in Sheep Fed Stylosanthes Hamata. Australian Journal of Agriculture Research 39: 235–244.

Melton-Celsa AR, O'Brien AD. Activation of Shiga-Like Toxins by Mouse And Human Intestinal Mucus Correlates with Virulence of Enterohemorrhagic *Escherichia Coli* O91:H21 Isolates in Orally Infected, Streptomycin-Treated Mice. Infect Immun 1996; 64:1569-76.

Metcalfe, R.J. Et Al. (2000) The Effect of Dose and Mobility on the Strength of Selection for Dmi Fungicide Resistance in Inoculated Field Experiments. Plant Pathology 49: 546-557.

Michael E. Peterson and Patricia A. Talcott.(2006). Small Animal Toxicology, Second Edition, Elsevier Saunders Inc, USA, Pp: 154-164.

Michael Kymisis, Konstantinos Hadjistavrou (2008). "Short-Term Effects of Air Pollution Levels on Pulmonary Function of Young Adults". The Internet Journal of Pulmonary Medicine 9 (2).

Molyneux, R.J., Stevens, K.L. and James, L.F. 1980. Chemistry of Toxic Range Plants. Volatile Constituents of Broomweed (Gutierrezia Sarothrae). Journal of Agriculture and Food Chemistry 28: 1332–1333.

Mond L, Langer K, Quincke F (1890). "Action of Carbon Monoxide on Nickel". Journal of the Chemical Society 57: 749–753.

Murray LJ, Habeshaw JA, Wiels J, Greaves MF. Expression of Burkitt Lymphoma-Associated Antigen (Defined by the Monoclonal Antibody 38.13) on both Normal and Malignant Germinal-Centre B Cells. Int J Cancer 1985;36:561-5.

Musch A: Dose-Time-Effect Relationships. In: Niesink Rjm, De Vries J, Hollinger Ma, Eds. Toxicology: Principles And Applications. pp.184-238. Boca Raton: CRC Press, 1996.

Nair GB, Takeda Y. The Heat-Stable Enterotoxins. Microb Pathog 1998; 24:123-31.

National Institutes of Health. The Jordan Report: Accelerated Development of Vaccines. 1998.

Needham Gr (1985). "Evaluation of Five Popular Methods for Tick Removal". Pediatrics 75: 997–1002.

Neer EJ. Heterotrimeric G Proteins: Organizers of Transmembrane Signals. Cell 1995; 80: 249-57.

O.R. Gilliam, C.M. Johnson and W. Gordy (1950). "Microwave Spectroscopy in the Region from Two to Three Millimeters". Physical Review 78 (2):

O'Brien AD, Kaper JB. Shiga Toxin-Producing *Escherichia Coli*: Yesterday, Today, and Tomorrow. In: Kaper JB, O'Brien AD, Editors. *Escherichia Coli* O157:H7 and Other Shiga Toxin-Producing *E. Coli* Strains. Washington: American Society for Microbiology; 1998. P. 1-11.

O'Brien AD, Lively TA, Chen M, Rothman SW, Formal SB. *Escherichia Coli* O157:H7 Strains Associated with Hemorrhagic Colitis in the United States Produce A *Shigella Dysenteriae* 1 (Shiga) Like Cytotoxin. Lancet 1983; I: 702.

O'Brien AD, Tesh VL, Donohue-Rolfe A, Jackson MP, Olsnes S, Sandvig K, *et al*. Shiga Toxin: Biochemistry, Genetics, Mode of Action, And Role in Pathogenesis. In: Sansonetti PJ, Editor. Pathogenesis of Shigellosis. 180th Ed. Berlin-Heidelberg: Springer-Verlag; 1992. P. 66-94.

Olea N, Olea-Serrano F, Lardelli-Claret P, Et Al., Inadvertent Exposure to Xenoestrogens in Children, Toxicol. Ind. Health, 15:151–158.

Omaye St. (2002). "Metabolic Modulation of Carbon Monoxide Toxicity". Toxicology 180 (2): 139–50.

Oswald E, Sugai M, Labigne A, Wu HC, Fiorentini C, Boquet P, Et Al. Cytotoxic Necrotizing Factor Type 2 Produced By Virulent *Escherichia Coli* Modifies the Small GTP-Binding Proteins Rho Involved In Assembly of Actin Stress Fibers. Proceedings of National Academy of Sciences USA. 1994; 91: 3814-8.

Osweiler G.A: Brief Guide to Clinical Toxicosis in Small Animals. In: Current Veterinary Therapy Ix.Edt.Krik,Rw;Philadelphia, WB Saunders. 1986:132-135.

Osweiler Gd, Carson Tl, Buck Wb, Van Gelder Ga. Clinical and Diagnostic Veterinary Toxicology, 3rd Edition. Dubuque: Kendall/Hunt, 1985; 3-32.

Osweiler Gd. General Toxicologic Principles. In: Peterson Me and Talcott Pa, Eds. Small Animal Toxicology: Philadelphia, WB Saunders, 2001; 2-14.

Osweiler Gd. Toxicology: The National Veterinary Medical Series for Independent Study. Philadelphia: Williams & Wilkins, 1996; 1-14.

Papageorgiou AC, Acharya KR. Superantigens as Immunomodulators: Recent Structural Insights. Structure 1997;5:991-6.

Pastan I. Targeted Therapy of Cancer With Recombinant Immunotoxins. Biochimica Et Biophysica Acta 1997; 1333:C1-6.

Pathak N. N (1997). A Text Book of Feed and Technology, Vikas Publishing Pvt.Ltd.

Pesticide Chemistry and Bioscience Edited by G.T Brooks and T.R Roberts. 1999. Published by the Royal Society of Chemistry Pollution - Definition from The Merriam-Webster Online Dictionary.

Poonam Pandey and J.S Arawal (2001). Nutrient Utilization and Growth Response in Crossbred Calves Fed Antibiotic and Probe Ionic Supplemented Diet. Indian Journal of Ani. Nutr 18(1):15-18.

Prakash,N (2003): Antibiotic and Pesticide Residues in Milk and Milk Products:- Toxicological Significance and Quality Assurance, National Seminar on Quality Up-Gradation and Safety Aspects of Dairy Products, Bidar, pp 21-24.

Prasad GS, Radhakrishnan R, Mitchell DT, Earhart CA, Dinges MM, Cook WJ, Et Al. Refined Structures of Three Crystal Forms of Toxic Shock Syndrome Toxin-1 and of A Tetramutant with Reduced Activity. Protein Sci 1997;6:1220-7.

Pravin Kumar (2004). Effect of Crop Residue Based Complete Feed Blocks on Nutrients Digestibility and Growth in Buffalo Calves. Indian Journal of Ani. Nutr. (30-32).

Pritchard, D.A., Stocks, D.C., O'sullivan, B.M., Martin, P.R., Hurwood, I.S. and O'rourke, P.K. 1988. The Effect of Polyethylene Glycol (Peg) on Wool Growth and Live Weight of Sheep Consuming Mulga (Acacia Aneura) Diet. Proceeding of Australian Society of Animal Production 17: 290–293.

Puri J.P and Gupta B.A (2001). Effect of Feeding Rice Straw Treated with Two Levels of Urea and Moisture on Growth, Nutrient Utilization in Crossbred Calves.Indian Journal of Ani. Nutr 18(1):54-59.

R. K. Thauer (1998). "Biochemistry of Methanogenesis: A Tribute to Marjory Stephenson. 1998 Marjory Stephenson Prize Lecture" (Free). Microbiology 144 (9): 2377–2406.

Raghavan, G.V. 1990. Availability and Use of Shrubs Tree Fodder in India. In: Shrubs and Tree Fodder for Farm Animals. C. Devendra (Ed.) pp. 196–210.

Rago JV, Schlievert PM. Mechanisms of Pathogenesis of Staphylococcal and Streptococcal Superantigens. Curr Top Microbiol Immunol 1998; 225:81-97.

Raharjo, Y.C., Cheeke, P.R. and Patton, N.M. 1990. Effect of Cecotrophy on The Nutrient Digestibility of Alfalfa and Black Locust Leaves. Journal of Applied Rabbit Research 613: 56–61.

Rao, N.P., Reddy, B.S. And Reddy, M.R. 1988. Utilization Of Autoclaved Castor Bean Meal In Cancentrate Ration For Sheep. Indian Journal Of Animal Nutrition 5: 121–128.

Reed, J.D., Soller, H. And Wood Ward, A. 1990. Fodder Tree and Straw Diets for Sheep: Intake, Growth, Digestibility and the Effect of Phenolics on Nitrogen Utilization. Animal Feed Science and Technology 30: 39–50.

Revised 1996 IPCC Guidelines For National Greenhouse Gas Inventories (Reference Manual) "Study Links Traffic Pollution to Thousands of Deaths" (In English), The Guardian (London, UK), Guardian Media Group (2008-04-15).

Roberts, G. P.; Youn, H.; Kerby, R. L. (2004). "Co-Sensing Mechanisms". Microbiology and Molecular Biology Reviews 68: 453–473.

Rothbard, Murray. "Conservation, Ecology, and Growth", for A New Liberty: The Libertarian Manifesto, 256-257

Roux E, Yersin A. Contribution A L'etude De La Diphtherie. Annales De l'Institut Pasteur 1888;2:629-61.

Russel, J.B. and Wilson, D.B. 1988. Potential Opportunities and Problems for Genetically Altered Rumen Microorganisms. Journal of Nutrition 118: 271–279.

Russell, R.W. and Lolley, J.R. 1989. Deactivation of Tannin in High Tannin Milo by Treatment with Urea. Journal of Dairy Science 72: 2427–2430.

Saiyed H, Dewan A, Bhatnagar V, et al., Effect of Endosulfan on Male Reproductive Development, Environ. Health Prospects., 2003, 111:1958-1962.

Sass J, Janssen S (2008). "Open Letter to Stephen Johnson, Administrator, U.S. Environmental Protection Agency: Ban Endosulfan". Int J Occup Environ Health 14 (3): 236–9. Erickson, Britt (May 21, 2008). "Groups Petition Epa To Ban Endosulfan". Chemical and Engineering News.

Saxena SK, O'Brien AD, Ackerman EJ. Shiga Toxin, Shiga-Like Toxin II Variant, and Ricin are All Single-Site RNA N-Glycosidases of 28 S RNA when Microinjected Into *Xenopus* Oocytes. J Biol Chem 1989;264:596-601.

Schiavo G, Montecucco C. The Structure and Mode of Action of Botulinum and Tetanus Toxins. In: Rood JI, Mcclane BA, Songer JG, Titball RW, Editors. The Clostridia: Molecular Biology and Pathogenesis. San Diego: Academic Press; 1997. p. 295-322.

Schlessinger D, Schaechter M. Bacterial Toxins. In: Schaechter M, Medoff G, Eisenstein BI, Editors. Mechanisms of Microbial Disease. 2nd Ed. Baltimore: Williams and Wilkins; 1993. p. 162-75.

Schlievert PM. Searching for Superantigens. Immunol Invest 1997;26:283-90.

Schmidt G, Sehr P, Wilm M, Selzer J, Mann M, Aktories K. Gln63 Of Rho Is Deamidated By *Escherichia Coli* Cytotoxic Necrotizing Factor-1. Nature 1997;387:725-9.

Schmidt WF, Bilboulian S, Rice CP, Fettinger JC, Mcconnell Ll, and Hapeman CJ, J. Ag. Food Chem., 2001, 49(11): 5372–5376.

Schmidt WF, Hapeman CJ, Fettinger JC, Rice CP, and Bilboulian S, J. Ag. Food Chem., 1997, 45(4): 1023–1026.

Schmitt N, Bowmer Ej, Gregson Jd (1969). "Tick Paralysis In British Columbia".

Schnabel, G., And Jones, A. L. 2001. The 14a-Demethylase (Cyp51a1) Gene Is Overexpressed In V. Inaequalis Strains Resistant To Myclobutanil. Phytopathology 91:102.

Sharma, J.K(2001):Antibiotic Residues in Milk and Milk Products:- Its Public Health Significance. CSIR Winter School, Oct16-Nov.5, PAU, Ludhiana, Pp176-79

Shqueir, A.A., Brown, D.L., Taylor, S.J., Rivkin, I., Klasing, K.C. 1989. Effects of Solvent Extraction, Heat Treatments and Added Cholesterol on Sesbania Sesban Toxicity in Growing Chicks. Animal Feed Science and Technology 27: 127–135.

Sierotzki, Helge (2000) Mode of Resistance to Respiration Inhibitors at the Cytochrome Bc1 Enzyme Complex of Mycosphaerella Fijiensis Field Isolates Pest Management Science 56:833-841.

Simi Chakrabarti. "20th Anniversary of World's Worst Industrial Disaster", Australian Broadcasting Corporation.

Singer, Siegfried Fred (1975). The Changing Global Environment, pp. 90.

Singh BR, Li B, Read D. Botulinum Versus Tetanus Neurotoxins: Why Is Botulinum Neurotoxin But Not Tetanus Neurotoxin A Food Poison? Toxicon 1995;33:1541-7.

Singh Nd, Sharma Ak, Dwivedi P, Patil Rd, Kumar M (2007). "Citrinin and Endosulfan Induced Teratogenic Effects in Wistar Rats". J Appl Toxicol 27 (2): 143–51.

Singh, R.V. 1982. Fodder Trees of India pp. 303. Oxford & IBH Publishing Co., New Delhi

Singhal, L.K. and Chauhan, R.S. 2000. Environmental Pollution by Agrochemicals and Its Impact on Epidemics of Animal Diseases. Pashudhan. 15: 1-8.

Sixma TK, Kalk KH, Van Zanten BA, Dauter Z, Kingma J, Witholt B, et al. Redefined Structure of *Escherichia Coli* Heat-Labile Enterotoxin, A Close Relative of Cholera Toxin. J Mol Biol 1993;230:890-918.

Snider DP. The Mucosal Adjuvant Activities of ADP-Ribosylating Bacterial Enterotoxins. Crit Rev Immunol 1995;15:317-48.

So M, Boyer HW, Betlach M, Falkow S. Molecular Cloning of An *Escherichia Coli* Plasmid Determinant That Encodes for the Production of Heat-Stable Enterotoxin. J Bacteriol 1976;128:463-72.

So M, Mccarthy BJ. Nucleotide Sequence of Transposon Tn1681 Encoding A Heat-Stable Toxin (ST) and its Identification in Enterotoxigenic *Escherichia Coli* Strains. Proceedings of National Academy of Sciences, U S A 1980;77:4011-5.

Song L, Hobaugh MR, Shustak C, Cheley S, Bayley H, Gouaux JE. Structure of Staphylococcal Alpha-Hemolysin, A Heptameric Transmembrane Pore. Science 1996;274:1859-66.

Songer JG. Bacterial Phospholipases and Their Role in Virulence. Trends Microbiol 1997;5:156-61.

Sorheim, S, Nissena, H, Nesbakken, T (1999). "The Storage Life of Beef and Pork Packaged in an Atmosphere with Low Carbon Monoxide and High Carbon Dioxide". Journal of Meat Science 52 (2): 157–64.

Soto Am, Chung Kl, Sonnenschein C, The Pesticides Endosulfan, Toxaphene, and Dieldrin Have Estrogenic Effects on Human Estrogensensitive Cells, Environ. Health Prospects., 1994, 102(4):380-383.

Spoo W. Concepts and Terminology. In: Plumlee KH, Ed. Clinical Veterinary Toxicology. St. Louis: Mosby Inc, 2003; 2-12.

Srivastava., D.N and Soni, J.L(1987). Veterinary Toxicology and Jurisprudence pp:18-73. First Edition, Anubha Prakashan, Jabalpur,

Staatz C.G,Bloom A.S.Lech J.J,A Pharmacological Study of Pyrethroid Neuronal Toxicity in Mice. Pest Biochem Physiol 1982;17:287-92.

Stein PE, Boodhoo A, Armstrong GD, Cockle SA, Klein MH, Read RJ. The Crystal Structure of Pertussis Toxin. Structure 1994;2:45-57.

Stein PE, Boodhoo A, Tyrell GT, Brunton J, Read RJ. Crystal Structure of the Cell-Binding B Oligomer of Verotoxin-1 From *E. Coli.* Nature 1992;355:748-50.

Stevens DL. Superantigens: Their Role in Infectious Diseases. Immunol Invest 1997; 26:275-81.

Stryer, Lubert (1995). Biochemistry, 4th Edition. W.H. Freeman and Company, Pp. 670.

Suh J-K, Hovde CJ, Robertus JD. Shiga Toxin Attacks Bacterial Ribosomes as Effectively as Eukaryotic Ribosomes. Biochemistry 1998;37:9394-8.

Sure V.K. (1996). Improving Nutritional Status of Rice Husk Through Chemical Biological Treatments. Journal of Agricultural Research. 30(10):15-10.

Taga S, Mangeney M, Tursz T, Wiels J. Differential Regulation of Glycosphingolipid Biosynthesis in Phenotypically Distinct Burkitt's Lymphoma Cell Lines. Int J Cancer 1995;61:261-7.

Tangendijaja, B., Rahardjo, Y.C. and Lowry, J.B. 1990. Leucaena Leaf Meal in the Diet of Growing Rabbits: Evaluation and Effect of A Low Mimosine Treatement. Animal Feed Science and Technology 29: 63–72.

Tanner, J.C., Reed, J.D. and Owen, E. 1990. The Nutritive Value of Fruits (Pods With Seeds) From Four Acacia Spp. Compared With Nong (Guizotia Abssinica) Meal as Supplements of Maize Stover for Ethiopian High Land Sheep. Animal Production 51: 127–133.

Tesh VL, O'Brien AD. The Pathogenic Mechanisms of Shiga Toxin and The Shiga-Like Toxins. Mol Microbiol 1991;5:1817-22.

Thakur M.L. and Verma T.C. (2000)…Effect of Nh3 / Urea Treatment of Baled Wheat Straw on its Nutritive Value. Indian Journal of Ani. Nutr.17 (1): 8-12.

Tomita T, Kamio Y. Molecular Biology of the Pore-Forming Cytolysins From *Staphylococcus Aureus,* A- and Gamma-Hemolysins and Leukocidin. Bioscience, Biotechnology, and Biochemistry 1997; 61:565-72.

Turner, D.B. (1994). Workbook of Atmospheric Dispersion Estimates: An Introduction to Dispersion Modeling, 2nd Edition, CRC Press.

Unnikrishnan,V.,Surendranath,B.,Gyathri,V.,Sampath K,T.& Rama Murthy,M.K(1998): Organochlorine Pesticide Residue Contents in Feeds and Feedstuffs. Indian J.Dairy Bio.Sci., 9:59-64.

Vaithiyanathan, S. and Singh, M. 1989. Seasonal Changes in Tannin Contents in Some Top Feeds in Arid Region. Indian Journal of Animal Science 59: 1565–1567.

Varayoud J, Monje L, Bernhardt T, Muñoz-De-Toro M, Luque EH, Ramos JG (August 2008). "Endosulfan Modulates Estrogen-Dependent Genes Like A Non-Uterotrophic Dose of 17beta-Estradiol". Reproductive Toxicology (Elmsford, N.Y.).

Wheeler AH. Therapeutic Uses of Botulinum Toxin. Am Fam Physician 1997;55:541-8.

Wick MJ, Iglewski BH. In: Moss J, Vaughan M, Editors. ADP-Ribosylating Toxins and G Proteins. Washington: American Society for Microbiology; 1990. P. 31-43.

Wilson Vs, Leblanc Ga (January 1998). "Endosulfan Elevates Testosterone Biotransformation and Clearance in Cd-1 Mice". Toxicol. Appl. Pharmacol. 148 (1): 158–68. Doi:10.1006/Taap.1997.8319.

Winkler U, Barth S, Schnell R, Diehl V, Engert A. The Emerging Role of Immunotoxins in Leukemia and Lymphoma. Ann Oncol 1997;8:139-46.

World Health Organization (Geneva).Alfa Cypermethrin.In:Environmental Health Criteria-142, WHO. Geneva: Library Cataloguing in Publishing Data1992.p.20-43

World Health Organization, Environmental Health Criteria 40, 1984.

World Health Organization, The WHO Recommended Classification of Pesticides by Hazard, 2005.

Zoidis, John D. (1999). "The Impact of Air Pollution on COPD". Rt: for Decision Makers in Respiratory Care.

Zwiers, L.H. *et al.* (2003) Abc Transporters of the Wheat Pathogen Mycosphaerella Graminicola Function as Protectants Against Biotic and Xenobiotic Toxic Compounds Molecular Genetics and Genomics 269:499-507.

INDEX

B

C

D

E

M

N

O

P

Q

R

S

T

❑❑❑